Editors

G. Marino and G. Sannia
Dipartimento di Chimica Organica e Biologica
Università di Napoli "Federico II"
Via Mezzocannone 16
I-80134 Napoli
Italy

F. Bossa
Dipartimento di Scienze Biochimiche
Università di Roma "La Sapienza"
P. le Aldo Moro 5
I-00185 Roma
Italy

A CIP catalogue record for this book is available from the Library of Congress,
Washington D.C., USA

Deutsche Bibliothek Cataloging-in-Publication Data
Biochemistry of vitamin B$_6$ and PQQ / ed. by G. Marino ... –
Basel ; Boston ; Berlin : Birkhäuser, 1994
    (Advances in life sciences)
    ISBN 3-7643-5067-9 (Basel ...)
    ISBN 0-8176-5067-9 (Boston)
NE: Marino, Gennaro [Hrsg.]

© 1994 Birkhäuser Verlag, PO Box 133, CH-4010 Basel, Switzerland
Camera-ready copy prepared by the authors
Printed on acid-free paper produced from chlorine-free pulp
Printed in Germany
ISBN 3-7643-5067-9
ISBN 0-8176-5067-9

9 8 7 6 5 4 3 2 1

In memory of Vincenzo Scardi 1924-1992

CONTENTS

Tryptophan-synthase and decarboxylases

X

Amine oxidases

Quinoprotein dehydrogenases

Molecular physiology

Molecular pathology

Preface

The International Meeting on Vitamin B_6 and Carbonyl Catalysis took place on Capri, Italy from 22nd to 27th May 1994 and was organized in conjunction with the 3rd Symposium on PQQ and Quinoproteins.

It was an extraordinary occasion for scientists from all over the world to meet and discuss new developments in these overlapping fields. Several sessions were dedicated to the molecular aspects of Vitamin B_6 and Quinone dependent enzymes, as well as to the cellular, biomedical and nutritional aspects. The congress was inaugurated by Paolo Fasella in his capacity as General Director of Science, Research and Development of the Commission of the European Communities, with an overview on International Scientific Collaboration. The scientific sessions started with a talk on the History of Vitamin B_6 given by David Metzler who at the very last minute presented Esmond Snell's paper adding some personal remarks. Unfortunately, both Esmond Snell and Alton Meister had to unexpectedly cancel the trip to Capri.

These proceedings contain the papers presented as oral contributions and a few selected poster presentations. The limited number of pages meant we could not publish many interesting poster presentations, including those selected for the three lively and exciting evening poster discussion sessions called by the organizers "Vino, taralli and ... discussion".

The first meeting on the chemical and biochemical aspects of Vitamin B_6 Catalysis was organized in 1962 in Rome. A book of proceedings was published at that time. Among the Vitamin B_6 club members it goes by the name of "The Old Testament".

The aim of the editors was not to provide the readers with a version of "The New Testament", but to give a wide overview of the problems and interests going on in this field.

The editors wish to thank all the Institutions and Companies which sponsored the meeting, the International Advisory Board and the colleagues of the Organizing Committee. Finally, and most important of all, our warmest thanks go to the authors of the articles, who made our task as easy as possible, and to all participants who contributed to turn this meeting into a stimulating, worthwhile and, for some of them, unforgettable event.

The Editors

Acknowledgement

HONORARY COMMITTEE

ANTHONY, Christopher (*U.K.*)
FASELLA, Paolo (*Italy*)
MEISTER, Alton (*USA*)
SNELL, Esmond E. (*USA*)
WADA, Hiroshi (*Japan*)

INTERNATIONAL ADVISORY BOARD

ADACHI, Osao (*Japan*)
BEREZOV, Temir T. (*Russia*)
CHRISTEN, Philipp (*Switzerland*)
CHURCHICH, Jorge E. (*USA*)
DAKSHINAMURTI, K. (*Canada*)
DANZIN, Charles (*France*)
DOONAN, Shawn (*Ireland*)
DUINE, J. A. (*The Netherlands*)
EVANGELOPOULOS, A. E. (*Greece*)
FUKUI, Toshio (*Japan*)
JANSONIUS, Johan (*Switzerland*)
JOHN, Robert (*UK*)
KAGAMIYAMA, Hiroyuki (*Japan*)
KAGAN, Herbert (*USA*)

KIRSCH, Jack F. (*USA*)
KLINMAN, Judith (*USA*)
KORPELA, Timo (*Finland*)
MANNING, James M. (*USA*)
MARTINEZ-CARRION, M. (*USA*)
McCORMICK, Donald B. (*USA*)
METZLER, David E. (*USA*)
MILES, Edith W. (*USA*)
MORINO, Yoshimasa (*Japan*)
SCHIRCH, Verne (USA)
SCHNACKERTZ, K.D. (*Germany*)
SODA, Kenji (*Japan*)
TORCHINSKY, Y. M. (*Israel*)

ORGANIZING COMMITTEE

MARINO, Gennaro (*Naples*)   President
MONDOVI', Bruno (*Rome*)   Co-President
SANNIA, Giovanni (*Naples*)   General Secretary
BONAVITA, Vincenzo (*Naples*)
BORRI VOLTATTORNI, Carla (*Verona*)
BOSSA, Francesco (*Rome*)
FINAZZI AGRO', Alessandro (*Rome*)
PASSARELLA, Salvatore (*Bari*)
ROSSI, Gian Luigi (*Parma*)
SILANO, Vittorio (*Rome*)

SPONSORS

International Union of Biochemistry and Molecular Biology (IUBMB), Commission of the European Communities, International Science Foundation, Italian Society of Biochemistry (SIB), National Research Council (CNR), University of Naples "Federico II", 2nd University of Naples, University of Rome "La Sapienza", University of Molise, Banco di Napoli, Beckman Analytical, DSM Research, Hoffmann-La Roche, Marion Merrell Dow, Mead Johnson Nutritionals, Microglass, Perkin Elmer, Tecnogen, Wallac Oy.

Contributors

Adachi, O., 215
Aggerbeck, M., 79
Agostinelli, E., 220
Ahmed, S. A., 103
Akhtar, M., 132
Anthony, C., 245
Antson, A. A., 167, 170
Arnone, A., 46
Artigues, A., 68
Azzariti, A., 74
Banik, U., 103
Barouki, R., 79
Becker, S., 145
Bender, D.A., 269
Birolo, L., 56
Blazquez, M., 200, 205
Borri Voltattorni, C., 137
Bossa, F., 21
Brown, D. E., 225
Brzovic, P. S., 108
Buckel, W., 195
Cai, K., 180
Carroll, D., 122
Chen, H., 175
Chen, L., 175, 257
Cho, S.-W., 308
Choi, E. Y., 308
Choi, S. Y., 308
Christen, P., 11
Churchich, J. E., 200
Cidlowski, J.A., 281
Cook, P. F., 185
Dakshinamurti, K., 293
Davidson, V. L., 257
Davies, D. R., 103
de Vries, S., 250
Dean, D. R., 190
Dementieva, I., 167
Demidkina, T. V., 170
Dodson, G. G., 167, 170
Dominici, P., 137
Dooley, D. M., 225
Duine, J. A., 250
Dunn, M. F., 108

Durley, R. C. E., 257
Esaki, N., 16
Feilleux-Duché, S., 79
Freebort, I., 215
Fukui, T., 151, 233
Funai, T., 85, 298
Gani, D., 132
Garcia-Blanco, F., 205
Garlatti, M., 79
Genovesio-Taverne, J.-C., 29
Ghosh, R., 122
Giannattasio, S., 74
Giartosio, A., 220
Gollnick, P., 175
Grabowski, R., 195
Greenaway, F. T., 230
Grimm, B., 90, 95
Hackert, M. L., 122
Hamasaki, N., 46
Hanoune, J., 79
Harutyunyan, E. G., 167, 170
Harwood, J. L., 95
Hayashi, H., 41, 51
He, Z., 230
Hennig, M., 29
Hidalgo, C., 205
Higaki, T., 51
Hiraga, K., 119
Hirotsu, K., 51
Hofmeister, A. M., 195
Hohenester, E., 29, 127
Huang, H., 230
Hyde, C. C., 103
Ichiyama, A., 85, 298
Iriarte, A., 68
Ishii, S., 41
Ishikawa, K., 298
Isupov, M., 167
Itoh, S., 262
Jang, S. H., 308
Jansonius, J.N., 29, 127
Jenny, M., 29
John, R. A., 95
Jongejan, J. A., 250

Biochemistry of Vitamin B$_6$ and PQQ
G. Marino, G. Sannia and F. Bossa (eds.)
© 1994 Birkhäuser Verlag Basel/Switzerland

History of Vitamin B6

Esmond E. Snell

Departments of Chemistry & Microbiology, The University of Texas, Austin, Texas, 78712, U. S. A.

Advances in our knowledge of the nature, function, metabolism, and medical importance of vitamin B-6 during the sixty years since its discovery are such that a proper history would require a book rather than the few pages at my disposal. I shall therefore discuss chiefly early studies of its nature and function, with which I am familiar, and to save space frequently cite summaries or reviews rather than the original literature.

Detection of the vitamins depended initially on the occurrence of certain unexplained diseases in man or domestic animals (eventually found to result from nutritional deficiencies), and also upon use of small laboratory animals, especially rats and chicks, as assay organisms. The chronology of these developments is documented in various treatises on the vitamins (e.g., Friedrich, 1988; Wagner & Folkers, 1964; Robinson, 1951; Williams, et al., 1950). Concurrent studies showed that some microorganisms also required addition of certain vitamins or vitamin-like compounds to their medium for growth and provided sensitive and specific assay procedures for these "growth factors". These alternative approaches to the study of vitamins are well illustrated by the history of vitamin B6.

Animal Assays for Vitamin B6: Pyridoxine

Early experimental diets for animals were of necessity crude, and deficiency symptoms (poor growth, dermatitis, etc.) produced by feeding them were rarely specific for a single substance. In 1934, however, György (1934, 1964) described a specific type of florid dermatitis in rats fed a partially purified ration to which concentrates of two newly available B-vitamins, vitamins B1 and B2, were added. The condition was prevented by yeast extract or other crude supplements; György called the new dietary essential *vitamin B6*. This assay, and improved versions of it, permitted isolation of a pure curative compound, announced over a five month period in 1938, by five different laboratories: Lepkovsky (Feb.), Kerestesy & Stevens (Feb.), György (April), Kuhn & Wendt (May) and Ichibi & Michi (see Snell, 1981). This compound was characterized and synthesized the following year in Heidleberg, in the Merck laboratories, and in Japan; it was a pyridine derivative, and György (1964) named it *pyridoxine*. An ironic twist was provided by Ohdake, who had crystallized this same compound seven years earlier (in 1932) as a side fraction in the isolation of vitamin B1 (Williams, et al., 1950). There was then no reason to suspect that it, too, was a vitamin.

Microbiological Assays for Vitamin B6: Pyridoxal and Pyridoxamine

Almost immediately following its isolation, pyridoxine (PN) was shown to promote growth of various yeasts (Schultz, et al., 1939; Eakin & Williams, 1939) and lactic acid bacteria (Moeller, 1938) in media that lacked this vitamin. I confirmed Moeller's result but found that the growth response of *Lactobacillus casei* and *Streptococcus faecalis* to PN was highly variable from day to day, and values for the "PN" content of natural products obtained by their use (but not by use of yeast) as assay organisms were impossibly high. Eventually we showed (see Snell, 1958, 1981) that unheated PN was essentially inactive as a vitamin for these bacteria, and that chemical treatments such as heating with the growth medium or, more effectively, mild oxidation or amination procedures, transformed PN in part to substances that were highly effective in promoting growth of lactic acid bacteria. Similar transformations of PN occurred when this vitamin was ingested by rats or men. Their mode of formation and their chemical properties pointed conclusively to an aldehyde and an amine as the active products and led directly to the synthesis of *pyridoxal* (PL) and *pyridoxamine* (PM). These compounds were thousands of times more active than PN for lactic acid bacteria; for fungi and animals the three compounds were about equally active. A differential assay for the three compounds based upon these different activities showed that PL and PM were present in natural materials and fully accounted for the discrepancies in assay values for vitamin B6 obtained with various test organisms when only PN was used as the standard (reviews: Snell, 1958, 1981). Thus, vitamin B6 is a complex of three compounds, PN, PL, and PM, and their combined forms; it is misleading and erroneous to use "pyridoxine" and "vitamin B6" as synonyms.

Discovery of Phosphorylated Forms of PL, PM, and PM

György (in 1936) and Kuhn & Wendt (in 1938) recognized that vitamin B6 occurred naturally in combined form, possibly as part of some enzyme, and used dialysis to remove low molecular weight compounds as the first step in their purification of the vitamin from yeast juice. Braunstein & Kritsman (1937) found that their transaminase preparations contained an apparently essential carbonyl group, and Uzawa (1943) reported that tryptophanase from *E. coli* required an unidentified coenzyme. None of these observations was pursued; the track leading to identification of pyridoxal 5'-phosphate (PLP) began with Gale's observations beginning about 1940 (see Gale, 1946) that a number of bacterial amino acid decarboxylases required a heat stable coenzyme.

Gunsalus et al. (1944) related this coenzyme to vitamin B6 when they showed that *S. faecalis* grown in media low in B6 contained almost no tyrosine decarboxylase activity, but that this activity appeared when the dried cells were incubated with PL plus ATP. This finding indicated that the coenzyme was a phosphorylated PL. A crude active coenzyme was then prepared by phosphorylation of PL with $POCl_3$. The position of the phosphate group was established by unequivocal synthesis of PLP by Baddiley in 1952 (see Snell, 1958).

Comparative microbiological assays with *S. faecalis* and yeast led Rabinowitz and Snell (1947) to the conclusion that pyridoxamine 5'-phosphate (PMP, prepared by non-enzymatic transamination between PLP and glutamate) also occurs naturally, and comprises much of the combined vitamin in natural products such as yeast extract. Wada et al. (1959) first showed that pyridoxine 5'-phosphate (PNP), later found to be an intermediate in the biosynthesis of PLP and PL by *E. coli* (Dempsey, 1966), also occurs naturally.

Functions of Vitamin B6

Observation of the model reactions (Eq. 1-3) led Snell (1944) to suggest that PL and PM might function as amino group carriers in enzymic transamination. Schlenk & Snell (1945) and Lichstein et al. (1945) demonstrated a decrease in transaminase activity (GOT) in vitamin B6-deficient cells

1. Glutamate + PL <---> α-Ketoglutarate + PM
2. Oxaloacetate + PM <---> Aspartate + PL
3. (Sum of 1 + 2): Glutamate + Oxaloacetate <--->
α-Ketoglutarate + Aspartate

of rat tissues or of *S. faecalis* respectively, that was restored to near "normal" by addition of PLP, thus validating the role of PLP as the coenzyme. Its postulated role as an amino group carrier elicitated sporadic denials that were largely quelled by (a) the isolation of pure GOT by Jenkins & Sizer (1957) and the demonstration that it exists in two specrophotometrically distinct forms, as predicted by Eqs. 1 and 2, (b) the demonstration (Meister et al., 1954) that pure apoGOT was activated equally by either PLP or PMP, and (c) the later finding that apoGOT, but not holoGOT, catalyzes reactions 1 and 2, i. e., that PL and PM can serve as poorly bound analogues of PLP or PMP (Wada and Snell, 1962). Thus *both* PLP and PMP serve as coenzymes of GOT, whereas only PLP serves this function in tryptophanase and the amino acid decarboxylases studied earlier. The azomethine link between PLP and an ϵ-amino group of a lysine residue, now recognized as a feature common to almost all PLP enzymes, was first discovered by Jenkins & Sizer (1957) in GOT and further characterized by Fischer, et al. (1958).

Subsequent studies have established PLP as the principal coenzyme in almost all reactions of the primary amino acids, and the subject has been reviewed frequently (cf. Meister, 1965). However,

4

PLP also has other functions: as the coenzyme for phosphorylase (Baranovski, et al. 1957), a function only recently explained in mechanistic terms (Palm, et al., 1991); as part of a coenzyme complex in lysine-2,3-aminomutase (Song & Frey, 1991); and perhaps in formation of some deoxy sugars (Gonzales-Porque and Strominger, 1972). For unknown reasons a pyruvoyl residue replaces PLP as coenzyme in a few decarboxylases (van Poelje & Snell, 1990).

Mechanism of Action of Vitamin B6

In addition to transamination, PL catalyzes a variety of other reactions of amino acids in non-enzymic systems. These reactions model most of the reaction types catalyzed by PLP enzymes and permitted convenient determination of the functional groups of the PL molecule necessary for catalysis. The heterocyclic nitrogen, the 3'-phenolic group, and the 4'-formyl group supplied the *minimum* essentials for such reactions (see Snell, 1958). Functional roles in catalysis were assigned to these groups in our initial formulation of a general mechanism for pyridoxal catalysis (Metzler, et al., 1954). Unbeknownst to us because of wartime disruption of communications, Braunstein & Shemyakin (1953) had published a similar mechanism a few months earlier based upon Braunstein's wide-ranging studies of PLP enzymes. An important extension to these proposals by Dunathan (35) provided insight into the stereochemistry of catalysis. These proposals provided the framework for the numerous subsequent studies of mechanism.

Concluding Remarks

While history never ends, one's space allotment does. For this reason (and a lack of personal involvement that equates to insufficient knowledge) I have mentioned, all too briefly, only some of the seminal accomplishments from the discovery of vitamin B6 to about 1960. Whole categories of important findings--most egregiously, those dealing with the metabolism, physiological role, and medical importance of this vitamin, as well as the tremendous contributions of crystallographic determinations of three-dimensional structures of PLP enzymes to understanding of mechanism--have been omitted. I hope some of these gaps will be filled at future conferences.

References

Baranowski, T., Illingworth, B., Brown, D. H. & Cori, C. H. (1957) Isolation of pyridoxal 5'-phosphate from crystalline muscle phosphorylase. *Biochim. Biophys. Acta* 25: 16-21.
Braunstein, A. E. & Kritsman, M. G. (1937) Formation and breakdown of amino acids by intermolecular transfer of the amino group. *Nature* 140: 503-504.
Braunstein, A. E. & Shemyakin, M. M. (1953) Theory of processes of amino acid metabolism catalyzed by pyridoxal enzymes. *Biokhimiya* 18: 393-411.
Dempsey, W. B. (1966) Synthesis of pyridoxine by a pyridoxal auxotroph of *Escherichia coli. J. Bacteriol.* 92: 333-337.
Dunathan, H. C. (1971) Stereochemical aspects of pyridoxal phosphate catalysis. *Advan. Enzymol.* 35: 79-134.

Fischer, E. H., Kent, A. B., Snyder, E. R. & Krebs, E. G. (1958) The reaction of sodium borohydride with muscle phosphorylase. *J. Am. Chem. Soc.* 80: 2906-2907.

Friedrich, W. (1988) *Vitamins.* de Gruyter, Berlin, New York.

Gale, E. F. (1946) The bacterial amino acid decarboxylases. *Advan. Enzymol.* 6: 1-32.

Gonzales-Porque, P. and Strominger, J. L. (1972) Introduction of the 3-deoxy group in 3, 6-dideoxyhexoses. Novel cofactor function for pyridoxamine 5′-phosphate. *Proc. Nat. Acad. Sci. U.S. A.* 69: 1625-1628.

Gunsalus, I. C., Bellamy, W. D. & Umbreit, W. W. (1944) A phosphorylated derivative of pyridoxal as the coenzyme of tyrosine decarboxylase. *J. Biol. Chem.* 155:685-686.

György, P. (1934) Vitamin B_2 and the pellagra-like dermatitis of rats. *Nature* 133: 448-449.

György, P. (1964) History of vitamin B_6. Introductory remarks. *Vitamins & Hormones* 22: 361-365.

Jenkins, W. T. & Sizer, I. W. (1957) Glutamic aspartic transaminase. *J. Am. Chem. Soc.* 79: 2655-2656.

Lichstein, H. C., Umbreit, W. W., & Gunsalus, I. C. (1945) Function of the vitamin B_6 group: Pyridoxal phosphate (codecarboxylase) in transamination. *J. Biol. Chem.* 161: 311-320.

Meister, A. (1965) *Biochemistry of the Amino Acids.* 2nd ed., vol. 1 & 2, Academic Press, New York.

Meister, A., Sober, H. A., & Peterson, E. A. (1954) Studies of the coenzyme activation of glutamic aspartic transaminase. *J. Biol. Chem.* 206: 89-100.

Metzler, D. E., Ikawa, M. & Snell, E. E. (1954) A general mechanism for vitamin B_6-catalyzed reactions. *J. Am. Chem. Soc.* 76: 639-644.

Moeller, E. F. (1938) Vitamin B-6 (Adermin) als Wuchsstoff fur Milchsäurebakterien. *Z. Physiol. Chem.* 254: 285-286.

Palm, D., Klein, H. W., Schinzel, R., Buehner, M. & Helmreich, E. J. M. (1991) The role of pyridoxal 5'-phosphate in phosphorylase. *Biochemistry* 29: 1099-1107.

Rabinowitz, J. C. & Snell, E. E. (1947) The vitamin B-6 group. XII. Microbiological activity and natural occurrence of pyridoxamine phosphate. *J. Biol. Chem.* 169: 643-650.

Robinson, F. A. (1951) *The Vitamin B Complex.* Wiley, New York.

Schlenk, F. & Snell, E. E. (1945) Vitamin B_6 and transamination. *J. Biol. Chem.* 157: 425-426.

Snell, E. E. (1944) The vitamin activities of pyridoxal and pyridoxamine. *J. Biol. Chem.* 154: 313-314.

Snell, E. E. (1958) Chemical structure in relation to biological activities of vitamin B_6. *Vitamins and Hormones* 16: 77-125.

Snell, E. E. (1981) Vitamin B-6 analysis: Some historical aspects. In: J. E. Leklum & R. D. Reynolds (eds.): *Methods in Vitamin B-6 Nutrition.* Plenum, New York, pp. 1-19.

Song, K. B. & Frey, P. A. (1991) Molecular properties of lysine-2,3-amino-mutase. *J. Biol. Chem.* 266: 7651-7655.

Uzawa, S. (1943) Formation of indole from L-tryptophan (VII). Separation of apo- and co-tryptophanase. *J. Osaka Med. Assoc.* 42: 1637.

van Poelje, P. D. & Snell, E. E. (1990) Pyruvoyl-dependent enzymes. *Ann. Rev. Biochem.* 59: 29-59.

Wada, H. & Snell, E. E. (1962) Enzymatic transamination of pyridoxamine. I. With oxaloacetate and α-ketoglutarate. *J. Biol. Chem.* 237: 127-132.

Wada, H., Morisue, T., Nishimura, W., Morino, Y., Sakamota, Y., & Ichihara, K. (1959) Enzymatic studies on pyridoxine metabolism. *Proc. Japan Acad.* 35: 299-304.

Wagner, A. F. & Folkers, K. (1964) *Vitamins & Coenzymes.* Wiley, New York.

Williams, R. J., Eakin, R. E., Beerstecher, E. & Shive, W. (1950) *Biochemistry of the B Vitamins.* Reinhold, New York.

MOLECULAR EVOLUTION

Biochemistry of Vitamin B$_6$ and PQQ
G. Marino, G. Sannia and F. Bossa (eds.)
© 1994 Birkhäuser Verlag Basel/Switzerland

Molecular evolution of pyridoxal-5'-phosphate-dependent enzymes

P. Christen, P.K. Mehta and E. Sandmeier

Biochemisches Institut der Universität Zürich,
Winterthurerstr. 190, CH-8057 Zürich, Switzerland

Summary

The pyridoxal-5'-phosphate-dependent enzymes (B$_6$ enzymes) that act on amino acid substrates are of multiple evolutionary origin. Database searches with sequence profiles indicate that the B$_6$ enzymes can be subdivided into several families of homologous proteins of which the α family is by far the largest. The α family includes enzymes that catalyze, with few exceptions, transformations of amino acids in which the covalency changes are limited to Cα. Enzymes of the β or γ families mainly catalyze replacement and elimination reactions at Cβ or Cγ, respectively. Apparently, the primordial pyridoxal-5'-phosphate-dependent enzymes were regio-specific catalysts, which first specialized for reaction specificity and then for substrate specificity. Part of the amino acid decarboxylases belong to the α family, the other decarboxylases constitute three different evolutionarily independent families. A few other B$_6$ enzymes appear to represent additional families of B$_6$ enzymes.

This short review recapitulates extensive studies on the evolutionary relationships among the B$_6$ enzymes that catalyze transformations of amino acids. Amino acid sequences of these enzymes were compared by computer-assisted algorithms. To date, more than 300 sequences of more than 50 different B$_6$ enzymes have been determined. Related sequences were multiply aligned and their homology verified by profile analysis. This database-searching program (Gribskov et al., 1990) is based on a position-specific scoring table, the profile, which is constructed from a set of homologous amino acid sequences and an amino acid substitution matrix. The profile is thus specific for a given set of homologous proteins and particularly suited to detect distant evolutionary relationships.

Table I. The α family of B₆ enzymes, comprehensive list of member enzymes

Enzyme	Reference
Aminotransferases of all substrate specificities except subgroup III (branched-chain and D-amino acid aminotransferase)	Mehta et al., 1989, 1993
Serine hydroxymethyltransferase	Alexander et al., 1994
Glycine-C-acetyltransferase	
5-Aminolevulinate synthase	
8-Amino-7-oxononanoate synthase	
Tryptophanase	Antson et al., 1993
Tyrosine phenol-lyase	
1-Aminocyclopropane-1-carboxylate synthase	Mehta & Christen, 1994
2-Amino-6-caprolactam racemase	
Glutamate-1-semialdehyde 2;1-aminomutase	
Isopenicillin-N-epimerase	
2,2-Dialkylglycine decarboxylase	
4-Amino-4-deoxychorismate synthase (*pabC* gene product)	Green et al., 1992; Mehta & Christen, 1993
Cysteine desulfurase (*nifS* gene product)	Mehta & Christen, 1993; Zheng et al., 1994
cobC gene product (cobalamin synthesis)	
malY gene product (abolishing endogenous induction of the maltose system)	Reidl & Boos, 1991
Amino acid decarboxylases of group II (see Table III)	Sandmeier et al., 1994

Profile analyses of their amino acid sequences showed that the B₆ enzymes are of multiple evolutionary origin, i.e. constitute several different families of homologous proteins. The largest family is the α family (Alexander et al., 1994) which includes by now a total of 34 enzymes (Table I). In the multiple alignment of the sequences of the α enzymes, the only residues remaining invariant out of the four invariant residues in the comprehensive alignment of aminotransferases (Mehta et al., 1993) appear to be the pyridoxal-5'-phosphate-binding lysine residue and the aspartate residue interacting with the pyridine N of the coenzyme. The enzymes of the α family, with few exceptions (Table II), catalyze reactions in which the covalency changes of the amino acid substrate are restricted to the same carbon atom that carries the amino group forming the imine linkage with the coenzyme. These enzymes use not only the same coenzyme but also a similar protein scaffold to catalyze quite different transformations of amino acids. It thus seems feasible to change the substrate or even the reaction specificity of a given enzyme by substitution of a limited number of critical amino acid residues. Indeed, substitutions

Table II. Lack of correlation between evolutionary affiliation and reaction type

Family	Enzyme	Reaction catalyzed
α	Tryptophanase	β-Elimination
	Tyrosine phenol-lyase	β-Elimination
	1-Aminocyclopropane-1-carboxylate synthase	α, γ-Replacement
β	Threonine synthase	β, γ-Replacement
γ	Cystathionine β-lyase	β-Elimination

of four single apolar active-site residues by histidine have increased the ratio between the activities of aspartate aminotransferase toward dicarboxylic and aromatic substrates by one to two orders of magnitude (Vacca et al., 1993; Pan et al., 1994), and re-engineering of the substrate binding site of the same enzyme has resulted in newly generated β-decarboxylase activity toward L-aspartate (Graber et al., 1993).

The β family includes L- and D-serine dehydratase, threonine dehydratase, the β subunit of tryptophan synthase, threonine synthase and cysteine synthase. These enzymes catalyze β-replacement or β-elimination reactions. The γ family incorporates *O*-succinylhomoserine (thiol)-lyase, *O*-acetylhomoserine (thiol)-lyase, and cystathionine γ-lyase, which catalyze γ-replacement or γ-elimination reactions, as well as cystathionine β-lyase. Thus, the affiliation of a given enzyme with one of the three families, which have been defined by structural criteria only, correlates in most cases with its regio-specificity. Profile analyses suggest that the α and γ families might be distantly related with one another, but are clearly not homologous with the β family (Alexander et al., 1994). Apparently, the earliest pyridoxal-5'-phosphate-dependent enzymes were regio-specific enzymes, which first diverged into reaction-specific catalysts and then specialized for substrate specificity.

Table III. Evolutionarily unrelated groups of amino acid decarboxylases

Group I	Glycine decarboxylase
Group II (belongs to α family)	Glutamate decarboxylase Tyrosine decarboxylase Aromatic-L-amino-acid decarboxylase Tryptophan decarboxylase (α-Methyldopa-hypersensitive gene product)
Group III	Ornithine decarboxylase (*E. coli*) Lysine decarboxylase (eubacteria) Arginine decarboxylase (*E. coli*, biodegradative)
Group IV	Ornithine decarboxylase (eucaryotes) Arginine decarboxylase (*E. coli*, biosynthetic; plants) Diaminopimelate decarboxylase (eubacteria)

In contrast to the aminotransferases which, with very few exceptions (see Table I), are members of the α-family, i.e. of a single family of homologous proteins, the amino acid decarboxylases appear to be of multiple evolutionary origin and belong to at least four mutually unrelated groups (Table III; Sandmeier et al., 1994). In some cases, amino acid decarboxylases are evolutionarily unrelated with each other even if they have the same substrate specificity and - in the case of arginine decarboxylase - occur in the same species. The amino acid decarboxylases thus provide a particularly impressive example of molecular functional convergence of B_6 enzymes. Conceivably, amino acid decarboxylases have evolved along even more than four different lineages; as yet, the amino acid sequences of only half of the known decarboxylases have been determined.

In addition to the amino acid decarboxylases of groups I, III and IV, a few other B_6 enzymes seem to be unrelated with the α, β or γ families by the criterion of profile analysis: alanine racemase, alliin lyase and selenocysteine synthase (which is perhaps related to the α or γ family). These enzymes may represent yet other families of B_6 enzymes. None of the B_6 enzymes analyzed seems to be related with any of the 36,000 non-B_6 protein sequences in the database. The specialization of the various B_6 enzymes for reaction and substrate specificity appears to have occurred in most cases already in the universal ancestor cell. This notion is based on the few instances in which sequences of the same enzyme of archaebacterial, eubacterial and eucaryotic species are known and are found to be much more similar among each other than to any other B_6 enzyme.

Acknowledgements

This work was supported by the Swiss National Science Foundation (grant 31-36542.92) and by the Bundesamt für Bildung und Wissenschaft as part of the EU program "Human Capital and Mobility" (grant BBW 93.0304, EU No. CHRX-CT93-0179).

References

Alexander, F.W., Sandmeier, E., Mehta, P.K. and Christen, P. (1994) Evolutionary relationships among pyridoxal-5'-phosphate-dependent enzymes. Regio-specific α, β and γ families. *Eur. J. Biochem. 219*, 953-960.

Graber, R., Sandmeier, E., Berger, P. and Christen, P. (1993) Changing the reaction specificity of a B_6 enzyme. Newly generated beta-decarboxylase activity in aspartate aminotransferase R 386A/Y225R. 25th Annual Meeting of the Swiss Societies for Experimental Biology (USGEB/USSBE), Basel, Abstracts, *Experientia 49*, A37.

Gribskov, M., Lüthy, R. and Eisenberg, D. (1990) Profile Analysis. *Methods Enzymol. 183*, 146-159.

Mehta, P.K. and Christen, P. (1993) Homology of pyridoxal-5'-phosphate-dependent aminotransferases with the *cobC* (cobalamin synthesis), *nifS* (nitrogen fixation), *pabC* (*p*-aminobenzoate synthesis) and *malY* (abolishing endogenous induction of the maltose system) gene products. *Eur. J. Biochem. 211*, 373-376.

Mehta, P.K. and Christen, P. (1994) Homology of 1-aminocyclopropane-1-carboxylate synthase, 8-amino-7-oxononanoate synthase, 2-amino-6-caprolactam racemase, 2,2-dialkylglycine decarboxylase, glutamate-1-semialdehyde 2,1-aminomutase and isopenicillin-*N*-epimerase with aminotransferases. *Biochem. Biophys. Res. Commun. 198*, 138-143.

Mehta, P.K., Hale, T.I. and Christen, P. (1989) Evolutionary relationships among aminotransferases: Tyrosine aminotransferase, histidinol-phosphate aminotransferase, and aspartate aminotransferase are homologous proteins. *Eur. J. Biochem. 186*, 249-253.

Mehta, P.K., Hale, T.I. and Christen, P. (1993) Aminotransferases: Demonstration of homology and division into evolutionary subgroups. *Eur. J. Biochem. 214*, 549-561.

Pan, P., Jaussi, R., Gehring, H., Giannattasio, S. and Christen, P. (1994) Shift in pH-rate profile and enhanced discrimination between dicarboxylic and aromatic substrates in mitochondrial aspartate aminotransferase Y70H. *Biochemistry 33*, 2757-2760.

Reidl, J. and Boos, W. (1991) The *malX malY* operon of *Escherichia coli* encodes a novel enzyme II of the phosphotransferase system recognizing glucose and maltose and an enzyme abolishing the endogenous induction of the maltose system. *J. Bacteriol. 173*, 4862-4876.

Sandmeier, E., Hale, T.I. and Christen, P. (1994) Multiple evolutionary origin of pyridoxal-5'-phosphate-dependent amino acid decarboxylases. *Eur. J. Biochem. 221*, 997-1002.

Vacca, R.A., Christen, P. and Sandmeier, E. (1993) Introduction of a histidine residue at position 17, 37 or 140 of aspartate aminotransferase. Effects on reaction and substrate specificity. 25th Annual Meeting of the Swiss Societies for Experimental Biology (USGEB/USSBE), Basel, Abstracts, *Experientia 49*, A36.

Zheng, L., White, R.H., Cash, V.L. and Dean, D.R. (1994) Mechanism for the desulfurization of L-cysteine catalyzed by the *nifS* gene product. *Biochemistry 33*, 4714-4720.

Biochemistry of Vitamin B$_6$ and PQQ
G. Marino, G. Sannia and F. Bossa (eds.)
© 1994 Birkhäuser Verlag Basel/Switzerland

Stereospecificity of aminotransferases for C-4' hydrogen transfer and enzyme evolution

K. Soda, T. Yoshimura and N. Esaki

Institute for Chemical Research, Kyoto University, Uji, Kyoto 611, Japan

Summary

D-Amino acid aminotransferase and branched-chain L-amino acid aminotransferase show a significant homology in amino acid sequence each other, but little similarity to all other aminotransferases. They are also unique in the stereospecificity for hydrogen transfer at the C-4' of external Schiff base intermediates: show the *pro-R* specificity in contrast to other various aminotransferases catalyzing the *pro-S* hydrogen transfer. This suggests that their topographical situations of the external Schiff base and the catalytic base in the active site are similar to each other, but different from those of other aminotransferases. X-Ray chrystallographic data of D-amino acid aminotransferase support this hypothesis: The structure of D-amino acid aminotransferase is different from those of other aminotransferases so far studied. Based on the structure, and stereospecificity for C-4' hydrogen transfer, D-amino acid aminotransferase and branched-chain L-amino acid aminotransferase probably evolved from the common ancestral protein, which was different from that of other aminotransferases.

Introduction

In all the reactions of aminotransferases studied so far, a proton is added or removed on the *si* face at C-4' of the plane of the conjugated π-system of the pyridoxal 5'-phosphate (PLP) -substrate imine (external Schiff base intermediate). This suggests the similar orientation of the catalytic base and the bound cofactor in the active sites of enzymes, and also their molecular evolution from a common ancestral protein (Dunathan and Voet, 1974). Recently, Christen and his cowarkers (Metha et al., 1993) classified the aminotransferases into four subgroups on the basis of comparison of their amino acid sequences: (I) aspartate aminotransferase and a few others, (II) ornithine aminotransferase and a few others (III) D-amino acid aminotransferase and branched-chain L-amino acid aminotransferase, (IV) serine aminotransferase and phosphoserine aminotransferase. Aminotransferases belonging to subgroups (I), (II), and (IV) are considerably homologous in the sequences, but D-amino acid aminotransferase (D-AAT) of *Bacillus* sp. YM-1 and branched-chain L-amino acid aminotransferase (BCAT) of *Escherichia coli* show a significant homology with each other in their primary structures, but are different from all other aminotransferases. The hydrogen transfer stereospecificities of only aspartate aminotransferase and alanine aminotransferase (subgroup I) have been determined among various aminotransferases. We were interested in stereospecificity of aminotransferases belonging to other subgroups. We established a simple method for determination of the stereospecificity for the C-4' proton transfer, and studied the stereochemistry of the reactions catalyzed by D-AAT and BCAT of subgroup III (Yoshimura et al., 1993), and L-ornithine aminotransferase (OAT) of *Bacillus* sp. YM-2 of subgroup II.

Materials and Methods

Materials. D-AAT was purified as described previously (Tanizawa, et al., 1989). BCAT of *E. coli* K-12 (Kuramitsu, et al., 1985) was kindly supplied by Dr. K. Inoue and Dr. H. Kagamiyama of Osaka Medical College, Takatsuki, Japan. Ornithine aminotransferase was purified from *Bacillus* sp. YM-2 as described elsewhere.

Apo-AspAT and apo-BCAT, and apo-DAT were prepared as described previously (Yoshimura, 1993). Apo-OAT was prepared by dialysis of the pyridoxamine 5'-phosphate (PMP) form of enzyme against 2M guanidium HCl for 12 hr followed by dialysis against 10 mM HEPES buffer (pH 8.0) at 4°C for 16 hr.

4'-*RS* -[4'-^{3}H]PMP was prepared as follows. The reaction mixture (pH 4.5) containing 16.5 μmol of PMP and 5.7 μmol of PLP in 150 μL of ^{3}H$_2$O (555 MBq) was incubated at room temperature in the dark for 4 days. The reaction mixture was then applied onto a Dow 1 column (acetate form, 1 x 7 cm) equilibrated with 0.1 M NaOH. After the column was washed with 0.1 M NaOH and water, PMP was eluted with 0.1 M HCl. PMP was further purified by reversed-phase column chromatography with an Ultron SC-18 column (Shinwa-Kako, Japan, 0.46 x 15 cm) equipped on a Shimadzu LC-6A HPLC system. PMP was eluted at 4.3 min with 0.1 % trifuluoroacetic acid with a flow rate of 1 mL/min.

4'-*S* and 4'-*R*-[4'-^{3}H]PMP were prepared by incubation of 4'-*RS* -[4'-^{3}H]PMP with apo-BCAT and apo-AspAT, respectively. The reaction mixture (0.5 mL) containing 50 mmol of Tris-HCl buffer (pH 8.0), 87.9 μmol of [4'-^{3}H]PMP, and 147 μmol of apo-AspAT or 176 nmol of apo-BCAT was incubated at 30°C for 15 hr. Under the conditions, AspAT (Tobler et al., 1986) and BCAT (Yoshimura et al., 1993) catalyze the exchange of C-4' pro-*S* and pro-*R* tritium with hydrogen of the solvent, respectively . The unlabeled PMP (8.9 nmol) was added to the mixture as a carrier, and the reaction was stopped by addition of 18 mL of 12 M HCl. The mixture was further incubated at 30°C for 3 hr followed by incubation at 75°C for 15 min.

After centrifugation, the supernatant solution was dried with a Speed Vac Concentrator (Savant, U.S.A.), and the residue was dissolved in 0.5 mL of H_2O. 4'-S -[4'-^{3}H]PMP (1.20 x 10^6 dpm/mmol) and 4'-R -[4'-^{3}H]PMP (1.08 x 10^6 dpm/mmol) thus obtained were purified by reversed-phase column chromatography.

Stereochemistry of the C-4' hydrogen abstraction from PMP in the half and overall reactions of D-AAT, BCAT, and OAT was studied as described below. The reaction mixture (100 μL) for the half reaction contained 10 mmol of Tris-HCl buffer (pH 8.0), 0.5 mmol of α-ketoglutarate, 1.98 nmol of 4'-S -[4'-^{3}H]PMP or 4'-R -[4'-^{3}H]PMP, and 5 nmol of apo-enzymes. The reaction was carried out at 30°C for 15 min and terminated by addition of 100 μL of 1 M HCl. The mixture was immediately frozen in liquid nitrogen and dried with a Speed Vac Concentrator. The residue was dissolved in 200 μL of H_2O and subjected to radioactivity assay. The tritium released from PMP was expressed as a vaporable radioactivity, which was obtained by subtraction of the radioactivity finally found from the radioactivity initially added to the reaction mixture. The reaction conditions for the overall transamination reactions were the same as those for the half reactions except that the reaction mixture of AspAT, D-AAT, BCAT, and OAT contained 3 μmol of L-aspartate, 1 μmol of D-alanine, 1μmol of L-valine, and 1 μmol of L-ornithine, respectively.

Results and Discussion

When a PMP form of aminotransferase is converted to a PLP-form by incubation with an amino acceptor (a half reaction), one hydrogen is withdrawn from C-4' of PMP. We examined the stereospecificities of D-AAT, BCAT, and OAT for the hydrogen abstraction by measurement of ^{3}H released in the reaction of an apo-form of enzyme with the stereospecifically tritiated PMP and α-ketoglutarate. The stereospecificities of D-AAT, BCAT, and OAT for the hydrogen abstraction in the overall reactions were also determined in the presence of D-alanine, L-valine, L-ornithine, respectively (Table I). In the half and overall reactions of D-AAT and BCAT, ^{3}H was released exclusively from 4'-R-[4'-^{3}H]PMP, whereas was released from only 4'-S-[4'-^{3}H]PMP by OAT and AspAT. Thus, D-AAT and BCAT specifically abstract the pro-R C-4' hydrogen from PMP in both half and overall reactions, and OAT and AspAT abstract the pro-S C-4' hydrogen.

The results obtained demonstrated for the first time that the pro-R hydrogen is added or withdrawn at C-4' of the bound cofactor in the aminotransferase reactions; aminotransferases of subgroup III catalyze the *re*-face transfer of the C-4' proton. The stereochemistry of this hydrogen transfer reflects the geometrical relations between the external Schiff base interemediate and a catalytic base of the enzyme. The result of stereochemistry suggests that the geometrical relations in D-AAT and BCAT are opposit to that of AspAT: the catalytic residue of D-AAT (K145) is probably located on the *re* -face of the external Schiff base intermediate. This was recently confirmed by crystallography. The identity of stereospecificity of D-AAT with that of BCAT indicates that their structures of active sites are homologous with each other, but different from those of other aminotransferases. This is compatible with the classification of aminotransferases according to their primary structures: both enzyme belong to the same subgroup (III), and differ from other three groups of aminotransferases.

Table I. Stereochemistry of hydrogen withdrawal from PMP in the half and overall reactions by AspAT, OAT, D-AAT and BCAT. Under the conditions no tritium was released in the absence of enzyme. Percentage given is ratio of radioactivity released to that initially added in the reaction mixture. (KG: α-ketoglutarate)

	4'-S--[4'-^{3}H]PMP		4'-R-[4'-^{3}H]PMP		
	^{3}H-released		^{3}H-released		
	dpm	%	dpm	%	
apo-AspAT + KG + L-Asp	1210	51	0	0	*si*
apo-OAT + KG	1472	72	0	0	*si*
apo-OAT + KG + L-Orn	1156	57	0	0	*si*
apo-D-AAT + KG	36	1.5	1681	78.6	*re*
apo-D-AAT + KG + D-Ala	0	0	1657	75.9	*re*
apo-BCAT + KG	229	9.6	1233	57.6	*re*
apo-BCAT + KG + L-Val	0	0	1506	70.4	*re*

Recently, three-dimensional structure of ω-amino acid: pyruvate aminotransferase (ω-APT), which falls under subgroup II as like OAT was shown (Watanabe et al., 1990). Its structure resembles that of the AspAT. The structure of D-AAT is quite different from those of AspAT and ω-APT (Sugio, personal communication). These results suggest that AspAT (subgroup I) and ω-APT (subgroup II) evolved divergently from the common ancestral protein, but the ancestral protein of D-AAT (subgroup III) is probably different from that of AspAT and ω-APT. Characteristics of aminotransferases on stereospecificity for the C-4' hydrogen transfer are compatible with those on based on their three-dimensional structures and the primary structures.

References

Dunathan, H. C. and Voet, J. G. (1974) Stereochemical evidence for the evolution of pyridoxal-phosphate enzymes of various function from a common ancestors. *Proc.Natl.Acad.Sci. U.S.A.* 71, 3888 - 3891.

Kuramitsu, S., Ogawa, T., Ogawa, H., Kagamiyama, H. (1985) Branched-chain amino acid aminotrans-ferase of *Escherichia coli*: Nucleotide Sequence of *ilvE* Gene and the deduced amino acid sequence. *J. Biochem. (Tokyo)* 97: 993-999.

Metha, P., Hale, T.I., and Christen, P. (1993) Aminotransferases: Demonstration of homology and division into evolutionary subgroups. *Eur. J. Biochem.* 214: 549 - 561.

Tobler, H.P., Christen, P., Gehring, H. Stereospecific labilization of the C-4' *pro-S* hydrogen of pyridoxamine 5'-phosphate in aspartate aminotransferase. (1986) *J.Biol.Chem.*, 261: 7105 - 7108.

Tanizawa, K., Asano, S., Masu, Y., Kuramitsu, S., Kagamiyama, H., Tanaka, and H., Soda, K. (1989) The primary structure of Thermostable D-amino acid aminotransferase from a Thermophilic *Bacillus* spiecies and its correlation with L-amino acid aminotransferase. *J. Biol. Chem.* 264: 2450-2454.

Watanabe, N., Yonaha, K., Sakabe, K., Sakabe, N., Aibara, S., and Morita, Y. (1990) Cryatal structure of ω-amino acid: pyruvate aminotransferase. In: Fukui,T., Kagamiyama, H., Soda, K., and Wada, H. (eds.): *Enzymes Dependent on Pyridoxal Phosphate and Other Carbonyl Compounds as Cofactors*, Pergamon Press, Oxford, pp.121-124.

Yoshimura, T., Nishimura, K., Ito, J., Esaki, N., Kagamiyama, H., Manning, J. M., and Soda, K. Unique Stereospecificity of D-amino acid aminotransferase and branched-chain L-amino acid aminotransferase for C-4' hydrogen transfer of the coenzyme. *J. Am. Chem. Soc.* 115: 3897 - 3900.

Biochemistry of Vitamin B$_6$ and PQQ
G. Marino, G. Sannia and F. Bossa (eds.)
© 1994 Birkhäuser Verlag Basel/Switzerland

Detection of weak structural similarities among PLP dependent enzymes

S. Pascarella and F. Bossa

Dipartimento di Scienze Biochimiche and Centro di Biologia Molecolare del C.N.R., Università La Sapienza, 00185 Roma, Italy

Summary

A multiple sequence alignment among homologous and distant PLP enzymes was constructed on the basis of three dimensional structure superposition. The profile calculated from this alignment was able to detect similarities to the serine hydroxymethyltransferase family and to PLP/PMP dependent enzymes involved in the biosynthesis of dideoxy and aminosugars. Sequence alignments between the profile and these sequences showed the conservation of some essential residues.

Introduction

We are studying the mechanism of action of the pyridoxal-P (PLP) dependent enzyme serine hydroxymethyltransferase (SHMT) with a site directed mutagenesis approach (Schirch et al., 1993). However, the lack of information on the spatial architecture of SHMT from crystallographic data limited severely a rational application of this approach as well as the interpretation of results. Detection of similarities to other PLP dependent enzymes for which a structural and functional characterization is available, could alleviate this handicap. Aminotransferases (AAT; McPhalen et al., 1992) are among the best characterized group of PLP dependent enzymes. Unfortunately, sequences of PLP enzymes which catalyze different reaction types are very distant and not easily comparable. This research is aimed at the detection of weak but significant structural similarities between SHMT and AAT.

Methods

Profile analysis in the GCG package (Gribskov et al., 1990) and an advanced version incorporating a weighting scheme (Lüthy et al., 1994) were used in the research. Secondary structure predictions of multiple sequence alignments were calculated with PHD (Rost et al., 1994). Structural superpositions were performed with the program HOMO (Rossmann and Argos, 1976) and verified and modified with an Indigo SiliconGraphics station. Crystallographic structures from cytosolic aspartate aminotransferase (PDB code: 7AAT; McPhalen et al., 1992), tyrosine phenol-lyase (1TPL; Antson et al., 1993) and dialkylglycine decarboxylase (DGD; Toney et al., 1993) were considered. The SWISS-PROT data bank was used for sequence searching. Secondary structure and side chain accessibility were calculated on the base of crystal coordinates with the program DSSP (Kabsch and Sander, 1983).

Results and Discussion

The sequences of 7AAT, 1TPL and DGD are rather distant (about 10% pairwise identity), and, therefore, were aligned by structural superposition. The resulting multiple sequence alignment (DAT) is the query profile for the SWISS-PROT search. A few members of the SHMT family were given a meaningful score, higher than those attributed to other sequences related to the input probe (Pascarella et al., 1993). The weighted profile, built from the sequence alignment of 14 SHMT sequences, detected a significant score for a few PLP enzymes (Table I) related to aminotransferases. The SHMT sequences were aligned to the DAT profile with the GCG routine PROFILEGAP. The alignment (Fig. 1) shows the conservation of three of the four residues conserved in all the aminotransferases of the α family (Mehta et al., 1993; Alexander et al., 1994), Asp222, Lys258, and Arg386 according to the AAT numbering system. The SHMT predicted secondary structure generally agrees with the experimentally observed structures for the three enzymes. Also, the alignment matches 80% of the core residues buried in all three structures (fractional side chain accessibility less than 5%) with conserved hydrophobic side chains in the 14

Table I. Top Z-scores assigned by the weighted profile based on the alignment of 14 SHMTs to some PLP dependent enzymes

SWISS-PROT code	enzyme	source	score
BIOF_BACSH	8-amino-7-oxononanoate synthase	*Bacillus sphaericus*	7.28
KBL_ECOLI	2-amino-3-ketobutyrate coenzyme A ligase	*Escherichia coli*	6.13
TNA1_SYMTH	tryptophanase 1	*Symbiobacterium thermophilum*	5.34
TNA2_SYMTH	tryptophanase 2	*Symbiobacterium thermophilum*	4.51
BIOF_ECOLI	8-amino-7-oxononanoate synthase	*Escherichia coli*	3.94
HEM1_RHOSH	5-aminolevulinic acid synthase	*Rhodobacter sphaeroides*	3.81

```
                  222                    258                  386
      1tpl     IKVFYDATRC.V         DGCTMSGKKDCLV        KLETVRLTIP...RRVY
      7aat     LLAYFDMAYQ.G         VVLSQSYAKNMGL        ...DGRISV........
       dgd     MLLILDEAQTGV         DILTLS..KTLGA        MGGVFRIAPP...LTV.
 glya_ecoli    AYLFVDMAHVAG         HVVTTTTHKTLAG        VTSGIRVGTPAITRRGF
 glya_camje    AYLFADIAHIAG         HVVSSTTHKTLRG        ITSGLRLGTPALTARGF
 glya_salty    AYLFVDMAHVAG         HVVTTTTHKTLAG        VTSGIRIGSPAVTRRGF
 glya_bacst    AYLMVDMAHIAG         HFVTTTTHKTLRG        VTSGIRIGTAAVTTRGF
 glya_hypme    AIFLVDMAHFAG         HVVTTTTHKTLRG        VTSGIRLGSPAGTTRGF
 glya_braja    AYLLVDMAHFAG         HVTTTTTHKSLRG        VTSGLRLGTPAATTRGF
 gly1_neucr    AYLVVDMAHISG         DVVTTTTHKSLRG        TPGGLRIGTPAMTTRGF
 gly1_rabit    AYLMADMAHISG         HVVTTTTHKTLRG        RPSGLRLGTPALTSRGF
   cs_shmt     AYLMADMAHISG         HVVTTTTHKTLRG        RPSGLRLGTPALTSRGL
 gly1_human    AYLMADMAHISG         HVVTTTTHKTLRG        RPSGLRLGTPALTSRGL
 gly2_human    AHLLADMAHISG         DIVTTTTHKTLRG        TPGGLRLGAPALTSRQF
 gly2_rabit    AHLLADMAHISG         DVVTTTTHKTLRG        TPGGLRLGAPALTSRQF
   gly2_pea    AVLLADMAHISG         DVVTTTTHKSLRG        VPGGIRMGTPALTSRGF
 glya_actac    AYLFVDMAHVAG         HVVTTTTHKTLGG        ITSGIRVGTPSVTRRGF
```

Figure 1. Alignment among SHMT sequences and the DAT profile in the regions containing the essential residues Asp222, Lys258 and Arg386. Codes for SHMTs are: GLYA_ECOLI: *Escherichia coli*; GLYA_CAMJE: *Campilobacter jejuni*; GLYA_SALTY: *Salmonella typhimurium*; GLYA_BACST: *Bacillus stearothermophilus*; GLYA_HYPME: *Hyphomicrobium methylovorum*; GLYA_BRAJA: *Bradyrhizobium japonicum*; GLY2_HUMAN: *Homo sapiens* (mit.); GLY2_RABIT: Rabbit (mit.); GLY1_HUMAN: *Homo sapiens* (cyt.); GLY1_RABIT: Rabbit (cyt.); GLY1_NEUCR: *Neurospora crassa* (cyt); GLY2_PEA: *Pisum sativum* (mit.); GLYA_BACST: *Bacillus stearothermophilus*; CS_SHEEP: sheep (cyt.). The other SHMT conserved arginine close to that equivalent to the AAT Arg386 is boldfaced. AAT numbering system is adopted.

SHMT sequences. These observations strongly support the structural similarity between SHMT and AAT. The residues predicted by the alignment to be catalytically relevant (in particular Asp222 and Arg386) were mutated by site directed mutagenesis. Results for Asp222 are preliminary while the results for Arg386 confirm the theoretical prediction (Delle Fratte et al., in preparation). Another arginine conserved in all SHMTs was mutated and showed little, if any, influence on activity (Fig. 1) .

The DAT profile based on structural superpositioning proved to be sensitive enough to localize some of the essential residues in SHMT. The profile assigned a meaningful score also to a group of homologous bacterial sequences belonging to a group of putative enzymes involved in the biosynthesis of antibiotics or surface antigens (Table II). The profile built with these sequences

Table II. Group of homologous bacterial sequences. DAT profile assigned to some of these sequences a score > 3.0

Sequence denominations and available SWISS-PROT codes in parentheses	putative function
eryC1 (ERBS_SACER)	erythromycin synthesis
degT (DEGT_BACSU)	pleiotropic regulatory gene
dnrJ (DNRJ_STRPE)	daunorubicin synthesis
prg1 (fragment)	puromycin synthesis
strS	streptomycin synthesis
orf10.4 in the *rfbG-rfbJ* intergenic region (YRF7_SALTY)	O antigen synthesis
o299 in the *rffE-rffT* region (YIFI_ECOLI)	enterobacterial common antigen synthesis
ascC	ascarylose synthesis
tylB	tylosin synthesis

24

```
                   222                                                             258
     1tpl  NMRAVRELTEAHGIKVFYDATRC.VENAYFIKEQEQGFENKSIAEIVHEMFSYA......DGCTMS.GKKDCLV.NI.GGF
     7aat  QWKELASVVKKRNLLAYFDMAYQ.GFASG............DINRDAWALRHFIEQGIDVVLSQS.YAKNMGLYGERAGA
      dgd  YMAALKRKCEARGMLLILDEAQTGVGRTG............TMFACQRDGVTP......DILTLS...KTLGA.GLPLAA
yifi_ecoli  EMDTIMALAKKHNLFVVEDAAQGVMSTYK.................GRALGTIGHIGCFSPH.ETKNYTAGGEGGAT
degt_bacst  DMEAIAAIAKRHGLVVIEDAAQAIGAKYN.................GKCVGELGTAATYSFF.PTKNLGAYGDGGMI
erbs_sacer  DLDALRAIADRHGLALVEDVAQAVGARHR.................GHRVGAGSNAAAFSFY.PGKNLGALGDGGAV
dnrj_strpe  DMTPVLELAAEHDLKVLEDCAQAHGARRH.................GRLVGTQGHAAAFSFY.PTKVLGAYGDGGAV
     prg1  DMDAILGVAERYGLRVLEDCSHAHGSRYK.................GKPVGTFGDAAVFSLQ.ANKAVYA.GEGGIL
     tylB  DLDPVGAFAEPHGLAVVEDAAQATARYRG................RRIGSGHRTAFSFY.PGKNLGALGDGGAV
     strS  DMAALTAVAAEAGVPVIEDAAQALGTEIG.................GRPIGGFGDLACVSLFFEQKVITSGGEGGAV
yrf7_salty  NLSEVRRIADKYNLWLIEDCCDALGTTYE.................GQMVGTFGDIGTVSFY.PAHHITM.GEGGAV
     ascC  DLAEVRRVADKYNLWLIEDCCDALGSTYD.................GKMAGTFGDIGTVSFY.PAHHITM.GEGGAV
```

Figure 2. Sequence alignment in the AAT active site region among DAT and the bacterial sequences involved in the biosynthesis of dideoxy and aminosugars. AAT numering system adopted.

also assigns to a few PLP enzymes a meaningful score, although not sufficiently high to prove a definitive structural homology (Pascarella and Bossa, 1994). Recently, Thorson *et al.* (1993), were able to purify and characterize the product of the gene *ascC*, which is highly homologous to YRF7_SALTY, and demonstrated that it is the pyridoxamine-P (PMP) dependent dehydrase responsible for the biosynthesis of ascarylose, a 3,6 dideoxysugar. They proposed also that the other homologous sequences are PLP dependent aminotransferases involved in the biosynthesis of the aminosugars contained in the molecule of some antibiotics and surface antigens. The alignment to the active site of DAT is reported in Fig. 2. The histidine at position 258 instead of the lysine which forms a Schiff base with the cofactor in the PLP and PLP/PMP dependent enzymes seems to occur only in the PMP dependent enzymes. This is compatible with the fact that the latter forms only an "external" Schiff base between the substrate and the PMP form of the cofactor. However, this enzyme still needs a base to catalyze a proton shift. This central event in PLP and PLP/PMP dependent enzymes is supposed to be catalyzed by the ε amino group of the same active site lysine residue (K258 in AAT, K87 in tryptophan synthase). Interestingly, site directed mutagenesis experiments on aspartate aminotransferases substituting the active site lysine with other polar amino acid residues, and in particular with histidine, showed that the mutated protein maintains the proper fold and the capacity of binding PLP/PMP. Catalytic activity was still measurable but significantly lower than that of the native enzyme (Fukaki et al., 1990; Ziak et al., 1990). Similarly, experimental evidence obtained after mutation of the active site lysine in serine hydroxymethyltransferase suggests that this residue is not the base which removes a proton from the α carbon of glycine in its conversion to serine (Schirch et al., 1993). This confirms the hypothesis formulated by Christen that the ubiquitous active site lysine in PLP dependent enzymes might "represent a consequence of the chemical reactivity of the cofactor rather than a mechanistic necessity" (Ziak et al., 1990). On the other hand, Asp222 is presumably required both by the PLP/PMP dependent aminotransferases and the exclusively PLP or PMP dependent enzymes (such as SHMT and dideoxysugar dehydrases, respectively) since it interacts with the pyridine N1 and stabilizes the required positive charge during catalysis. An arginine equivalent to AAT Arg386, which binds the α carboxylate of the amino acid substrate, cannot be localized by sequence alignment in the other Lys258 bearing enzymes. Its presence would be expected in the enzymes involved in amino sugar biosynthesis since the amino group donor in the transamination reaction is still an amino acid. Very likely, the active site area of these enzymes was changed significantly during evolution in order to accomodate and bind sugar substrates.

Acknowledgments

We are indebted to Dr. Michael D. Toney and Prof. Johan H. Jansonius for kindly providing the DGD coordinates before the release in the PDB. Computer services provided by the Italian EMBnet node in Bari and by Progetto VAXRMA at University La Sapienza in Rome were essential. We are grateful to Prof. Verne Schirch for helpful discussions and comments. This work has been in part supported by a CNR grant in the framework of Progetto Speciale Bioinformatica and by a grant from the Commission of the European Communities (Human Capital and Mobility, contract ERBCHRXCT930179).

References

Alexander F. W., Sandmeier E., Mehta P. K. and Christen P. (1994) Evolutionary relationship among pyridoxal -5'-phosphate-dependent enzymes: regio specific α, β and γ families. *Eur. J. Biochem.* 219: 953-960.

Antson A. A., Demidkina T. V., Gollnick P., Dauter Z., Von Tersch R. L., Long J., Berezhnoy S. N., Phillips R. S., Harutyunyan E. H. and Wilson K. S. (1993). Three-dimensional structure of tyrosine phenol-lyase. *Biochemistry* 32: 4195-4206.

Fukaki S., Ueno H., Martinez del Pozo A., Pospishil M. A., Manning J. M., Ringe D., Stoddard B., Tanizawa K., Yoshimura T., Soda K. (1990). Substitution of glutamine for lysine at the pyridoxal phosphate binding site of bacterial D-amino acid transaminase. *J. Biol. Chem.* 265: 22306-22312.

Gribskov M., Lüthy R. and Eisenberg D. (1990). Profile analysis. *Methods Enzymol.* 183: 146-159.

Kabsch W. & Sander C. (1983). Dictionary of protein secondary structure: pattern recognition of hydrogen-bonded and geometrical features. *Biopolymers* 22: 2577-2637.

Lüthy, R, Xenarios I. and Bucher P. (1994) Improving the sensitivity of the sequence profile method. *Prot. Sci.* 3: 139-146.

McPhalen C. A., Vincent M. G. and Jansonius J. N. (1992). X-ray structure, refinement and comparison of three forms of mitochondrial aspartate aminotransferase. *J. Mol. Biol.* 225: 495-517.

Mehta P. K., Hale T. I. and Christen P. (1993). Aminotransferases: demonstration of homology and division into evolutionary subgroups. *Eur. J. Biochem.* 214: 549-561.

Pascarella S., Schirch V. and Bossa F. (1993) Similarity between serine hydroxymethyltransferase and other pyridoxal phosphate dependent enzymes. *FEBS Lett.* 331: 145-149.

Pascarella S. and Bossa F. (1994) Similarity between piyridoxal/pyridoxamine phosphate-dependent enzymes involved in dideoxy and deoxyaminosugar biosynthesis and other pyridoxal phosphate enzymes. *Prot. Sci.* 3: 701-705.

Rossmann M. G. and Argos P. (1976) Exploring structural homology of proteins. *J. Mol. Biol.* 105: 75-95.

Rost B., Sander C. and Schneider R. (1994) PHD: an automatic mail server for protein secondary structure prediction. *Comp. Appl. Biosci.* 10: 53-60.

Schirch D., Delle Fratte S., Iurescia S., Angelaccio S., Contestabile R., Bossa F. and Schirch V. (1993). Function of the active-site lysine in *Escherichia coli* serine hydroxymethyltransferase. *J. Biol. Chem.* 268: 23132-23138.

Thorson J. S., Lo S. F., Liu H-w. and Hutchinson C. R. (1993). Biosynthesis of 3,6-didehoxyexoses: new mechanistic reflections upon 2,6-dideoxy, 4,6-dideoxy, and amino sugar construction. *J. Am. Chem. Soc.* 115: 6993-6994.

Toney M. D., Hohenester E., Cowan S. W. and Jansonius J. N. (1993). Dialkylglycine decarboxylase structure: bifunctional active site and alkali metal sites. *Science* 261: 756-759.

Ziak M., Jaussi R., Gehring H. and Christen P. (1990). Aspartate aminotransferase with the pyridoxal-5'-phosphate-binding lysine residue replaced by histidine retains partial catalytic competence. *Eur. J. Biochem.* 187: 329-333.

AMINOTRANSFERASES

Biochemistry of Vitamin B₆ and PQQ
G. Marino, G. Sannia and F. Bossa (eds.)
© 1994 Birkhäuser Verlag Basel/Switzerland

Crystallographic studies on the vitamin B₆-assisted enzymic transamination reaction

J.N. Jansonius, J.-C. Génovésio-Taverne, M. Hennig, E. Hohenester, M. Jenny, V.N. Malashkevich, M. Moser, R. Müller, B.W. Shen, W. Stark, A. von Stosch and M.D. Toney

Biozentrum, University of Basel, Department of Structural Biology, Klingelbergstrasse 70, 4056 Basel, Switzerland

Vitamin B_6-dependent enzymes involved in amino acid metabolism seem to belong to a small number of independent families. They catalyze a wide variety of reactions on numerous different substrates (Dolphin et al., 1986). The aminotransferases, included in the α-family in the classification of Alexander et al. (1994), have been assigned to one of four subgroups, three of which are evolutionarily related (Mehta et al., 1993). In the following, some aspects of the three-dimensional structures and/or functional properties of aspartate aminotransferase (AspAT; subgroup I), dialkylglycine decarboxylase (DGD; subgroup II), ornithine aminotransferase (OAT; subgroup II) and phosphoserine aminotransferase (PSAT; subgroup IV) will be discussed.

Mitochondrial AspAT (mAspAT). In a longterm joint project with P. Christen et al. (University of Zurich) structure-function relationships of this enzyme are being investigated. Crystal structures have been determined of most of the catalytic intermediates (Christen and Metzler, 1985), or of representative models thereof, in the reversible transamination half-reaction that converts L-aspartate into oxaloacetate (Table 1). No crystal structure of the quinonoid intermediate has been obtained, since even in the most favourable case, with *erythro*-3-hydroxyaspartate as (pseudo) substrate it accumulates to no more than 20 % of the total intermediates. In crystals of the mAspAT-maleate complex at pH 7.5, a simple soak in solutions of

L-Asp or L-Glu caused maleate to be replaced by the substrate. Since the oxo acid product did not leave the active site, an equilibrium mixture of catalytic intermediates resulted, in which the ketimine dominated, with about 80 %. Accordingly, these structures could be determined (Malashkevich et al., 1993). The same procedure, applied to *erythro*-3-hydroxyaspartate, unexpectedly caused accumulation of the carbinolamine intermediate (A. von Stosch, J.-C. Génovésio-Taverne et al., unpublished results). This phenomenon could be explained by a favourable network of hydrogen bonds in the carbinolamine involving the α- and β-hydroxyl groups of the (pseudo) substrate, Tyr70* and Lys258. Steric hindrance between the β-OH and C4' of the cofactor apparently causes the ketimine intermediate to be of higher energy. These structures demonstrated: 1) The catalyzed reaction steps take place in the closed active site under exclusion of bulk water, as had been expected. 2) The structural rearrangements in the covalent cofactor-substrate adduct from one intermediate to the next are minimal. 3) The hypothesis of Ivanov and Karpeisky (1969) that, upon completion of each reaction step, optimal conditions for the next step are created holds not only in chemical but also in structural terms. 4) H.C. Dunathan's (1966) hypothesis applies to the external aldimine as well as to the ketimine intermediates.

Table I. Crystal structures representing catalytic intermediates in the half-reaction of the PLP-form of mAspAT with L-aspartate to produce the PMP-form and oxaloacetate: structures in space group P1 have the open, those in $C222_1$ the closed conformation. References, a, McPhalen et al., 1987; b, McPhalen et al., 1992a; c, Génovésio-Taverne, Picot, Vincent and Jansonius, in preparation; d, McPhalen et al., 1992b; e, Malashkevich et al., 1993; f, Génovésio-Taverne et al., unpublished

Catalytic intermediate	Crystal structure	pH	Space group	Resolution (Å)	Reference
PLP-enzyme, unliganded	PLP-enzyme, unliganded	7.5	P1	1.9	a,b
	idem	5.1	P1	2.3	a,b
+ L-Asp, Michaelis complex	+ maleate	7.5	$C222_1$	2.15	a,c
+ L-Asp, external aldimine	+ 2-methylaspartate	7.5	$C222_1$	2.3	a,c,d
PMP-enzyme + oxaloacetate, ketimine	+ L-aspartate	7.5	$C222_1$	2.4	e
idem, carbinolamine	+ *erythro*-3-hydroxyaspartate	7.5	$C222_1$	2.0	f
idem, Michaelis complex	PMP-enzyme + maleate	7.5	$C222_1$	2.1	c
PMP-enzyme, unliganded	PMP-enzyme, unliganded	7.5	P1	2.2	a,b

Escherichia coli AspAT (eAspAT) has now also been studied crystallographically in considerable detail in Basel, both the wild type (Jäger et al., 1994a) and mutant enzymes (Jäger et al., 1994b; Malashkevich et al., 1994). In collaboration with J.F. Kirsch et al. (this Volume), the structure of a hexamutant (V39L/K41Y/T47I/N69L/T109S/N297S) was solved as unliganded enzyme and in complexes with the competitive inhibitors maleate, hydrocinnamic acid (HCA) and indolepropionic acid. This hexamutant was designed to modify eAspAT into an enzyme with properties as close as possible to those of *E.coli* tyrosine aminotransferase (eTyrAT), an enzyme that shares the same catalytic, cofactor- and substrate binding residues with eAspAT, but has the curious property to be 10^2 - 10^4 times more active towards aromatic substrates, while being equally active towards dicarboxylic substrates. The hexamutant of Kirsch et al. exhibits 10 % of the activity of eTyrAT towards phenylalanine without loss of activity towards aspartate. It was a challenge to explain these facts in structural terms.

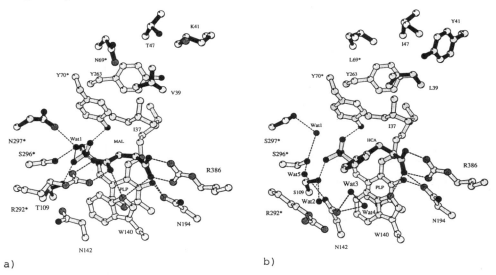

a)   b)

Figure 1. The substrate binding site and the "hydrophobic patch" in (a) wild type eAspAT with maleate bound and (b) the hexamutant /V39L/K41Y/T49I/N69L/T109S/N297S/ eAspAT with HCA bound. The atoms are coloured in grey tones according to their atomic number. Wat, water molecule. Hydrogen bonds are indicated by dashed lines. Asterisks label residues from the adjacent subunit and dark bonds emphasize the side chains of the six (to be) mutated residues. Note the ejection of R292* from the active site upon binding of an aromatic ligand to the hexamutant enzyme and the different water structures in the substrate side chain-binding site in the w.t. and hexamutant enzyme, respectively.

The first surprise was that the crystalline unliganded hexamutant eAspAT was found in the closed conformation, a so far unique situation. Thus, the open/closed conformational equilibrium in this mutant clearly favours the closed structure, thereby reducing the K_m values of the substrates. This is especially important for the aromatic ones. A hydrophobic patch that glues the small domain to the neighbouring subunit in the closed conformation is more extensive and compact in the hexamutant than in w.t. eAspAT (Figure 1). This is brought about by the mutations V39L/K41Y/T47I/N69L. The mutations T109S/N297S are favourable selectively for aromatic

32

substrates. This can also be explained by comparing Figures 1a and 1b. The water structure in the substrate side chain-binding pocket favours dicarboxylates (here maleate) in the w.t. enzyme, but leaves more space for aromatic side chains in the hexamutant, while presumably also favouring the "ejection" of Arg 292*. The latter would be physically in the way and lack a countercharge in the conformation it has in the maleate complexes of both w.t. eAspAT and the hexamutant. Thus, Arg292* acts as a switch that enables either dicarboxylic or aromatic substrates to bind productively in the closed hexamutant eAspAT active site, and, presumably, in *E.coli* tyrosine aminotransferase as well.

Dialkylglycine decarboxylase from *Pseudomonas cepacia*. The three-dimensional structure of this α_4-tetrameric enzyme was recently solved as part of a joint project with J.W. Keller, University of Alaska, Fairbanks (Toney et al., 1993). DGD has two very interesting unusual features. First of all, it catalyzes both α-decarboxylation and transamination in the same active site, a feature that already intrigued H.C. Dunathan (1971). Secondly, the X-ray study revealed two alkali ion binding sites per monomer. Site 1 is adjacent to the active site and contains in the native enzyme a K^+ ion, which is needed for activity. It can be replaced by Na^+, which inhibits the enzyme. The second site contains a strongly bound Na^+ ion which locally stabilizes the structure, but seems to have no other functional role. Structure and catalytic mechanism will be discussed by M.D. Toney et al. in this Volume. Here we briefly report on more recent additional metal binding studies (E. Hohenester et al., to be submitted). 2.8 Å resolution structures have been determined of DGD with either Rb^+ or Li^+ bound in site 1. These structures are isomorphous with the active K^+- containing, and the Na^+- inhibited enzyme, respectively. Since Rb^+ activitates and Li^+ inhibits DGD, there seems to be a unique catalytically active structure with K^+ or Rb^+ bound and an inactive structure in which K^+ is replaced by Na^+ or Li^+. The small size of these ions causes the K^+ ligand Ser80* to rotate away from the metal and to replace the active site residue Tyr301* in a hydrogen bond to Gln52. This causes the Tyr301* phenyl ring to reorient, which, presumably, inactivates the enzyme.

Phosphoserine aminotransferase from *Escherichia coli*. PSAT is an α_2-dimer with 362 amino acid residues per chain. It lacks significant sequence identity with other aminotransferases (Mehta et al., 1993). Crystals of space group $P2_12_12_1$ with one dimer per asymmetric unit (Kallen et al., 1987) diffract to 2.3 Å resolution. With the multiple isomorphous replacement (MIR) technique, preliminary phases were obtained that are of sufficient quality to discern the dimer in electron density maps, to determine position and orientation of its molecular twofold axis and to trace the polypeptide chain in a number of, mostly helical, regions. A partial structure was reported (Stark et al., 1991). More recently, the model was further extended but the structure could not be refined. Attempts to improve the phases by iterative molecular averaging either with or without combination with MIR phases are currently underway. Also histogram matching (Zhang, 1993) is being applied.

Human recombinant ornithine aminotransferase. L-ornithine:2-oxoacid aminotransferase (EC 2.6.1.13) is a mitochondrial matrix enzyme. It is nuclear-encoded as a 439-residue precursor which is processed to its mature form upon entrance into the mitochondrion (Inana et al., 1986; Ramesh et al., 1986). Malfunction or absence of the enzyme causes gyrate atrophy, a recessive genetic disease which leads to blindness. The enzyme was expressed in *Escherichia coli*. After purification it easily crystallized in space group $P3_221$ with a = b = 116.3 Å, c = 190.0 Å, $\alpha = \beta = 90°$, $\gamma = 120°$ as an α_6 hexamer with three subunits per asymmetric unit. Self rotation function calculations revealed the presence of both threefold and twofold non-crystallographic symmetriy, suggesting the point group 32 for the hexamer (Shen et al., 1994). The structure of OAT was recently solved by molecular replacement, using a truncated DGD model (≈ 30 % sequence identity) as a search model (Shen et al., to be published). The local threefold axis of the resulting hexamer unexpectedly has a screw component of 17 Å between successive dimers. After rigid body refinement at 6 Å resolution with XPLOR, molecular averaging and phase extension to 3.0 Å resolution (program RAVE; G. Kleywegt and T.A. Jones, Uppsala), a complete model of the subunit could be built into the averaged map with the help of the program "O" (T.A. Jones). Continued phase extension to 2.5 Å resulted in a map that showed all side chains, the orientations of the peptide groups and a number of structural water molecules, including several that bind to the PLP phosphate.

The overall folding of the polypeptide chain is very similar to that of DGD despite some large local deviations, mainly in surface loops, including the regions involved in the different dimer-dimer interactions in the two enzymes. Figure 2 displays some key residues in the OAT active site, which is delimited by stretches of polypeptide chain in essentially the same conformation as in DGD. The cofactor PLP-Lys292 aldimine (numbering according to the 439 residue precursor sequence) has exactly the same conformation as in DGD. The following active site residues are conserved (in brackets the DGD sequence number): D263 (243); Q266 (246); K292 (272); T322* (303*, not shown); R413 (406).

34

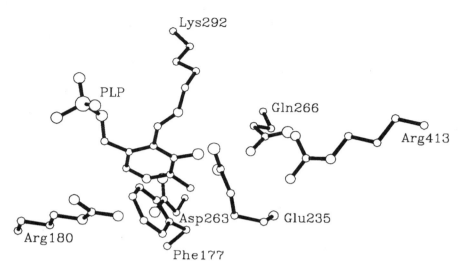

Figure 2. Cofactor and selected side chains in the active site of human ornithine aminotransferase (precursor numbering). C, N, O and P are indicated by circles of increasing size in that order. Pyridoxal-5'-phosphate makes a (protonated) Schiff base with Lys292, which has the same side chain conformation as in dialkylglycine decarboxylase. Asp263 stabilizes a proton on the pyridine N1. Gln266 stabilizes through a hydrogen bond the negative charge on O3'. The putative substrate binding site is in front of PLP, above Phe177. Arg180, Glu235 and Arg413 are the probable substrate-binding residues (see text).

Important exchanges include: Y85 (Q52 in DGD, not shown); F177 (W138); R180 (M141); E235 (S215). These last two new charged residues seem to be the logical candidates to bind the substrate ornithine in a productive Michaelis complex for transamination of its δ-amino group. In fact, mutation of R180 to threonine causes gyrate atrophy (Mitchell et al., 1989), confirming that R180 is essential for activity. Thus, a first quite cursory inspection of the active site of this "in the last minute" solved OAT structure already seems to give a clue to the ornithine binding mode. For binding of glutamate, which is transaminated to 2-oxoglutarate, Glu235 may have to rotate out of the active site. Arg413 and Arg180 would then be responsible for binding the substrate α- and ω-carboxylate groups, respectively.

Acknowledgment

Support by the Swiss National Science Foundation grants 31-25712.88; 31-25713.88 and 31-36432.92 (to J.N. Jansonius) and by the U.S. National Institutes of Health grant HL 33254-9 (to B.W. Shen) is gratefully acknowledged.

References

Alexander, F.W., Sandmeier, E., Mehta, P.K. and Christen, P. (1994) Evolutionary relationships among pyridoxal-5'-phosphate-dependent enzymes. Regio-specific α, β and γ families. *Eur. J. Biochem.* 219: 953-960.

Christen, P. and Metzler, D.E. (eds.) (1985) *Transaminases*, John Wiley & Sons, New York.

Dolphin, D., Poulson, R. and Avramovic, O. (eds.) (1986) *Vitamin B6 pyridoxal phosphate, Part B*, John Wiley & Sons, New York.

Dunathan, H.C. (1966) Conformation and reaction specificity in pyridoxal phosphate enzymes. *Proc. Natl. Acad. Sci. USA* 55: 712-716.

Dunathan, H.C. (1971) Stereochemical aspects of pyridoxal phosphate catalysis. *Adv. Enzymol.* 35: 79-134.

Inana, G., Totsuka, S., Redmond, M., Dougherty, T., Nagle, J., Shiono, T., Ohura, T., Kominami, E. and Katunuma, N. (1986) Molecular cloning of human ornithine aminotransferase mRNA. *Proc. Natl. Acad. Sci. USA* 83: 1203-1207.

Ivanov, V.I. and Karpeisky, M.Ya. (1969) Dynamic three-dimensional model for enzymic transamination. *Adv. Enzymol.* 32: 21-53.

Jäger, J., Moser, M., Sauder, U. and Jansonius, J.N. (1994a) Crystal structures of *Escherichia coli* aspartate aminotransferase in two conformations. *J. Mol. Biol.* 239: 285-305.

Jäger, J., Pauptit, R.A., Sauder, U. and Jansonius, J.N. (1994b) Three-dimensional structure of a mutant *E.coli* aspartate aminotransferase with increased enzymic activity. *Protein Engineering* 7: 605-612.

Kallen, J., Kania, M., Markovic-Housley, Z., Vincent, M.G. and Jansonius, J.N. (1987). In: Korpela, T. and Christen, P. (eds.): *Biochemistry of Vitamin B6*, Birkhäuser Verlag, Basel, pp. 157-160.

Malashkevich, V.N., Toney, M.D. and Jansonius, J.N. (1993) Crystal structures of true enzymatic reaction intermediates: Aspartate and glutamate ketimines in aspartate aminotransferase. *Biochemistry* 32: 13451-13462.

Malashkevich, V.N., Jäger, J., Ziak, M., Sauder, U., Gehring, H., Christen, P. and Jansonius, J.N. (1994) Structural basis for the catalytic activity of aspartate aminotransferase K258H lacking the pyridoxal-5'-phosphate-binding lysine residue. *Biochemistry*, submitted for publication.

McPhalen, C.A., Vincent, M.G., Picot, D. and Jansonius, J.N. (1987). In: Korpela, T. and Christen, P. (eds.): *Biochemistry of Vitamin B6*, Birkhäuser Verlag, Basel, pp. 99-102.

McPhalen, C.A., Vincent, M.G. and Jansonius, J.N. (1992) X-ray structure refinement and comparision of three forms of mitochondrial aspartate aminotransferase. *J. Mol. Biol.* 225: 495-517.

McPhalen, C.A., Vincent, M.G., Picot, D., Jansonius, J.N., Lesk, A.M. and Chothia, C. (1992) Domain closure in mitochondrial aspartate aminotransferase. *J. Mol. Biol.* 227: 197-213.

Mehta, P.K., Hale, T.I. and Christen, P. (1993) Aminotransferases: demonstration of homology and division into evolutionary subgroups. *Eur. J. Biochem.* 214: 549-561.

Mitchell, G.A., Brody, L.C., Sipila, I., Looney, J.E., Wong, C., Engelhardt, J.F., Patel, A.S., Steel, G., Obie, C., Kaiser-Kupfer, M. and Valle, D. (1989) At least two mutant alleles of ornithine δ-aminotransferase cause gyrate atrophy of the choroid and retina in Finns. *Proc. Natl. Acad. Sci. USA* 86: 197-201.

Ramesh, V., Shaffer, M.M., Allaire, J.M., Shih, V.E., Gusella, J.F. (1986) Investigation of gyrate atrophy using a cDNA clone for human ornithine aminotransferase. *DNA* 5: 493-501.

Shen, B.W., Ramesh, V., Müller, R., Hohenester, E., Hennig, M. and Jansonius, J.N. (1994) Crystallization and preliminary X-ray diffraction studies of recombinant human ornithine aminotransferase. *J. Mol. Biol.*, submitted for publication.

Stark, W., Kallen, J., Markovic-Housley, Z., Fol, B., Kania, M. and Jansonius, J.N. (1991). In: Fukui, T., Kagamiyama, H., Soda, K. and Wada, H. (eds.): *Enzymes dependent on pyridoxal phosphate and other carbonyl compounds as cofactors*, Pergamon Press, Oxford, pp. 111-115.

Toney, M.D., Hohenester, E., Cowan, S.W. and Jansonius, J.N. (1993) Dialkylglycine decarboxylase structure: bifunctional active site and alkali metal sites. *Science* 261: 756-759.

Zhang, K.Y.J. (1993) SQUASH - Combining constraints for macromolecular phase refinement and extension. *Acta Crystallogr.* D49: 213-222.

Biochemistry of Vitamin B_6 and PQQ
G. Marino, G. Sannia and F. Bossa (eds.)
© 1994 Birkhäuser Verlag Basel/Switzerland

Redesign of aspartate aminotransferase specificity to that of tyrosine aminotransferase

Jack F. Kirsch and James J. Onuffer[1]

Molecular and Cell Biology Department, University of California, Berkeley, CA 94720, USA
[1]*Present address: Parnassus Pharmaceuticals, Inc. 1501 Harbor Bay Parkway, Alameda, CA 94502*

Summary

The values of k_{cat}/K_m are strongly correlated with chain length for the reactions of *E. coli* tyrosine aminotransferase, but are nearly independent of this variable for aspartate aminotransferase. Both enzymes exhibit nearly equal reactivity with dicarboxylic acid substrates. Six key amino acid differences were identified that were found to be responsible for 80% of the specificity difference. It is postulated that a major role for Arg292 in aspartate transaminase is to exclude nonspecific substrates by keeping the enzyme in an open inactive form. The free energy to close the enzyme into its active conformation derives from association with specific ligands.

Introduction

The ultimate objective of enzyme design is to acquire the knowledge to prepare a polypeptide sequence that would fold to form a protein that is an efficient catalyst for an arbitrarily chosen chemical reaction, encompassing controlled regio and stereo chemistry. The realization of such an objective, if it can be attained at all, appears to lie in the distant future as the conceptually simpler problem of how a given sequence will fold, let alone form an enzyme-like active site, as yet escapes our comprehension.

To help to advance our understanding of the principles required for ultimate *de novo* protein design, less ambitious experiments in "enzyme redesign" have been undertaken as heuristic way stations with realizable objectives. Here, an enzyme of known activity, and usually with a known three dimensional structure, is mutated in an attempt to recruit the catalytic power to a different activity or substrate specificity by rational selection of relatively few mutations. Recent successful examples include the engineering of changes in the substrate specificity of subtilisin (Estell *et al.*, 1986; Wells *et al.*, 1987); the transformation of glutathione reductase to a trypanothione reductase (Bradley *et al.*, 1991; Henderson *et al.*, 1991); and the conversion of lactate dehydrogenase to phenylpyruvate and L-hydroxyisocaproate dehydrogenases (Dunn *et al.*, 1991). At times significantly larger than anticipated numbers of mutations have to be introduced to achieve what superficially appears to be a modest goal. For example, Hedstrom *et al.* (1992) were only able to introduce significant chymotrypsin specificity into recombinant trypsin after several mutations including the replacement of two surface loops of trypsin with those found in chymotrypsin, as well as by changing four additional residues in the S1 binding site.

The reactions catalyzed by the *E. coli* aspartate (eAATase)- and tyrosine (eTATase) aminotransferases are shown in Equation 1.

$$RCH(NH_2)COOH + PLP\text{-transaminase} \rightleftharpoons R(CO)COOH + PMP\text{-transaminase} \quad (1)$$

$$R = -(CH_2)_{1-2}COO^-$$ aspartate and tyrosine aminotransferases
$$R = -(CH_2)Aryl$$ tyrosine aminotransferase

Materials and Methods

These are described in Onuffer and Kirsch (in preparation) and in the legends to Tables I and II.

Results and Discussion

Aspartate aminotransferase kinetics have been exhaustively characterized (*e. g.* Velick and Vavra, (1962), Kiick and Cook, (1983), Julin and Kirsch, (1989), L. M. Gloss and J. F. Kirsch, unpublished results), but those of tyrosine aminotransferase have been less extensively explored (Powell and Morrison, 1978; Hayashi *et al*, 1993). The two enzymes exhibit overlapping substrate specificities. The rates of transamination of L-aspartate and L-glutamate do not differ significantly, but those for the aromatic amino acids are 10^2 -10^4 greater for eTATase (J. J. Onuffer, B. Ton, and J. F. Kirsch, unpublished results). Table I shows the dependence of the rate constants for the transamination of a series of n-alkyl and dicarboxylic α-amino acids, by eAATase and eTATase. Both enzymes are very effective catalysts of the rates of transamination of the dicarboxylic amino acids; however, eTATase shows a strong linear dependence of k_{cat}/K_m ($\Delta G/CH_2 = 1.4$ kcal/mol) on alkyl chain length, that is absent in eAATase. These and other studies with natural substrates suggest a model in which the two enzymes share a common binding mode for the dicarboxylic amino acids, but eTATase has an additional means for accommodation of nonpolar substrates.

Table I. Dependence of free energies of activation on substrate side chain length for the transamination reactions of aspartate and tyrosine aminotransferases: Conditions 0.2 M TAPS, 140 mM KCl, pH 8.0, 25°C. $\Delta G^{=,|} = RT(\ln(k_b T/h) - \ln(k_{cat}/K_m))$. $\Delta\Delta G^{=,|} = \Delta G^{=,|}_{eTATase} - \Delta G^{=,|}_{eAATase}$

Substrate $^{-}OOC\diagdown^{(CH_2)_n}\diagup CH_3$ $^{+}H_3N$	$\Delta G^{=,\|}$ (k_{cat}/K_m) kcal mol^{-1}	$\Delta G^{=,\|}$ (k_{cat}/K_m) kcal mol^{-1}	$\Delta\Delta G^{=,\|}$ kcal mol^{-1}
n =	eAATase	eTATase	eTATase - eAATase
0	17.8	17.0	-0.8
1	17.8	16.0	-1.8
2	17.4	14.5	-2.9
3	16.5	12.6	-3.9
5	17.5	10.3	-7.2

$^{-}OOC\diagdown^{(CH_2)_n}\diagup COO^{-}$
$^{+}H_3N$

n =	eAATase	eTATase	eTATase - eAATase
1	10.2	11.0	0.8
2	11.9	12.1	0.2
3	16.4	16.5	0.1

Although high resolution X-ray crystallographic structures have been determined for eAATase, efforts to crystallize eTATase have not yet been successful. Sequence alignments of eTATase and eAATase show *ca.* 43% sequence identity and 72% similarity; therefore both enzymes must share close secondary and tertiary structure. Six active site residues of eAATase were targeted by homology modeling as likely determinants of aromatic amino acid reactivity with eTATase. Two of these (Thr109 and Asn297) are invariant in all known aspartate aminotransferase enzymes, but differ in eTATase (Ser109 and Ser297). The other four (Val39, Lys41, Thr47, and Asn69) line the active site pocket of eAATase, and are replaced by amino acids with more nonpolar side chains in eTATase (Leu39, Tyr41, Ile47, and Leu69). The testing of each of the six substitutions in all possible combinations would have required the construction of $2^6 = 64$ possible proteins; therefore, a series of progressively larger combinations of mutants was chosen with a certain degree of arbitrariness. The values of k_{cat}/K_m for the mutant construct containing all six mutations, Hex, are compared with those of the two wildtype enzymes in the transamination of phenylalanine and aspartate in Table II. The Hex mutant has more eTATase-like properties than does any of the other mutant constructs containing fewer substitutions.

Table II: Dependence of free energies of activation for the transamination reactions of aspartate, tyrosine, and redesigned aminotransferases: Conditions 0.2 M TAPS, 140 mM KCl, pH 8.0, 25°C. $\Delta G^{\neq,|} = RT(\ln(k_b T/h) - \ln(k_{cat}/K_m)$. $\Delta\Delta G^{\neq,|} = \Delta G^{\neq,|}_{eTATase} - (\Delta G^{\neq,|}_{eAATase}$ or $\Delta G^{\neq,|}_{Hex})$. Values are in kcal/mol

	$\Delta G^{\neq,\|}$ (k_{cat}/K_m)	$\Delta G^{\neq,\|}$ (k_{cat}/K_m)	$\Delta G^{\neq,\|}$ (k_{cat}/K_m)	$\Delta\Delta G^{\neq,\|}$ (eTATase - eAATase)	$\Delta\Delta G^{\neq,\|}$ (eTATase - Hex)
	eAATase	Hex	eTATase	*predesign*	*postdesign*
aspartate	10.2	9.9	11.0	0.8	1.1
phenylalanine	14.1	9.8	8.7	-5.4	-1.1

The data show that most of the objective of redesigning AATase to transaminate phenylalanine has been achieved in the Hex mutant (*i.e.*. about 80% of the total $\Delta\Delta G$ of 5.4 kcal/mol differentiating eAATase from eTATase in this characteristic has been claimed by the six mutations, $\Delta\Delta G$ = 4.3 kcal/mol). However, in work to be published elsewhere (Onuffer, *et al* in preparation), it is shown that the design is still imperfect, in that the Hex mutant has much greater affinity for both dicarboxylic and aromatic inhibitors than does either of the two wildtype enzymes. For example, the values of the dissociation constants for the maleate complexes with eAATase, eTATase and Hex are 19, 140, and 0.44 mM respectively. Maleate binds to Hex much more tightly than it does to either its parent eAATase or to its targeted eTATase. Moreover the value of k_{cat}/K_m for the transamination of aspartate is much closer to that of eAATase than to that of eTATase (Table II). Some combinations of the remaining amino acid differences in the two wildtype enzymes must be responsible for the transduction of this excess binding energy to catalysis.

The structural basis for the engineered change in specificity effected by the Hex mutant of AATase is described in the contribution from the Jansonius Laboratory in this volume. Briefly, they find that the mutations in AATase shift the conformational equilibrium from the open to the closed form of the enzyme, and that these substitutions make it possible for the side chain of aromatic amino acid substrates to displace Arg292 to solvent.

The new structural and kinetic investigations combine to define more fully the role of Arg292 in transamination. This residue is primarily responsible for association with the ω-carboxylate of dicarboxylic acid substrates. Interpretations of early crystallographic investigations focused on its role in controlling the equilibrium between the open unliganded and the closed conformation formed when dicarboxylic substrates are bound (Kirsch *et al*, 1984). We do not know the free energy required to close the unliganded enzyme, but Malashkevich *et al* (1993) have recently determined that the equilibrium constant for the conformational transition from the open to the closed liganded aldehyde form is approximately unity. The open form is very unlikely to have significant transaminase activity as witnessed by the very low rates of transamination by AATases exhibited for substrates such as alanine and aromatic amino acids that do not effect conformational closure. The mitochondrial AATase, for example, crystallizes in the open form when complexed with N-phosphopyridoxyl -L-tyrosine (Kirsch *et al*, 1984). We would like to suggest that Arg292 acts as a gatekeeper in AATase to exclude unwelcome substrates by maintaining the enzyme in the relatively inactive open form. Part of the endogenous free energy of interaction of reactive dicarboxylic acid substrates must be expended to close the enzyme to its active conformation. The mechanism is one of ion pairing through interaction of the ω-carboxylate of the substrate with the guanidino moiety of Arg292. The six mutations that are described in this study shift the conformation of the unliganded eAATase from open to closed with the consequence that the enzyme is in an active conformation and a wider variety of substrates is accepted.

Acknowledgments
This work was supported by NIH Grant GM-35393. J. J. O. was supported in part by NIH Molecular Biophysics Training Grant GM-08295.

References

Bradley, M., Bücheler, U. S., and Walsh, C. T. (1991) Redox enzyme engineering: conversion of human glutathione reductase into a trypanothione reductase. *Biochemistry* 30: 6124-6127.

Dunn, C. R., Wilks, H. M., Halsall, D. J., Atkinson, T., Clarke, A. R., Muirhead, H., and Holbrook, J. J. (1991) Design and synthesis of new enzymes based on the lactate dehydrogenase framework. *Phil. Trans. R. Soc. Lond. B* 332: 177-184.

Estell, D. A., Graycar, T. P., Miller, J. V., Powers, D. B., Burnier, J. P., Ng, P. G., and Wells, J. A. (1986) Probing steric and hydrophobic effects on enzyme-substrate interactions by protein engineering. *Science* 233: 659-663.

Hayashi, H., Inoue, K., Nagata., T., Kuramitsu, S., and Kagamiyama, H. (1993) *Escherichia coli* aromatic amino acid aminotransferase: characterization and comparison with aspartate aminotransferase. *Biochemistry* 32: 12229-12239.

Hedstrom, L., Szilagyi, L., Rutter, W. J. (1992) Converting trypsin to chymotrypsin: the role of surface loops. *Science* 255: 1249-1253.

Henderson, G. B., Murgolo, N. J., Kuriyan, J., Osapay, K., Kominos, D., Berry, A., Scrutton, N. S., Hinchliffe, N. W., Perham, R. N., and Cerami, A. (1991) Engineering the substrate specificity of glutathione reductase toward that of trypanothione reduction. *Proc. Natl. Acad. Sci.* 88: 8769-8773.

Julin, D. A., and Kirsch, J. F. (1989) Kinetic isotope effect studies on aspartate aminotransferase: evidence for a concerted 1,3 prototropic shift mechanism for the cytoplasmic isozyme and L-aspartate and dichotomy in mechanism. *Biochemistry* 28: 3825-3833.

Kiick, D. M. and Cook, P. F. (1983) pH studies toward the elucidation of the auxiliary catalyst for pig heart aspartate aminotransferase. *Biochemistry* 22: 375-382.

Kirsch, J. F., Eichele, G., Ford, G. C., Vincent, M. G., Jansonius, J. N., Gehring, H., and Christen, P. (1984) Mechanism of action of aspartate aminotransferase proposed on the basis of its spatial structure. *J. Molec. Biol* . 174: 497-525.

Powell, J. T. and Morrison, J. F. (1978) The purification and properties of the aspartate aminotransferase and aromatic-amino-acid aminotransferase from *Escherichia coli*. *Eur J. Biochem.* 87:391-400.

Malashkevich, V. N., Toney, M. D., and Jansonius, J. N. (1993) Crystal structures of true enzymatic reaction intermediates: aspartate and glutamate ketimines in aspartate aminotransferase. *Biochemistry* 32:13451-13462.

Velick, S. G. and Vavra, J. (1962) A kinetic and equilibrium analysis of the glutamic oxaloacetate transaminase mechanism. *J. Biol. Chem.* 237: 2109-2122.

Wells, J. A., Powers, D. B., Bott, R. R., Graycar, T. P., and Estell, D. A. (1987) Designing substrate specificity by protein engineering of electrostatic interactions. *Proc. Natl. Acad. Sci. U. S. A.* 84: 1219-1223.

Biochemistry of Vitamin B$_6$ and PQQ
G. Marino, G. Sannia and F. Bossa (eds.)
© 1994 Birkhäuser Verlag Basel/Switzerland

Enzyme–substrate interactions modulating protonation and tautomerization states of the aldimines of pyridoxal enzymes

H. Kagamiyama, H. Hayashi, T. Yano, H. Mizuguchi and S. Ishii

Department of Biochemistry, Osaka Medical College, 2-7 Daigakumachi, Takatsuki 569, Japan

Summary
    The mechanism of activation of PLP-Lys aldimines of Aspartate aminotransferase (AspAT), aromatic amino acid aminotransferase (ArAT), and aromatic L-amino acid decarboxylase (AADC) to the ketoenamine form was studied. In AspAT and ArAT the aldimines exist as the nonprotonated form. Upon binding of substrate amino acids, the pK_a of these aldimines are increased and the aldimines become the protonated, ketoenamine form, which is considered to be favorable for transaldimination. The increase in pK_a by binding of amino acids was proved by mutagenesis studies to be mediated mainly by interaction of α-carboxylate group of the substrate and Arg386 of the enzymes. In AADC, the aldimine is protonated, but it exists as the enolimine tautomer and is not favorable for transaldimination. In the presence of a substrate amino acid, it undergoes tautomerization to the ketoenamine form. Pyridoxal enzymes show a variety of spectra, and PLP-Lys aldimines exist as several protonated/deprotonated forms. However, it is proposed that all these forms are converted to the protonated, ketoenamine form upon binding of substrate amino acids, either by altering the pK_a values of the PLP-Lys aldimines or by changing the polarity of the microenvironment around the aldimines.

Introduction

    Pyridoxal 5'-phosphate (PLP) enzymes catalyzes a variety of reactions: transamination, decarboxylation, racemization, β- and γ-replacement/elimination, aldol cleavage etc. These reactions are promoted by the electron-withdrawing ability of the pyridine ring of PLP which is connected via a conjugated C=N double bond of PLP-amino acid aldimine to one of the three σ-bonds around the α-carbon atom of the amino acid (Snell, 1985; Metzler, 1977). Therefore, formation of the PLP–amino acid aldimine, i.e., the "external" aldimine, by transaldimination between the PLP-Lys "internal" aldimine and the substrate amino acid, is a prerequisite step of the reactions catalyzed by PLP enzymes. To allow the transaldimination step to proceed efficiently, the substrate amino group must be deprotonated (from $-NH_3^+$ to $-NH_2$), and the internal aldimine should be protonated (-CH=NH$^+$-). The protonated internal aldimine absorbs at around 430 nm, and this is the wavelength of the main absorption band of most PLP enzymes (Kallen et al., 1985). However, the absorption spectra of a number of PLP-enzymes are different from the "typical" absorption spectrum. These spectroscopically "unusual" PLP enzymes include aspartate aminotransferase (AspAT), aromatic amino acid aminotransferase (ArAT), histidinol phosphate aminotransferase (HPAT), tryptophanase, glutamate decarboxylase (GluDC), and aromatic L-amino acid decarboxylase (AADC) (Kallen et al., 1985; Martin, 1970; Metzler et al., 1991; O'Leary, 1971; Voltattorni et al., 1979). AspAT and ArAT have low values of the internal aldimine pK_a, and at neutral pH these enzymes have significant fraction of deprotonated internal aldimine structure (Fig. 1:I), with absorption at around 360 nm (Kallen et al., 1985). HPAT and AADC show enhanced absorption at around 335 nm. This absorption band is generally ascribed to the enolimine structure (Fig. 1:II), which exists in only small amount in "usual" PLP enzymes. Tryptophanase and GluDC show pH-dependent change in absorption spectra; the absorption maxima of both enzymes shift from 420–430 nm to 330–340 nm with increasing pH. The nature of the 330–340 nm absorption is still controversial in both enzymes .

The deprotonated aldimine structure and the enolimine structure are both supposed to be unfavorable for nucleophilic attack of the amino group of substrate amino acid. Therefore, in the above "spectroscopically unusual" PLP enzymes, the aldimines must undergo structural transition to the protonated, ketoenamine form (Fig. 1:III) before they are attacked by the substrate amino acids. In this paper, we analyzed the spectroscopic properties of the PLP–Lys aldimines of AspAT, ArAT, and AADC, and their interaction with substrates and substrate analogs, for the purpose of elucidating the transaldimination process in these PLP enzymes.

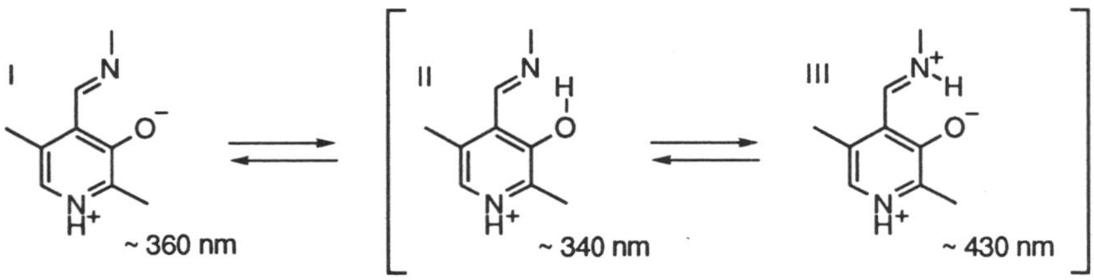

Figure 1. Structures of deprotonated aldimine (I), and ketoenamine (II) and enolimine (III) form of protonated aldimines

Materials and Methods
    E. coli AspAT and ArAT, and rat liver AADC were prepared as describe previously (Kamitori et al., 1987; Hayashi et al., 1993ab). All the spectroscopic measurements were performed at 25°C in buffer solutions containing 50 mM Good buffer components, and 0.1 M KCl (for the measurements of AspAT and ArAT).

Results and Discussion

Aspartate and aromatic aminotransferases

The spectra of the PLP-form of AspAT and ArAT have absorption bands at around 360 nm which is prominent at low pH, and at around 430 nm which is prominent at high pH. The spectral transition from 360 nm to 430 nm is a protonation event at the aldimine nitrogen of PLP-Lys258 Schiff base (Kallen et al., 1985), and the pK_a of the aldimine nitrogen was obtained to be 6.85 for AspAT, and 6.65 for ArAT.

The above pK_a values are unusually low as compared to the PLP-amine aldimines in aqueous solutions (pK_a = 10–11; Kallen et al., 1985). The pK_a of the aldimine of AspAT is considered to be lowered by interaction of the pyridine ring of the PLP–Lys258 aldimine with several active site residues, Asp222, Tyr225, and Asn194. Asp222 stabilizes the protonation at pyridine nitrogen of

PLP, thus lowering the pK_a of the PLP–Lys258 aldimine (Yano et al., 1992). Both Tyr225 and Asn194 form hydrogen bonds to 3'-O of PLP, and these H-bonds prevent the electrons of the phenolic 3'-O from flowing into the aldimine double bond; this also lowers the pK_a of the aldimine (Goldberg et al., 1991; Yano et al, 1993). In addition, the two positively charged arginine residues, Arg292 and Arg386, are expected to promote deprotonation at the aldimine nitrogen. Arg292 and Arg386 have been identified as the residues responsible for binding the ω- and α-carboxylate groups, respectively, of dicarboxylic substrates, and it has been postulated that the binding of dicarboxylic substrates to AspAT increases the pK_a of the PLP-Lys258 aldimine, and causes a proton transfer from the substrate amino group to the aldimine nitrogen. The free amino group then attacks the polarized aldimine carbon atom, and transaldimination from the internal aldimine to the external aldimine proceeds efficiently (Kirsch et al., 1984). In accordance with this hypothesis, R292L and R386L AspATs showed increased internal aldimine pK_a values as compared with WT enzyme. The effect of mutation at Arg386 was, however, 3 times larger than that at Arg292 (0.46 versus 0.14), although crystallographic studies indicated that both arginine residues are situated at 8 Å from the internal aldimine nitrogen (Kamitori et al., 1990). Asn194 is located within the hydrogen bonding distance from the side chain of Arg386 and from the 3'-O of PLP. Therefore Asn194 was supposed to be involved in the larger electrostatic effect of Arg386 on the aldimine, because the electron withdrawal ability of Asn194 appears to be enhanced by the presence of the positive charge on the Arg386. We have introduced mutations at position 194 and 386. Mutation of WT AspAT to R386L results in the loss of both the Coulombic interaction and Asn194-medicated interaction of Arg386 with the aldimine nitrogen, whereas making the same mutation R386L on N194A AspAT loses only the Coulombic interaction of Arg386 and the aldimine nitrogen. Therefore the Asn194-mediated interaction may be obtained if we compare the pK_a shift on [WT→R386L] mutation with that on [N194A→N194A/R386L] mutation. It was estimated that neutralization of Arg386 increases the pK_a of the internal aldimine by 0.12 pH unit through Coulombic interaction, and by 0.34 pH unit through Arg386–Asn194–PLP hydrogen bonding network. The idea that Asn194 functions to electrically link Arg386 and PLP was also supported by analog-binding studies. When maleate binds to the enzyme, the increase in the pK_a value was 2.0 units for the wild-type enzyme and 1.0 unit for the N194A enzyme (Yano et al., 1993). It was supposed that without Asn194, the effect of neutralization of the charge of Arg386 on the aldimine nitrogen through the above hydrogen-bonding network was diminished.

The reactions of ArAT with dicarboxylic amino acids and aromatic amino acids were similar to the mechanism described above for the reaction of AspAT with dicarboxylic amino acids (Iwasaki et al., 1994). Analysis on the acid-base chemistry of binding of dicarboxylic and aromatic substrate analogs to ArAT showed that the internal Schiff base pK_a increased by these analogs. This suggests that the pK_a of the ArAT Schiff base is increased by aromatic amino acid substrates to the extent that proton transfer from the substrate amino group to the imine nitrogen and subsequent transaldimination efficiently proceeds. That Arg386 has larger effect than Arg292 on the pK_a value of aldimine via a hydrogen-bonding linkage involving Asn194 was also proven in ArAT, using similar mutation analyses as those used for AspAT (Mizuguchi et al., unpublished results). The residues involved in the hydrogen bonding network, Arg386 and Asn194, are strictly conserved among Subgroup I aminotransferases. It is reasonable that Arg386 is the more committed residue in modulating the aldimine pK_a than Arg292, because Arg386 is the residue which interacts with the α-carboxylate group—the "conserved" group of all the substrates for Subgroup I aminotransferases.

Aromatic L-amino acid decarboxylase

Rat liver AADC has been successfully expressed in *E. coli* enough to be analyzed enzymologically (Hayashi et al., 1993a). Rat liver AADC, like pig kidney enzyme, has an intense absorption at 335 nm and a weaker one at 425 nm. The 425-nm and 335-nm absorption bands represent the ketoenamine form and enolimine form, respectively, of a protonated internal aldimine. On the reaction of AADC with dopa, the absorption in the coenzyme region of AADC showed biphasic changes before reaching a steady state. Pre-steady-state and steady-state kinetic investigations showed that the catalytic reaction of AADC proceeds as shown in the equation: $E + S \leftrightarrow X_1 \leftrightarrow X_2 \rightarrow E + P$. The rate constant was determined for each step, and the absorption spectra of the two intermediates were postulated from the calculation of the absorption changes during the reaction. The structures of X_1 and X_2 were assigned to the Michaelis complex and the external aldimine, respectively, from comparison of the predicted absorption spectra of X_1 and X_2 to those of AADC complexed with substrate analogs. In each intermediate, the absorption at 335 nm was greatly decreased. These results indicate that the PLP-Lys303 aldimine is placed in an apolar environment in AADC, and on binding of the substrate the enolimine structure is rapidly converted to the ketoenamine structure, which is thought to be the "active" form of the PLP-Lys aldimine.

In conclusion, AspAT and ArAT increases its aldimine pK_a on binding of substrates, thus converting the nonprotonated form of the aldimine to the protonated (ketoenamine) form. The aldimine of AADC changes from the enolimine form to the ketoenamine form, probably by altering the polarity of the active site environment. In all cases, the resultant ketoenamine form of aldimine is the form favorable for transaldimination. The amino group of the substrate amino acid must be deprotonated before attacking the aldimine. In AspAT and ArAT, the deprotonated aldimine acts as the proton acceptor. However, the aldimine of AADC does not undergo pH-dependent change in structure, hence it cannot function as the proton acceptor. Efforts are now being made to identify the possible proton-accepting base in AADC.

47

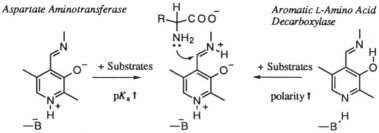

Figure 2. Changes in the structure of the aldimines of AspAT (ArAT) and AADC on binding of substrates.

References

Goldberg, J.M., Swanson, R.V., Goodman, H.S. and Kirsch, J.F. (1991) Structure of the complex between pyridoxal 5'-phosphate and the tyrosine 225 to phenylalanine mutant of *Escherichia coli* aspartate aminotransferase determined by isotope-edited classical Raman difference spectroscopy. *Biochemistry* 30:305-312.

Hayashi, H., Mizuguchi, H. and Kagamiyama, H. (1993a) Rat liver aromatic L-amino acid decarboxylase: Spectroscopic and kinetic analysis of the coenzyme and reaction intermediates. *Biochemistry* 32:812-818.

Hayashi, H., Inoue, K., Nagata, T., Kuramitsu, S. and Kagamiyama, H. (1993b) *Escherichia coli* aromatic amino acid aminotransferase: Characterization and comparison with aspartate aminotransferase. *Biochemistry* 32:12229-12239.

Iwasaki, M., Hayashi, H. and Kagamiyama, H. (1994) Protonation state of the active-site Schiff base of aromatic amino acid aminotransferase: Modulation by binding of ligands and implications for its role in catalysis. *J. Biochem.* 115:156-161.

Kallen, R.G., Korpela, T., Martell, A.E., Matsushima, Y., Metzler, C.M., Metzler, D.E., Morozov, Yu.V., Ralston, I.M., Savin, F.A., Torchinsky, Yu.M. and Ueno, H. (1985) Chemical and spectroscopic properties of pyridoxal and pyridoxamine phosphates. in *Transaminases* (Christen, P., & Metzler, D.E., Eds.) pp 37-108, John Wiley & Sons, New York.

Kamitori, S., Hirotsu, K., Higuchi, T., Kondo, K., Inoue, K., Kuramitsu, S., Kagamiyama, H., Higuchi, Y., Yasuoka, N., Kusunoki, M., H. and Matsuura, Y. (1987) Overproduction and preliminary X-ray characterization of aspartate aminotransferase from *Escherichia coli*. *J. Biochem.* 101:813-816.

Kamitori, S., Okamoto, A., Hirotsu, K., Higuchi, T., Kuramitsu, S., Kagamiyama, H., Matsuura, Y. and Katsube, Y. (1990) Three-dimensional structure of aspartate aminotransferase from Escherichia coli and its mutant enzyme at 2.5 Å resolution. *J. Biochem.* 108:175-184.

Kirsch, J.F., Eichele, G., Ford, G.C., Vincent, M.G., Jansonius, J.N., Gehring, H. and Christen, P. (1984) Mechanism of action of aspartate aminotransferase proposed on the basis off its spatial structure. *J. Mol. Biol.* 174:497-525.

Martin, R.G. (1970) Imidazolylacetolphosphate: L-glutamate aminotransferase—Mechanism of *Action. Arch. Biochem. Biophys.* 138:239-244.

Metzler, D.E. (1977) *Biochemistry*, pp. 444-461, Academic Press, New York.

Metzler, C. M., Viswanath, R. and Metzler, D. E. (1991). Equilibria and absorption spectra of tryptophanase. *J. Biol. Chem.* 266:9374-9381.

O'Leary, M.H. (1971) A proposed structure for the 330-nm chromophore of glutamate decarboxylase and other pyridoxal 5'-phosphate dependent enzymes. *Biochim. Biophys. Acta* 242:484-492

Snell, E.E. (1985) Pyridoxal phosphate in nonenzymic and enzymic reactions. in *Transaminases* (Christen, P., & Metzler, D.E., Eds.) pp 19-35, John Wiley & Sons, New York.

Voltattorni, C.B., Minelli, A., Vecchini, P., Fiori, A. and Turano, C. (1979) Purification and characterization of 3,4-dihydroxyphenylalanine decarboxylase from pig kidney. *Eur. J. Biochem.* 93:181-188.

Yano, T., Kuramitsu, S., Tanase, S., Morino, Y. and Kagamiyama, H. (1992) Role of Asp222 in the catalytic mechanism of *Escherichia coli* aspartate aminotransferase: The amino acid residue which enhances the function of the enzyme-bound coenzyme pyridoxal 5'-phosphate. *Biochemistry* 31:5878-5887.

Yano, T., Mizuno, T. and Kagamiyama, H. (1993) A hydrogen-bonding network modulating enzyme function: asparagine-194 and tyrosine-225 of *Escherichia coli* aspartate aminotransferase. *Biochemistry* 32:1810-1815.

Biochemistry of Vitamin B$_6$ and PQQ
G. Marino, G. Sannia and F. Bossa (eds.)
© 1994 Birkhäuser Verlag Basel/Switzerland

Functional role of the mobile stretch Gly36-Val37-Gly38 of porcine cytosolic aspartate aminotransferase

Y. Morino, S. Tanase, Q-W., Pan, N. Hamasaki, M. Mayumi, S. Rhee[1], P. H. Rogers[1], A. Arnone[1]

Department of Biochemistry, Kumamoto University School of Medicine, Kumamoto 860 Japan; [1]Department of Biochemistry, College of Medicine, The University of Iowa, Iowa City, Iowa 52242, USA

Summary

According to X-ray studies of porcine cytosolic aspartate aminotransferase, Val37 and Gly38, which are part of a flexible loop, are shown to interact directly with bound substrate. Gly36 is not adjacent to substrate but within hydrogen bonding distance to the side chain of Arg386 either in the absence or presence of substrate ligand. To probe the functional roles of the residues 36-38, mutant enzymes at these positions were prepared by the site-directed mutagenesis. From X-ray and solution experiments we find that the V37A, G38A, and G38S mutations do not cause significant perturbations to the unliganded enzyme. Replacing Val37 with Ala increased significantly K_m for substrates but did not affect k_{cat}. On the other hand, replacing Gly38 with Ala or Ser resulted in striking decreases in both k_{cat} and K_m, (1 or 0.02% in k_{cat}/K_m, respectively). Replacement of Gly36 by Ala led to a large decrease in k_{cat} and a small increase in K_m with consequent decrease in k_{cat}/K_m to 4%. Interestingly, the mutation resulted in a sharp rise in the internal aldimine pK_a to 7.5 compared to 6.3 for wild-type. Thus, Gly38 and Gly36 are probably required for proper function of the enzyme because they permit a high level of flexibility for the 36-38 peptide, which in turn allows the essential substrate-induced movement of the small domain.

Introduction

Recent crystallographic structural determinations of porcine cytosolic (Arnone *et al.*, 1985) and chicken mitochondrial (Jansonius *et al.*, 1985; McPhalen *et al.*, 1992) aspartate aminotransferase (AspAT) have shown that each subunit of these dimeric proteins is composed of a large domain (residues 50-326), and a small domain (residues 12-49 and 327-412). The active site pocket is positioned between the two domains. A conspicuous structural feature common to these AspATs is a dynamic "induced-fit" movement of the small domain toward the large domain upon binding a substrate. The conformational change is particularly remarkable in the mobile amino-terminal loop extending from residues 14 to 38. Residues 14 to 35 show a large translocation (3-5 Å in C$_\alpha$) while the peptide stretch from residue 36 to 38 exhibits a high degree of reorientation accompanied by a large change in the dihedral angles for the peptide bonds at Gly36 and 38. In the present study, the functional and structural roles of Gly36, Val37, and Gly38 in porcine cytosolic enzyme (cAspAT) were probed by applying the site-directed *in vitro* mutation technique for amino acid substitutions. Part of this paper has recently appeared in a publication (Pan *et al.*, 1993).

Materials and Methods

Enzyme preparation—Production and purification of wild-type and mutant enzymes were performed as previously described (Fukumoto *et al.*, 1991, Nagashima *et al.*, 1989). Each of mutant enzymes, G36A, V37A, G38A, and G38S, was obtained in a yield comparable to that of wild-type enzyme. Final preparations of these mutant enzymes exhibited homogeneity on sodium dodecylsulfate-polyacrylamide gel electrophoresis.

Kinetic Studies—The reaction was performed in the coupled assay with malate dehydrogenase and NADH, and the decrease in absorbance at 340 nm was recorded at 25°C. The reaction mixture contained, in 1 ml, 50 mM HEPES buffer (pH 8.0), 100 mM KCl, 0.01 mM EDTA, 0.1 mM NADH, 5 μg of pig heart mitochondrial malate dehydrogenase, and desired concentrations of L-aspartate and 2-oxoglutarate. The maximal catalytic constant (k_{cat}) and Michaelis constant (K_m) for substrates were determined by the method of nonlinear least squares.

Thermal Stability of cAspATs—A solution containing the PLP form of each enzyme sample in 50 mM MES buffer (pH 6.0) and 50 mM NaCl was divided into several 50-μl portions in reaction tubes with tight caps, and these tubes were kept at 76°C. At various times, each tube was serially withdrawn and immediately cooled on ice, then centrifuged to remove denatured protein. Remaining transamination activity in the supernatant was measured. A pseudo-first order rate constant for the inactivation, $k_{inactivation}$, was obtained by the relation, $k_{inactivation} = 0.693/t_{1/2}$, where $t_{1/2}$ is the half-time for inactivation.

Calorimetry—A difference scanning calorimeter, DSC120, Seiko Instrument Inc. (Tokyo), was used to record thermograms on 60-μl samples containing 1 mg of wild-type and mutant enzymes. All samples were dialyzed against a buffer (50 mM MES, pH 6.0, and 50 mM NaCl) which was used as reference solution. Temperature of denaturation (T_d) was obtained as a transition maximum in a thermogram.

Results and Discussion

Mutation of Gly 38 and V37

Spectral Properties of V37A, G38A and G38S Mutants—There was no detectable difference between the wild-type and mutant enzymes in circular dichroic spectra in the range from 200 to 250 nm, suggesting lack of gross conformational change upon mutation. Spectra at visible region also showed no significant differences between wild-type and mutant enzymes, suggesting that the amino acid substitution at position 37 or 38 may not affect the state of bound PLP.

X-ray Diffraction Studies—Electron density images at 1.8 Å resolution (not shown) clearly revealed the positions of the expected mutant side chains for all three cAspAT variants. When the structures of the G38A, G38S, and V37A enzymes were superimposed on the structure of wild-type cAspAT, it was found that the mutation-induced structural perturbations are small and confined to the immediate vicinity of the mutation site. The largest structural differences are barely significant for the G38A and G38S mutations. In the case of the V37A enzyme, the largest perturbations are less than 1 Å and are associated with residues 37 and 38. For both G38A and G38S, no noncovalent interactions are lost, and the addition of side chain atoms does not result in the formation of new noncovalent bonds of 4.0 Å or less. On the other hand, the loss of side chain atoms in the V37A enzyme does lead to the loss of a few very weak noncovalent interactions (contacts of 3.6 Å to 3.9 Å) with the side chains of Asn388 and Arg41.

Overall Transamination Reaction—Comparison of the kinetic parameters of reactions catalyzed by the mutant enzymes (Table 1) indicates that V37A can be characterized as a K_m mutant. In contrast, replacing Gly38 with alanine or serine results in very pronounced decreases in k_{cat} values as well as several fold increases in K_m values. Specifically, the ratio k_{cat}/K_m decreases by 3 orders of magnitude for the G38A mutant and by 4 orders of magnitude for the G38S mutant.

Table 1. Catalytic properties of wild-type and mutant cAspAT

	wild type	G36A	V37A	G38A	G38S
k_{cat}, s^{-1}	230	20	237	11.6	1.44
K_m, mM					
Aspartate	1.85	2.56	12.6	7.9	50
2-Oxoglutarate	0.08	0.16	0.34	0.96	5.0
k_{cat}/K_m, mutant/wild					
Aspartate	(1)	0.06	0.15	0.01	0.0002
2-Oxoglutarate	(1)	0.04	0.24	0.004	0.0001

These results show that the contribution of Gly38 to catalysis is much greater than that of Val37, and suggests that mutations at residue 38 may lead to the loss of structural flexibility for the 36-38 peptide stretch, which could prevent in turn the substrate-induced movement of the entire small domain. This notion is supported by our recent unpublished X-ray diffraction studies on the 2-methylaspartate complexes of the G38A and G38S enzymes. Preliminary analysis of these data indicates that while 2-methylaspartate binds at the active sites of both mutants, the binding does not induce the closure of the small domain. This finding appears to be consistent with the fact that V37A mutant enzyme showed upon the addition of the ligand a typical spectral change similar to that observed with wild-type enzyme but G38 mutant enzymes did not (data not shown).

Thermal Stability of Mutant Enzymes—The wild-type and mutant enzymes were allowed to stand at 76°C, and the remaining activity on the timed aliquots was measured. Inactivation of enzymes followed the pseudo-first order kinetics. Under the present conditions, the rate constants for inactivation were 0.0033, 0.0048, 0.0019, and 0.0014 min^{-1} for wild-type, mutant V37A, G38A, and G38S enzymes, respectively, indicating that mutations at position 37 would not appreciably affect the thermal stability of enzyme protein whereas the mutations at position 38 appear to increase slightly the protein stability. These findings were also supported by difference scanning calorimetric measurements of T_d values.

Mutation of Gly36

Replacement of Gly36 by Ala led to a large decrease in catalytic rate and a small increase in K_m with consequent decrease in k_{cat}/K_m to 4%, compared with that for wild-type (Table 1). Interestingly, the mutation resulted in a sharp rise of the internal aldimine pK_a value to 7.5 (6.3 for wild-type). Decrease in thermal stability upon the mutation was indicated by 170-fold enhancement in the inactivation rate at 76°C, and also by a drop of T_d value from 76.9°C (wild-type) to 75°C at pH 6.0. Structural reason for these changes is not clear until the X-ray structure of this mutant enzyme is solved. The heat stability was largely restored in the presence of 2-oxoglutarate, suggesting that the mutant enzyme may assume the closed conformation upon binding the ligand. Thus Gly36 represents one of the key residues that play an important role in a proper movement of the amino-terminal loop in the open to closed transition of the enzyme.

Structural and functional roles of the floppy aminot-erminal loop

The binding of a dicarboxylic substrate between Arg386 and Arg292 induces the small domain to shift toward the coenzyme and the large domain so as to seal off the active site and the bound substrate. Tethering of the small domain of one subunit to the other subunit *via* the amino-terminal peptide contributes significantly to the open-to-closed conformational transition (Fukumoto *et al.*, 1991). Comparison of the structures of the unliganded cAspAT and its complex with 2-methylaspartate complex reveals that the large ligand-induced shift/reorientation of residues 15-18 and 36-38 results in the sequestration of bound ligand within the active site cleft by a group of residues that includes Val17, Phe18, Gly 36, Val37 and Gly38 (Fig. 1). Specifically, the side chains of Val17 and Phe18 shift by over 5 Å to make *van der Waals* contacts with the ligand carboxylate sites: that of Val37, to make *van der Waals* contacts with the ligand α-carboxylate and β-carbon atom. The peptide bonds involving Gly38 are repositioned so that its peptide NH forms a strong hydrogen bond with the ligand α-carboxylate, and the main chain atoms make *van der Waals* contacts with the ligand α-methyl group. Gly36 O is positioned at 3.5 Å from Arg386

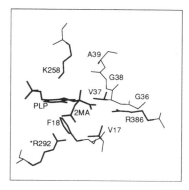 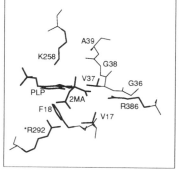

Fig. 1. A stereodiagram showing several active site residues, the 17-18, and 36-39 peptide stretches in the complex of porcine cytosolic aspartate aminotransferase with 2-methylaspartate (2MA).

guanidinium NH in the open form of enzyme and it is reoriented upon binding the ligand closer (3.1 Å) to the side chain of Arg386. Upon binding the ligand, fairly strong hydrogen bonds are thus formed between Gly38 N and the ligand α-carboxylate, on one hand, and, between Gly36 O and the side chain of Arg386, on the other. This is associated with bringing the bulky side chain of Val37 into *van der Waals* contacts with the ligand. Such multiple sets of interaction between the ligand molecule and several parts of the mobile stretch Gly36-Val37-Gly38 are involved in holding the ligand tightly within the active site. Particularly, the two glycine residues in this mobile stretch are conserved in all AspAT sequences so far described, suggesting a critical structural requirement for the enzyme function. Catalytic consequences of mutations of these residues to alanine appear to reflect functionally separate roles of individual residues; mutation of Val37 to alanine results in a large increase in K_m without affecting k_{cat}, whereas that of Gly36 or Gly38 leads to a marked decrease in k_{cat}.

The functional importance of flexible loop structures is an issue of central importance in enzymology. There are several well-documented examples of substrate-induced conformational changes that facilitate catalysis by bringing mobile residues into contact with the substrate ligand: *e.g.*, triose phosphate isomerase (Wierenga, R. K. *et al.*, 1992), hexokinase (Bennett, W. S. and Steiz, T. A., 1980), lactate dehydrogenase (Gerstein, M. and Chothia, C., 1991), etc. Thus, the mobile stretch 36-38 in the flexible loop of cAspAT represents a key structural element that serves to enhance substrate recognition by providing binding energy for the transition state.

References

Arnone, A., Rogers, P. H., Hyde, C. C., Briley, P. D., Metzler, C. M., and Metzler, D. E. (1985) Pig cytosolic aspartate aminotransferase: The structure of the internal aldimine, external aldimine, and ketimine and of the β subform. In: Christen, P. and Metzler, D. E. (eds.):*Transaminases,* John Wiley & Sons, New York, pp.138-155.

Bennett, W. S., and Steiz, T. A. (1980) Glucose-induced conformational change in yeast hexokinase. *J. Mol. Biol.* 140: 211-230.

Fukumoto, Y., Tanase, S., Nagashima, F., Ueda, S., Ikegami, K., and Morino, Y. (1991) Structural and functional role of the amino-terminal region of porcine cytosolic aspartate aminotransferase. *J. Biol. Chem.* 266: 4187-4193.

Gerstein, M., and Chothia, C. (1991) An analysis of protein loop closure: two types of hinges produce one motion in lactate dehydrogenase. *J. Mol. Biol.* 220: 133-149.

Jansonius, J. N., Eichele, G., Ford, G. C., Picot, D., Thaller, C., & Vincent, M. G. (1985) Spatial structure of mitochondrial aspartate aminotransferase. In: Christen, P. and Metzler, D. E. (eds.): *Transaminases*, John Wiley & Sons, New York, pp.110-138.

McPhalen, C. A., Vincent, M. G., Picot, D., Jansonius, J. N., Lesk, A. M., and Chothia, C. (1992) Domain closure in mitochondrial aspartate aminotransferase. *J. Mol. Biol.* 227: 197-213.

Nagashima, F. Tanase, S., Fukumoto, Y., Joh, T., Nomiyama, H., Tsuzuki, T., Shimada, K., Kuramitsu, S., Kagamiyama, H., and Morino, Y. (1989) cDNA cloning and expression of pig cytosolic aspartate aminotransferase in Escherichia coli: Amino-terminal heterogeneity of expressed products and lack of its correlation with enzyme function. *Biochemistry* 28: 1153-1160.

Pan, Q-W., Tanase, S., Fukumoto, Y., Nagashima, F., Rhee, S., Rogers, P. H., Arnone, A., and Morino, Y. (1993) Functional roles of Val37 and Gly38 in the mobile loop of porcine cytosolic aspartate aminotransferase. *J. Biol. Chem.* 268: 24758-24765.

Wierenga, R. K., Noble, M. E. M., and Davenport, R. C. (1992) Comparison of the refined crystal structures of liganded and unliganded chicken, yeast and trypanosomal triosephosphate isomerase. *J. Mol. Biol.* 224: 1115-1126.

Biochemistry of Vitamin B_6 and PQQ
G. Marino, G. Sannia and F. Bossa (eds.)
© 1994 Birkhäuser Verlag Basel/Switzerland

Using ^{1}H- and ^{15}N-NMR spectroscopy to observe active sites of porcine cytosolic and *Escherichia coli* aspartate aminotransferases

D.E. Metzler, C.M. Metzler, E.T. Mollova, R.D. Scott, A. Kintanar, S. Tanase[1], K. Kogo[1], T. Higaki[1], Y. Morino[1], H. Kagamiyama[2], T. Yano[2], S. Kuramitsu[2], H. Hayashi[2], K. Hirotsu[3], I. Miyahara[3]

Iowa State University, Dept. of Biochemistry and Biophysics, Ames, Iowa, 50011, USA,
[1]*Kumamoto University, Dept. of Biochemistry, 2-2-1, Honjo, Kumamoto 860, Japan,*
[2]*Osaka Medical College, Dept. of Medical Chemistry, 2-7 Daigakumachi, Takatsuki City, Osaka 269, Japan,*
[3]*Osaka City University, Dept. of Chemistry, Sugimoto, Sumiyoshi-ku, Osaka 558, Japan*

Summary

Studies of aspartate aminotransferases (AspAT) under a variety of conditions by ^{1}H NMR spectroscopy have allowed assignment of some downfield resonances. We report new results using specific active site mutants of porcine cytosolic and *E. coli* AspATs as well as HMQC - NMR spectroscopy on ^{15}N-containing *E. coli* AspAT.

Introduction

^{1}H NMR spectra of enzymes in H_2O often contain resonances in the 10-20 ppm range that arise from protons in the active site. These protons act as sensitive monitors that may provide insight into mechanisms of substrate binding, recognition, conformational change and catalysis.

Results and Discussion

The spectra of both porcine cytosolic aspartate aminotransferase (cAspAT) and aspartate aminotransferase from *Escherichia coli* (*E. coli* AspAT) in H_2O display a series of 17-20 distinct NMR resonances in the downfield 10-18 ppm region.(Kintanar et al., 1991; Scott et al., 1991; Metzler et al., 1994). Spectra of the apoenzymes (Fig. 1a) lack the most downfield peak A which represents the proton (H_a) on the ring nitrogen of pyridoxamine 5'-phosphate (PMP) or pyridoxal 5'-phosphate (PLP). Peak B (Fig.1,*b,c*) is missing from the spectra of the histidine

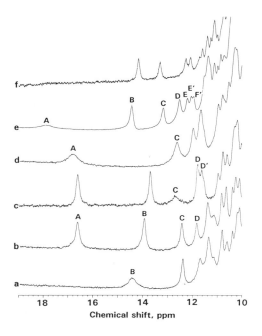

Figure 1. ¹H NMR spectra of porcine cAspAT and *E. coli* AspAT measured under the conditions described previously (Kintanar et al, 1991) at 35⁰ C. Chemical shifts are relative to sodium 2,2-dimethyl-2-silapentane-5 sulfonate (DSS) *a*, Apoenzyme form of cAspAT, pH 6.7; *b*, PMP form of cAspAT, pH 5.7; *c*, PMP form of *E. coli* AspAT, pH 6.7; *d*, H143A mutant of *E. coli* AspAT, pH 8.3; *e*, glutarate complex of cAspAT, pH 6.8; *f*, glutarate complex of the H189Q mutant of cAspAT produced in bacteria, pH 6.0.

mutant proteins H143Q of cAspAT and H143A or H143N of the *E. coli* enzyme (Fig. 1d). This confirms a previous suggestion based on a nuclear Overhauser effect (NOE; Fig. 2a) that peak B represents $HN^{\varepsilon 2}$ of H143 (H_b), a proton that is hydrogen-bonded to the same oxygen atom of the D222 carboxylate as is H_a. A weaker NOE from B to D suggested that the latter arises from $HN^{\varepsilon 2}$ of H189 (H_d). This conclusion was confirmed by the absence of peak D from spectra of the H189Q mutant (Fig. 1f). Spectra of the PMP forms of the enzyme are nearly constant from pH 5 to 9, but peak A of the PLP form moves from 15.4 to 17.4 ppm as the pH is lowered from pH 9 to 4.8 (not shown here). The change is centered around a pK_a of 6.15 for pig cAspAT and 6.5 for *E. coli* AspAT in dilute phosphate buffers. These values are exactly those observed spectrophotometrically for deprotonation of the Schiff base nitrogen. Peak B moves around the same pK_a in the opposite direction to peak A by nearly 1 ppm.

We interpret the pH-dependent shifts in peaks A and B as arising from the tight interaction of the Schiff base proton (H_s) with the phenolate oxygen. At low pH this localizes the negative charge on the phenolate group allowing the N^+H of the pyridine ring to form a strong hydrogen bond to the neighboring D222 oxygen atom, a condition favoring a downfield position for H_a.

At high pH the charge on the phenolate oxygen is delocalized and is centered within the ring near the pyridinium N^+H. This causes an increase in the microscopic pK_a of the N^+H of over 3 units in the free coenzyme. It also causes the hydrogen bond from D222 to H_b to be strengthened, leading to the observed 1 ppm downfield shift. A much smaller effect is propagated to H_d. Although the PMP ring is dipolar ionic, peak A is located at 16.6 ppm, closer to that in the low pH form of the PLP enzyme than in the high pH form. This suggests that in the PMP form the $-NH_3^+$ group of the coenzyme also interacts strongly with its phenolate oxygen atom. Peak A of the Michaelis complex with α-methylaspartate (360 nm form) is also at 16.6 ppm (Scott et al., 1991), indicating a similar tight ion pair between the substrate-NH_3^+ and the phenolate charge, which may be delocalized into the Schiff base group . Peak A of the external aldimine (430 nm form) is at 17.2 ppm for similar reasons.

Using the jump and return pulse sequence of Plateau and Gueron we have obtained useful one-dimensional NOE spectra as well as NOESY spectra (Metzler et al., 1994). The latter have revealed a number of cross-peaks, which have been investigated further by one-dimensional NOE measurements. These have yielded precise chemical shift values. Examples are shown in Fig. 2. The expected NOE from H_a of PMP to H_b is clearly seen as is that to HC6 of the coenzyme ring at 6.5 ppm in Fig. 2a. Upon irradiation of peak B of the succinate complex of the *E. coli* enzyme (Fig. 2b), a strong pair of closely spaced NOE peaks arise at 7.1 and 7.25 ppm. These doubtless represent the two CH protons of the imidazole ring of H143. Strong NOE peaks from D at 7.5 ppm and 8.4 ppm (Fig. 2c) must represent the CH protons of the H189 ring. Their positions agree well with those predicted for an uncharged imidazole ring from the X-ray coordinates of the protein. They are shifted downfield in the H193 mutant (Fig. 2d) as predicted. A third NOE peak at 7.25 ppm is aligned exactly with that of one of the CH protons of H143. This NOE must be from the H189 ring $NH^{\varepsilon 2}$ to the $HC^{\varepsilon 1}$ of the H143 ring. According to the X-ray structure these are only 2.8 Å apart. A similar result was observed for porcine cAspAT (Fig. 2,d,e) for which H_b and the H143 $HC^{\varepsilon 1}$ proton are 2.6 Å apart.

A weak cross-peak between peaks D and G of cAspAT suggested that one component of peak G is $HN^{\varepsilon 2}$ of H193, which is 3.4 Å away from H_d. NOE measurements (e.g. Fig. 2,c,e) showed that peak D (H189) of the *E. coli* enzyme is also at 11.8-11.9 ppm. By comparison of NOE spectra we conclude that peak D' of the *E. coli* enzyme, at 11.68 ppm in the PMP form, is probably the same as peak C of cAspAT, which is found at 12.4 ppm and probably represents the A192 peptide HN (C192 for *E. coli* AspAT). This peak has a strong NOE at 9.4 to 9.9 ppm, probably from the H193 peptide HN proton.

The binding of dicarboxylates leads to characteristic changes in the spectra of the PLP forms. Peak A is much broadened and for pig cAspAT peaks E, E', and F' (which is "buried" in the free enzyme), assume characteristic positions which vary from one inhibitor to another. Fig. 1e

58

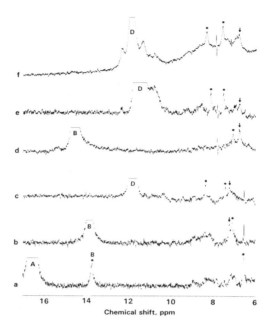

Fig. 2. One-dimensional NOE spectra at 35°C. The largest (truncated) peak in each curve is the one irradiated. Asterisks or arrows mark the major nuclear Overhauser effects. *a*, Irradiation of peak A of *E. coli* AspAT, PMP form, pH 6.9; *b*, Irradiation of peak B of the succinate complex of *E. coli* AspAT, pH 5.1; *c*, Irradiation of peak D of same sample; *d*, Irradiation of peak B of cAspAT, PLP form; *e*, Irradiation of peak D of the same sample; *f*, Irradiation of peak D of cAspAT, H193Q mutant, PLP form;   Arrows mark the H143 HC$^{\epsilon 1}$

shows the spectrum of the glutarate complex of pig cAspAT. Peaks D, E, E', and F' are all seen in well defined positions. We suggest that peak F' at 11.22 ppm ,which has moved downfield upon dicarboxylate binding, is the W140 indole NH, a proton known from X-ray structures to hydrogen-bond to the side chain carboxylate of substrates and inhibitors. It does not move downfield as much in the H189Q mutant (Fig. 1*f*). A similar peak is present in the succinate complex of *E. coli* AspAT but is absent from the spectrum of the W140F mutant.

Although the spectra of pig cAspAT have narrower resonances than those of *E. coli* AspAT, the latter enzyme has advantages. Mutant proteins can be isolated more easily and the cost of growing cells on an ^{15}NH$_3$-containing medium is low. From 4 liters of medium we obtained 135 mg of uniformly ^{15}N-labeled protein, only the coenzyme ring nitrogen lacking ^{15}N. With this enzyme we have recorded heteronuclear multiple quantum coherence (HMQC) spectra. Except for the most rapidly exchanging protons, each HN proton gives a single resonance. The plot in Fig. 3 shows amide and tryptophan resonances. Peak D' at 11.7 ppm (very weak peak at lower edge of figure is strong under some conditions) is confirmed as an amide HN. The histidine peaks are not seen in this plot but are in a more downfield region of ^{15}N chemical

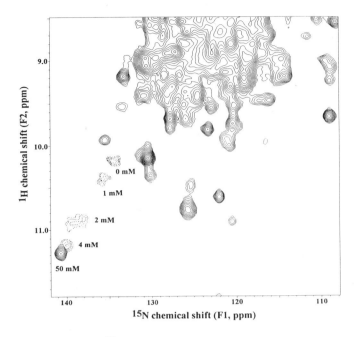

Figure 3. HMQC NMR spectrum of ^{15}N-containing *E. coli* AspAT in the presence of 50mM potassium succinate at pH 6 35°C. Dotted contours indicate positions of the resonance of W140 in the absence of succinate and with 1, 2, and 4 mM succinate.

shifts. Peaks B, D, and Peaks at 11.6-11.7 and at 10.2 ppm (H193) are confirmed as histidines. Two other histidines remain undetected. Indole NH protons tend to have ^{15}N chemical shift values of about 130-140 ppm. We have identified 4 peaks in this region as tryptophan. One of these moves downfield from 10.2 to 11.3 ppm upon titration with succinate at pH 6 (Fig. 3). This confirms its assignment to W140. The large change in chemical shift suggests formation of a strong hydrogen bond between succinate and the indole NH. Surprisingly, in the PMP form in phosphate buffer the ^{1}H shift is 11.5 ppm perhaps as a result of phosphate biding. The peak moves upfield when succinate is added.

Acknowledgement. Supported by NIH Grant DK01549.

References

Kintanar, A., Metzler, C. M., Metzler, D. E., and Scott, R. D. (1991) NMR Observations of Exchangeable Protons of Pyridoxal Phosphate and Histidine Residues in Cytosolic Aspartate Aminotransferase. *J. Biol. Chem.* **266**, 17222-17229.

Metzler, D.E., Metzler, C.M., Mollova, E.T., Scott, R. D., Tanase, S., Kogo, K., Higaki, T. and Morino, Y. (1994) NMR Studies of [1]H Resonances in the 10-18 ppm Range for Cytosolic Aspartate Aminotransferase. *J. Biol. Chem.* **269**, In press.

Scott, R.D, Jin, P., Miura, R., Chu, W.C., Kintanar, A.,Metzler, C. M.,Metzler, D. E. (1991) In: Fukui, T., Kagamiyama, H., Soda, K. and Wada, H. (eds): *Enzymes Dependent on Pyridoxal Phosphate and Other Carbonyl Compounds as Cofactors"* Pergamon Press, Oxford, pp. 129-143.

Biochemistry of Vitamin B₆ and PQQ
G. Marino, G. Sannia and F. Bossa (eds.)
© 1994 Birkhäuser Verlag Basel/Switzerland

Aspartate aminotransferases like it hot

Gennaro Marino, Leila Birolo and Giovanni Sannia

Dipartimento di Chimica Organica e Biologica, Università di Napoli "Federico II", Via Mezzocannone 16, Napoli, Italy[1]

A remarkable tendency towards thermophilicity and thermostability seems to be a general trend of aspartate aminotrasferases (AspAT). This was first discovered by Jenkins *et al.* (1959) who introduced a vigourous heating step into their purification protocol for pig heart cytosolic enzyme. AspATs from different microorganisms living in different habitats are inactivated at temperatures 30-40° above the optimum growth temperature of the organism (T_{opt}), as shown in Table I. Even AspAT from a *Moraxella* strain, which grows in the Antarctic, has a T_{inact} of 48°C where T_{inact} is the temperature at which after a 10 min incubation of the cell extracts, transaminase activity is 50% of the value before incubation.

Table I. **Tendency of aspartate aminotransferases towards thermostability.**
T_{opt}, optimum growth temperature; T_{inact}, inactivation temperature (see text for definitions)

Organism	T_{opt} (°C)	T_{inact}(°C)
Pyrococcus furiosus	100	>115
Sulfolobus solfataricus	87	105
Thermotoga maritima	80	115
Escherichia coli	37	62
Moraxella TAC II 125	10	48

[1] This paper is dedicated to the memory of our very much missed friend and colleague Gianpaolo Nitti.

Since 1985, the attention of this research group has focused on the characterization of AspAT from *S. solfataricus* (Marino *et al.*, 1991 and references within).

AspAT from *Sulfolobus solfataricus* (AspAT*Ss)* follows the general AspAT trend. It has been defined a hyperthermophilic enzyme since it has an optimum temperature for enzyme activity at 100°C and a T_{inact} of 105°C.

Expression of the gene coding for AspAT from *S. solfataricus* in the mesophilic host *E. coli* and characterization of the recombinant protein (Arnone *et al.*, 1992), demonstrated that all the thermal properties of AspAT*Ss* are exclusively determined by the primary structure of the protein. The recombinant AspAT*Ss* is functionally equivalent to the enzyme purified from the cell extract of the thermophilic organism indicating that post-translational modifications identified in the protein isolated from the thermophilic organism (Zappacosta *et al.*, 1994) as well as the temperature at which the protein folds *in vivo* have no influence on the thermal and catalytic properties of this enzyme.

It is worth noting that recombinant AspAT*Ss* as well as the enzyme purified from *S. solfataricus* show a non-linear Arrhenius plot of the catalytic constants for the transaminase reaction. It has now been demonstrated that this peculiar behaviour is a common feature of AspATs, even when isolated from mesophilic or psychrophilic organisms (data to be published) and it is under investigation in terms of an equilibrium between at least two conformations with different catalytic properties.

The hypothesis of a temperature-modulated molecular switch between two protein populations at equilibrium, with different functional and structural properties, was corroborated by limited proteolysis experiments carried out on AspAT*Ss* (Arnone *et al.*, 1992). The two conformational states experienced by AspAT*Ss* in the absence of substrates differed in the exposure and/or the flexibility of a peptide located in the amino-terminal region, as the non-linear Arrhenius plot of the inactivation rate constants in the presence of thermolysin suggests. The coincidence of the break points in the two Arrhenius plots (Fig. 1) suggests a common explanation for the similar behaviour of two completely independent experiments. Moreover, fluorescence anisotropy of a mutant of AspAT*Ss*, where the cysteine residue introduced by site-directed mutagenesis into position 31 of the amino-terminal region of the protein was labelled with the fluorescence probe trimethylamino bimane, has provided evidence for such a temperature-modulated conformational (data to be published).

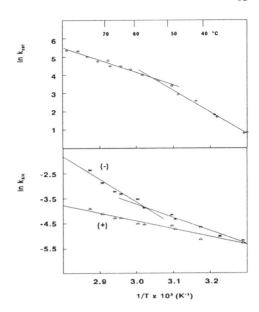

Fig. 1 - **Arrhenius plots of the catalytic constant of AspATSs and of thermolytic inactivation rates.** The k_{cat} values for the transaminase reaction were determined at different temperatures using a saturated concentration of L-cysteine sulphinate and 2-oxoglutarate as substrates. The values of the apparent constant of inactivation rates (k_{AH}) are calculated as the reciprocal of the half-lives.

This type of study has been extended to the *E. coli* enzyme and it was discovered that a break occurs at around 32°C. Fig.2 shows that, even in this case, the Arrhenius plots of the inactivation rate constants (k_{AH}) in the presence of trypsin is non-linear, suggesting a conformational change occurring at a temperature corresponding to the discontinuity observed in the Arrhenius plot of the catalytic constant (k_{cat}).

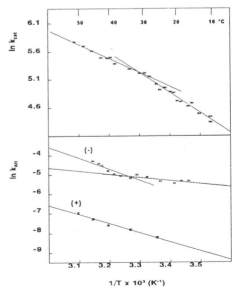

Fig. 2 - **Arrhenius plots of the catalytic constant of AspATEc and of tryptic inactivation rates.** The k_{cat} values for the transaminase reaction were determined at different temperatures using a saturated concentration of L-aspartate and 2-oxoglutarate as substrates. The values of the apparent constant of inactivation rates (k_{AH}) are calculated as the reciprocal of the half-lives.

The physiological meaning of such a conformational change might be to provide the cell with a sort of internal temperature controller that operates in the high temperature range. As a consequence, the change in the catalytic activity is less temperature dependent in the high than in the low temperature range. The effect of the reduced activation energy for the transamination reaction in the high temperature range meant a lower energetic barrier was needed for the reaction to proceed, but, at the same time, an increase in temperature within this range corresponded to a small increase in the catalytic activity. The fact that cells usually defend their metabolism against temperature changes is exemplified by the continuously decreasing slope between the minimum and optimum temperatures in the Arrhenius plot of bacterial growth (Ratkowsky et al., 1982). Bacterial growth is a complex biological process involving a variety of substrates and enzymes, and it is thus not surprising that the Arrhenius law does not adequately describe the effect of temperature on the growth of bacteria, but it is worth mentioning that the trend is in the direction of reducing the effects of small temperature changes near the T_{opt}, in a sort of "buffering effect". Considering the key role played by aspartate aminotransferase, the occurrence of a temperature-regulated conformational transition is not surprising: The question now is, which kind of structural change could explain such an effect?

It seemed interesting to investigate if proline residues play some kind of role. It was observed that this transition is a common feature of AspATs, and attention was therefore given to the proline residues which remain invariant in all AspATs characterized so far. This analysis, carried out on the basis of the sequence alignment reported by Metha et al. (1993) revealed that three proline residues are highly conserved in AspATs. In all the AspATs whose three dimensional structure has been studied so far, two out of three prolines were in the *cis* conformation, namely Pro138 and Pro195, following the numbering of the cytoplasmatic enzyme from pig heart, while the third one, Pro298, is in the *trans* conformation.

Some preliminary experiments carried out on a mutant of AspAT from *E. coli*, in which Pro298 was substituted with an Ala, showed an Arrhenius plot of the catalytic constant different from the one obtained for the wild-type enzyme in the position of the break point and in the activation energies which can be calculated in the two temperature ranges.

These preliminary experiments need further work in order to elucidate this intriguing aspect of the AspAT - temperature relationship.

Acknowledgements

This work was carried out with grants from the Ministero dell'Università e Ricerca Scientifica, Consiglio Nazionale delle Ricerche (Progetto Finalizzato Biotecnologie e Biostrumentazione) and from the Commission of the European Community, Human Capital and Mobilities Programme (contract ERB4050PL922141).

References

Arnone, M. I., Birolo, L., Cubellis, M. V., Nitti, G., Marino, G. and Sannia, G., (1992) Expression of a hyperthermophilic aspartate aminotransferase in *Escherichia coli. Biochim. Biophys. Acta* 1160, 206-212.

Arnone, M. I., Birolo, L., Giamberini, M., Cubellis, M. V., Nitti, G., Sannia, G. and Marino, G., (1992) Limited proteolysis as a probe of conformational changes in aspartate aminotransferase from *Sulfolobus solfataricus. Eur. J. Biochem.*, 204, 1183-1189.

Jenkins, W. T., Yphantis, D. A. and Sizer, I. W. (1959) Glutamic aspartic transaminase. I Assay, purification, and general properties. *J. Biol. Chem.* 234, 51-58.

Marino, G., Arnone, M. I., Birolo, L., Cubellis, M. V., Nitti, G., Pucci, P., Zappacosta, F. and Sannia, G. (1991) Aspartate aminotransferase from *Sulfolobus solfataricus*: a hyperthermophilic enzyme. In *Enzymes Dependent on Pyridoxal Phosphate and Other Carbonyl Compounds as Cofactors* (Eds. Fukui, T., Kagamiyama, H., Soda, K. and Wada, H.) pp. 43-55.

Metha, P. K., Hale, T. I. and Christen, P. (1993) Aminotransferases: demonstration of homology and division into evolutionary subgroups. *Eur. J. Biochem.*, 214, 549-561.

Ratkowsky, D. A., Olley, J., McMeekin, T. A. and Ball, A. (1982) Relationships between temperature and growth rate of bacterial cultures. *J. Bacteriol.*, 149, 1-5.

Zappacosta, F., Sannia, G., Savoy, L.A., Marino, G. and Pucci, P. (1994) Post-translational modifications in aspartate aminotransferase from *Sulfolobus solfataricus*. Detection of N-ε-methyl lysine by mass spectrometry. *Eur. J. Biochem.*, 222, 761-767.

Biochemistry of Vitamin B$_6$ and PQQ
G. Marino, G. Sannia and F. Bossa (eds.)
© 1994 Birkhäuser Verlag Basel/Switzerland

Studies on the mechanism of action of D-amino acid transaminase

James M. Manning

The Rockefeller University, New York 10021, USA

Summary

Bacterial D-amino acid transaminase catalyzes the synthesis of D-glutamate and D-alanine for the bacterial cell wall peptidoglycan. The enzyme is likely present in all bacteria but is absent in mammalian cells. The mechanism of action of several enzyme-activated inhibitors (suicide substrates) of bacterial D-amino acid transaminase is reviewed with the objective of defining an inhibitor that might be a useful antimicrobial agent. Site-directed mutagenesis is being used to elucidate the mechanism of action of the enzyme.

Introduction

In our studies on bacterial D-amino acid transaminase we have had two major objectives. One is to probe the mechanism of transaminases and the other is to develop an inactivator of an enzyme involved in bacterial cell wall biosynthesis. Such a compound might prove to be a novel antimicrobial agent.

All bacterial peptidoglycans contain L-alanine, D-alanine and D-glutamate (as D-isoglutamine). In view of the increasing problem with penicillin resistance, our strategy is to deplete the bacterial cell of free D-glutamate or D-alanine needed for cell wall biosynthesis. To accomplish this we have focused on a key bacterial enzyme, D-amino acid transaminase (Martinez-Carrion and Jenkins, 1965; Manning et al., 1974; Soper and Manning, 1976; Soper et al., 1977; Tanizawa et al., 1989). This pyridoxal 5'-phosphate enzyme is a homodimer of 30,000 Da subunits, which catalyzes the interconversion of D-glutamate and D-alanine as well as most D-amino acids from the corresponding α-keto acids.

Inactivation of D-Amino Acid Transaminase by Suicide Substrates

β-Chloro-D-alanine - This compound is the first suicide substrate that we studied with this enzyme (Manning et al., 1974; Soper et al., 1977). It is also an inhibitor of bacterial growth. Even though chloro-D-alanine will probably not be a useful drug, studies on it were important in showing that D-amino acid transaminase is a target worth considering for the development of future antimicrobial agents.

Inactivation by Cycloserine - This compound is a structural analogue of alanine and it has also been shown by Lambert and Neuhaus (1972) and by Wang and Walsh (1978) to be an inhibitor of alanine racemase. Paskihina (1964) and Churchich (1967) also studied cycloserine. We found that D-cycloserine is a very efficient inhibitor of D-amino acid transaminase (Soper and Manning, 1981). However, it is not used as an antimicrobial agent because it displays some toxicity.

Inactivation by Gabaculine - This compound inactivates the transaminase by immobilizing the coenzyme in a stable secondary amine structure (Soper and Manning, 1982). As a result of this inactivation, gabaculine is an antimicrobial agent. An important lesson from these studies was that even a minor event catalyzed by the enzyme, i.e. removal of β-protons, can make the enzyme susceptible to inactivation by a suicide substrate that bears very little resemblance to the natural substrate.

Inactivation by D-Serine - This compound is a relatively poor substrate; it is 1% as active as the best substrate (Tanizawa et al., 1989). D-Serine forms a significant amount of a quinonoid intermediate absorbing at 493 nm (Martinez del Pozo et al., 1989). As the 493 absorbance band slowly disappears, activity is lost. The finding that D-serine inactivates this transaminase may explain an early report that D-serine inhibits the growth of many different types of bacteria (Maas and Davis, 1951).

Site-Directed Mutagenesis Studies

Replacement of Cys Residues by Gly - The transaminase from B. sphaericus contains 4 SH groups per subunit, which are titratable by DTNB instantaneously in the denatured protein but slowly in the native state (Soper et al., 1979). When 1-2 of the SH groups are titrated, activity is lost. Inhibition could be due to the modification of SH groups near the active site but it could also result from the introduction of a large bulky DTNB group close to the active site of the enzyme. The thermostable enzyme has 3 SH groups per subunit (Tanizawa et al., 1989). By site-directed mutagenesis experiments we have replaced each of the three Cys residues per subunit separately with Gly (Merola et al., 1989). Each of the mutants has nearly full activity, indicating that none of the SH groups is important for enzymatic activity.

S146A - When the Ser next to the active site Lys-145, which binds PLP, is replaced by an Ala residue, there is no effect on activity (Merola et al., 1989). However, the sulfhydryl titration rate of this mutant in the native state is significantly increased, but the normal slow rate is restored in the presence of D-alanine.

W139F - When one of the 3 Trp residues, Trp-139, is replaced by a variety of other amino acids, only the Phe mutant (W139F) is stable (Martinez del Pozo et al., 1989). Studies on this W139F mutant showed that an aromatic residue at position 139 of D-amino acid transaminase is very important for the stability of this enzyme and perhaps indirectly for the binding of PLP.

K145Q (Attenuated Enzyme) - The Lys that binds coenzyme PLP was replaced by a Gln to remove the basic side chain at position 145 (Futaki et al., 1990). This Lys was considered to be the sole catalytic base. This active site mutant retains 2-3% the activity of the wild type enzyme but it still catalyzes transamination ten thousand times faster than the nonenzymic rate (Bhatia et al., 1993). A comparison of the kinetic constants for the entire reaction pathway of the wild-type and the K145Q mutant enzyme provided concrete evidence that the activity of the mutant enzyme was real and not due to contaminating wild-type enzyme (Bhatia et al., 1993). Studies in the presence of exogenous amines revealed that these additives affect mutant enzymes in various ways.

The K145Q mutant enzyme, which is referred to as "attenuated", reacts with substrates very slowly to permit study of some of the individual steps of the reaction - especially the transaldimination step and the step involving the formation of the ketimine and the PMP enzyme. Since this mutant had intrinsic activity, we proposed that there was an alternate catalytic base involved in the activity of these active-site mutant enzymes (Futaki et al., 1990; Yoshimura et al., 1992). Studies with the K145N mutant suggested Lys-267 as the possible alternate base (Yoshimura et al., 1992), although more studies are needed to confirm this assignment.

The findings on the K145Q mutant enzyme are reminiscent of those reported by Martinez-Carrion and his colleagues on L-aspartate transaminase that had been carbamylated or dimethylated at its active site Lys-258, which usually binds PLP (Martinez-Carrion et al., 1979; Roberts et al., 1988). The findings with the K145Q mutant enzyme of D-amino acid transaminase suggest that a network comprised of Lys-145 and other amino acid side chains acts in concert with the coenzyme PLP to promote highly efficient catalysis and stereochemically precise transamination.

Stereochemical Studies - The wild-type enzyme can slowly accept some L-amino acids to convert the PLP form of the enzyme to the PMP form but the efficiency of this transformation is much less than with D-amino acids (Martinez del Pozo, 1989). In the reverse or the second half reaction with added keto acid, the product amino acids have only the D configuration. Small amounts of an L-amino acid would likely be formed, but these amounts are beyond the limits of detection of our assay (0.1%). We interpret the results to indicate that the stereochemical fidelity of the overall reaction with D-amino acid transaminase is preserved. Thus, if the enzyme occasionally makes an error in the first half-reaction and accepts an L-amino acid, then the products, pyruvate and the PMP enzyme, are not optically active. In the second half-reaction, the protonation is stereospecific, so the overall stereochemical fidelity of the enzyme is maintained.

Recently, we have used a similar rationale to develop a general method for the detection of D-amino acids (Jones et al., 1994). If any D-amino acid (except D-proline) is added to α-ketocaproate in the presence of pure D-amino acid transaminase, it is converted nearly quantitatively to norleucine. This amino acid, which is not a normal constituent of biological materials, can be quantified by amino acid analysis since it elutes in a position different from that of any other amino acids. The identity of the D-amino acid(s) is established by a corresponding decrease in the susceptible amino acid(s).

A corollary to this principle is that α-ketocaproate can deplete the supply of bacterial D-amino acids needed for cell wall growth, as has recently been demonstrated (Jones et al., 1994).

In summary, D-amino acid transaminase and alanine racemase are targets for the development of new antimicrobial agents. However, our results show that it is not reasonable to design a suicide substrate based only on the structure of the natural substrate alone. More information is needed about the target enzyme in terms of its active site and its side reactions. Finally, with sufficient information on the structure of the target enzyme, perhaps a synthetic suicide substrate can be made to inactivate it with the specificity and efficiency of a penicillin.

Acknowledgements

The author is grateful to his many talented colleagues who participated in various aspects of these studies - Shiroh Futaki, Wanda Jones, Alvaro Martinez del Pozo, Marcello Merola, Maria Pospischil, Thomas Soper, Hiroshi Ueno, Peter Van Ophem, and Tohru Yoshimura. This work was supported in part by NSF grant DMB 91-06174).

References

Bhatia, M.B., Futaki, S., Ueno, H., Ringe, D., Yoshimura, T., Soda, K., and Manning, J.M. (1993) Kinetic and Stereochemical Comparison of Wild-type and Active-Site K145Q Mutant Enzyme of Bacterial D-Amino Acid Transaminase. J. Biol. Chem. 268: 6932-6938.

Churchich, J.E. (1967) The interaction of cycloserine with glutamate aspartate transaminase as measured by fluorescence spectroscopy. J. Biol. Chem. 242: 4414-4417.

Futaki, S., Ueno, H., Martinez del Pozo, A., Pospischil, M.A., Manning, J.M., Ringe, D., Stoddard, B., Tanizawa, K., Yoshimura, K. and Soda, K. (1990) Substitution of Glutamine for Lysine at the Pyridoxal Phosphate Binding Site of Bacterial D-Amino Acid Transaminse. J. Biol. Chem. 265: 22306-22312.

Jones, W.M., Ringe, D., Soda, K., and Manning, J.M. (1994) Determination of Free D-amino Acids with a Bacterial Transaminase: Their Depletion Leads to Inhibition of Growth. Anal. Biochem. 218: 204-209.

Lambert, M.P. and Neuhaus, F.C. (1972) Mechanism of D-Cycloserine Action: Alanine racemase from Escherichia coli W. J. Bacteriol. 110: 978.

Maas, W.K. and Davis, B.D. (1950) Pantothenate Studies: I. Interference by D-serine and L-aspartic acid with pantothenate synthesis in Escherichia coli. J. Bacteriol. 60: 733.

Manning, J.M., Merrifield, N.E., Jones, W.M., and Gotschlich, E.C. (1974) Inhibition of bacterial growth by β-chloro-D-alanine. Proc. Natl. Acad. Sci. U.S.A. 71: 417-421.

Martinez del Pozo, A., Merola, M., Ueno, H., Manning, J.M., Tanizawa, K., Nishimura, K., Asano, S., Tanaka, H., Soda, K., Ringe, D. and Petsko, G.A. (1989) Activity and Spectroscopic Properties of Bacterial D-Amino Acid Transaminase after Multiple Site-Directed Mutagenesis of a Single Tryptophan Residue. Biochemistry 28: 510-516.

Martinez del Pozo, A., Merola, M., Ueno, H., Manning, J.M., Tanizawa, K., Nishimura, K., Soda, K. and Ringe, D. (1989) Stereospecificity of Reactions Catalyzed by Bacterial D-Amino Acid Transaminase. J. Biol. Chem. 264: 17784.

Martinez del Pozo, A., Pospischil, M., Ueno, H., Manning, J.M., Tanizawa, K., Nishimura, K., Soda, K., Ringe, D., Stoddard, B. and Petsko, G.A. (1989) Effects of D-Serine on Bacterial D-Amino Acid Transaminase: Accumulation of an Intermediate and Inactivation of the Enzyme. Biochemistry 28: 8798-8803.

Martinez del Pozo, A., Ueno, H., Merola, M., Danzin, C. and Manning, J.M. (1989) γ-Acetylenic-γ-aminobutyrate as an enzyme-activated inhibition of D-amino acid transaminase. Biochimie 71: 505-508.

Martinez-Carrion, M. and Jenkins, W.T. (1965) D-Alanine-D-glutamate transaminase. J. Biol. Chem. 240:3538-3546.

Martinez-Carrion, M., Slebe, J.C. and Gonzalez, M. (1979) Sterepcje,ostru pf holoaspartate transaminase after modification of the active site Lys-258. J. Biol. Chem. 254: 3160-3162.

Merola, M., Martinez del Pozo, A., Ueno, H., Recsei, P., Di Donato, A., Manning, J.M., Tanizawa, K., Masu, Y., Asano, S., Tanaka, H., Soda, K., Ringe, D. and Petsko, G.A. (1989) Site-Directed Mutagenesis of the Cysteinyl Residues and the Active-Site Serine Residue of Bacterial D-Amino Acid Transaminse. Biochemistry 28: 505-509.

Paskihina, T.S. (1964) Vopr. Med. Khim. 10: 526.

Roberts, W.J., Hubert, E., Iriarte, A., and Martinez-Carrion, M. (1988) Site-specific methylation of a strategic lysyl residue in aspartate aminotransferase. J. Biol. Chem. 263: 7196-7202.

Soper, T.S. and Manning, J.M. (1976) Synergy in the antimicrobial action of penicillin and β-chloro-D-alanine in vitro. Antimicrob. Agents Chemotherap. 9: 347-349.

Soper, T.S. and Manning, J.M. (1981) Different modes of action of inhibitors of bacterial D-amino acid transaminase. J. Biol. Chem. 256: 4263-4268.

Soper, T.S. and Manning, J.M. (1982) Inactivation of pyridoxal phosphate enzymes by gabaculine. Correlation with enzymic exchange of β-protons. J. Biol. Chem. 257: 13930-13936.

Soper, T.S., Jones, W.M. and Manning, J.M. (1979) Effects of substrates on the selective modification of the cysteinyl residues of D-amino acid transaminase. J. Biol. Chem. 254: 10901-10905.

Soper, T.S., Jones, W.M., Lerner, B., Trop, M., and Manning, J.M. (1977) Inactivation of bacterial D-amino acid transaminase by β-chloro-D-alanine. J. Biol. Chem. 252:3170-3175.

Tanizawa, K., Masu, Y., Asano, S., Tanaka, H., and Soda, K. (1989) Thermostable D-amino acid aminotransferase from a Thermophilic Bacillus species. J. Biol. Chem. 264:2445-2449.

Ueno, H., Soper, T.S. and Manning, J.M. (1984) Enzyme-activated inhibition of bacterial D-amino acid transaminase by β-cyano-D-alanine. Biochim. Biophys. Res. Commun. 122: 485-491.

Wang, E. and Walsh, C.T. (1978) Suicide substrates for the alanine racemase of Escherichia coli B. Biochemistry 17: 1313-1321.

Yoshimura, T., Bhatia, M.B., and Manning, J.M. (1992) Partial Reactions of Bacterial D-Amino Acid Transaminase with Asparagine Substituted for the Lysine that Binds Coenzyme Pyridoxal 5'-Phosphate. Biochemistry 31: 11748-11754.

Biochemistry of Vitamin B₆ and PQQ
G. Marino, G. Sannia and F. Bossa (eds.)
© 1994 Birkhäuser Verlag Basel/Switzerland

Cytosolic factors and the twisting path from birth to berth in aspartate aminotransferases

A. Iriarte, A. Artigues, B. Lain, J.R. Mattingly, Jr. and M. Martinez-Carrion

Division of Molecular Biology and Biochemistry, School of Biological Sciences, University of Missouri-KC, Kansas City, MO 64110, USA

Summary

The two isozymes of AspAT can provide a suitable model system to analyze how different protein sequences end up adopting a nearly identical final three-dimensional structure either during spontaneous refolding in buffer or when folding is mediated by specific cellular components. The relationship of the folding process to the requirements for import of the mitochondrial form into the organelle, as well as the role of structural elements of the protein in the specificity of this biological process, are available to molecular analysis through the use of this isozyme system.

Introduction

Aspartate aminotransferases (AspAT) exist in eucaryotes as two isozyme forms that share extensive sequence homology. Even though both are encoded by the nuclear genome and synthesized in the cytoplasm, their final location differs since one of them remains in the cytoplasm (cytosolic, c) while the other is translocated to mitochondria (mitochondrial, m). The latter is synthesized as a precursor protein (pmAspAT), which in rat liver contains a 29 amino acid presequence peptide (Mattingly et al., 1987) which is excised by mitochondrial proteases prior to its final stages of folding in the matrix of mitochondria, where it resides. Despite the sequence discrepancies and different biological paths from synthesis to folded active enzymes, the isozymes are practically indistinguishable with respect to their overall three-dimensional structure (Malashkevich et al., 1990). Thus, these isozymes represent a nature-provided system of homologous proteins particularly well suited for the study of protein folding mechanisms and of the factors controlling folding following their synthesis in cytosolic polysomes. The latter aspect is of particular interest as it is widely believed (Glover and Lindsay, 1992) that fully folded proteins, including mAspAT (Mattingly et al., 1993a), cannot be imported by mitochondria. Thus, information on the cellular components interacting with the nascent isozymes can provide evidence as to the regulation of their folding reactions, the structural basis for such regulation, as well as a better understanding of the possible implications of their distinct folding processes for the selective import of only one isozyme. To approach these issues we have used four different enzyme constructs: mature and precursor mAspAT or cAspAT and a fusion protein containing the presequence peptide of pmAspAT covalently attached to the N-terminal residue of cAspAT (pcAspAT) as an artificial analogue of a true precursor protein.

Results and Discussion

In vitro Refolding Studies. It is well known that after unfolding, many proteins are capable of unassisted refolding when the denaturant is diluted out. The functional 3D structure of proteins is solely determined by their amino acid sequences. This process occurs spontaneously without the need for an input of energy. This action is driven by small differences in the Gibbs free energy between the unfolded and native states. The refolding of all four forms of mammalian AspAT after denaturation by guanidine hydrochloride (GnHCl) is achieved with high efficiency and speed under controlled experimental conditions (Reyes et al., 1993), with the cytosolic isozyme showing 2 to 3-fold faster rates of folding than the mitochondrial counterpart. The proteins fold properly in the absence of pyridoxal 5'-phosphate (PLP), although the coenzyme improves the yield of the reaction and when covalently attached to the active site lysine it also increases slightly the rate of the process (Reyes et al., 1993). On the other hand, the presequence peptide has no influence on either isozyme's refolding, whether followed by monitoring regain of activity or recovery of the fluorescence or circular dichroism native signals. Together, the information gathered on the spontaneous refolding of these proteins supports a mechanism of folding which includes a rapid formation of secondary structure, early fast dimerization, at least two slow isomerization steps and late binding of PLP.

Folding in cell-free extracts. We have also analyzed the folding of these proteins in an environment more closely resembling that encountered by a newly synthesized protein as it emerges from the ribosome. After the proteins are synthesized in rabbit reticulocyte lysate (RRL) programmed with the appropriate mRNA and in the presence of ^{35}S-methionine (Mattingly et al.,

1993a), we follow their folding by monitoring the change in the susceptibility of the translation product to trypsin over time, taking advantage of the fact that when fully folded these proteins are extremely resistant to proteolysis even in the presence of cellular extracts. The acquisition of protease resistance is one of the few sensitive experimental approaches suitable for this purpose (Mattingly et al., 1993a and 1993b). We have analyzed in this way the folding of the four variants of the isozymes introduced above, as well as of a deletion mutant lacking a 28-amino acid segment from the N-terminal end (Mattingly et al., 1993b). Folding of mAspAT is retarded in the lysate and this effect is more pronounced for the precursor form of the enzyme. By contrast, p or cAspAT fold extremely rapidly and the presence of the presequence peptide has no effect on the folding of this protein. Removal of the N-terminal segment of mAspAT impedes folding completely. This time-dependent gain in trypsin resistance has been previously documented to be due to the gain of a folded native-like conformation (Mattingly et al., 1993a). These observations suggest that molecular chaperones present in RRL may recognize elements in both the presequence peptide and the N-terminal region of mAspAT. The latter seems to be crucial for the protein to attain a fully folded conformation. This is in addition to the control caused by the limiting availability of the necessary pyridoxal phosphate, which in the cytosol is present in excess but in a non-free, possibly protein attached form (Mattingly et al., 1993a). These results support our proposed hypothesis that structural elements of the mature portion of the protein, including those residing in the N-terminal region, are important for chaperone recognition and control of folding of the mitochondrial isozyme (Mattingly et al., 1993b). Furthermore, there is a marked discriminatory recognition by cytosolic chaperones for structural segments of the mitochondrial isozyme which suggest that chaperones may be more selective in their interaction with incompletely folded proteins than originally believed. Certain elements in the primary structure and possibly in the secondary/tertiary structure of their "substrate" may act as targeting or recognition sites. These elements apparently are absent or masked very early in the folding process in the cytosolic isozyme and, hence, mute for chaperone recognition.

Relationship between protein folding state and import into mitochondria. The import of pmAspAT synthesized in RRL into isolated rat liver mitochondria is inversely related to its degree of folding (Mattingly et al., 1993a). As the folding of the translation product progresses following completion of the synthesis reaction, its uptake by functionally active mitochondria concomitantly decreases. By contrast mAspAT, even immediately after its synthesis, cannot be imported by these same mitochondria in a similar posttranslational import assay. These results are consistent with the specificity and need of the presequence peptide for import and contrast with reports on the import into isolated rat liver mitochondria of chicken mAspAT synthesized in a procaryotic transcription/translation system (Giannattasio et al., 1990). These contradictory observations stress the need of a careful and exhaustive analysis of the import reaction for true internalization of the protein into mitochondrial matrix, as folded mAspAT is both already trypsin resistant and can attach to mitochondrial surfaces. Overall, the behavior of mAspAT is consistent with that of most translocated mitochondrial proteins in its need for both a certain degree of protein unfolding and the presence of the presequence peptide for specific and efficient import. In addition, elements in the sequence of the mature component of the protein may play a significant role in this process, as mutants lacking the N-terminal peptide segment fail to fold and to be imported by mitochondria. Mature folded mAspAT or cAspAT, or even chemically unfolded mAspAT, fail to block the import of pmAspAT by isolated mitochondria.

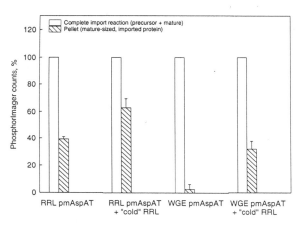

Figure 1. Import of *in vitro* synthesized pmAspAT into isolated mitochondria. Import reactions contained aliquots of translation reactions, after stopping protein synthesis by addition of cycloheximide, with freshly isolated mitochondria. The amount of radiolabeled mature-sized band associated with the mitochondrial pellet after centrifugation of the import reaction relative to the total intensity of the precursor plus mature bands was used to calculate the percentage of pmAspAT imported. "Cold" RRL was added at a ratio of 10:1 by volume. The intensity of the radiolabeled bands was determined using the Molecular Dynamics PhosphorImager[TM].

Association of hsp70 with nascent mAspAT. The ubiquitous molecular chaperone hsp70 is found associated with both pmAspAT and mAspAT during their synthesis in cell-free extracts.

However, this binding is mostly transitory as coimmunoprecipitation of radiolabeled mAspAT with hsp70 antibodies drops dramatically within minutes of stopping protein synthesis (Lain et al., 1994). Binding of the hsp70 chaperone, however, is not the only cytoplasmic component required for mitochondrial import, as pmAspAT is efficiently translocated long after its association with hsp70 has ended. Furthermore, mAspAT, which cannot be imported, also binds transiently to hsp70. This initial interaction of the mitochondrial enzyme with hsp70 may be required to prevent aggregation or undesirable interactions of the nascent protein as it emerges from the ribosome. Yet, a subsequent transfer to another cytosolic chaperone(s) may be necessary for further control of folding and presentation of the passenger protein to the mitochondrial surface prior to import. The need of other cytosolic factors besides hsp70 is illustrated in Fig. 1, which shows that the presence of complete RRL is required for import. Even though significant amounts of hsp70 remain bound to pmAspAT after its synthesis in wheat germ extract (WGE), the translation product is not translocated by viable mitochondria. Addition of complete RRL also partially restores folding of the protein in the absence of mitochondria (data not shown) or its import into the organelle when present in the medium. Thus, some of these cytosolic factors which support posttranslational import may be system-specific. Our results also show that the maintenance of the passenger protein in an incompletely folded conformation, although necessary, is not sufficient for mitochondrial import competency. Protein factors present in the RRL seem also to be required. Such factors and requirements may vary according to the protein being imported or the type of cell where import occurs.

Chaperone-mediated folding of AspAT. The folding of chemically denatured proteins promoted by GroEL, the *E. coli* member of the hsp60 or chaperonin family of molecular chaperones, requires a cochaperone, GroES, and MgATP. The presence of this complete chaperone system allows GnHCl-denatured mAspAT or pmAspAT to fold at 37 C with a 60% to 70% yield. At this high temperature neither protein can spontaneously refold in buffer in the absence of chaperones. The presence of GroEL alone arrests refolding of the mitochondrial proteins even at 0 C, whereas, at this low temperature, GroEL only slows down the refolding of the cytosolic isozyme. An extensive study of the refolding of these proteins as mediated by the GroEL/GroES system in the presence of MgATP has provided information that is consistent with the fact that the two homologous isozymes are not recognized equally by GroEL. Since the two isozymes do not differ significantly in hydropathy profiles (Mattingly et al., 1993b), it is likely that the targeting signals are constituted by epitope-like regions involving either specific sequences or

80

structural motifs in folding intermediates of each isozyme. In summary, the two isozymes of AspAT provide one of the best experimental systems presently available to identify and characterize the structural basis for the interaction of molecular chaperones with their intended unfolded substrates to fulfill their critical, and still obscure, role in the control of protein folding in the cell.

References

Giannattasio, S., Marra, E., Abruzzese, M.F., Greco, G. and Quagliariello, E. (1991) *In vitro* Synthesized Precursor and Mature Mitochondrial Aspartate Aminotransferase Share the Same Import Pathway into Isolated Mitochondria. *Arch. Biochem. Biophys.* 290: 528-534.

Glover, L.A. and Lindsay, J.V. (1992) Targeting Proteins to Mitochondria: A Current Overview. *Biochem J.* 284:609-620.

Lain, B., Iriarte, A. and Martinez-Carrion, M. (1994) Dependence of the Folding and Import of the Precursor to Mitochondrial Aspartate Aminotransferase on the Nature of the Cell-free Translation System, *J. Biol. Chem.*, in press.

Malashkevich, V.N., Torchinsky, Y.M., Strokopytov, B.V., Borisov, V.V., Genovesio-Taverne, J.-C. and Jansonius, J.N. (1990) The Structural Differences Between Chicken Cytosolic and Mitochondrial Aspartate Aminotransferases. In: T. Fukui, H. Kagamiyama, K. Soda and H. Wada (eds.): *Enzymes Dependent on Pyridoxal Phosphate and Other Carbonyl Compounds as Cofactors*, Pergamon Press, Tokyo, pp.99-105.

Mattingly, J.R., Jr., Rodriguez-Berrocal. F.J., Gordon, J., Iriarte, A. and Martinez-Carrion, M. (1987) Molecular Cloning and *In Vivo* Expression of a Precursor to Rat Mitochondrial Aspartate Aminotransferase. *Biochem. Biophys. Res. Commun.* 149:859-865.

Mattingly, J.R.,Jr., Youssef, J., Iriarte, A. and Martinez-Carrion, M. (1993a) Protein folding in a Cell-Free Translation System: The Fate of the Precursor to Mitochondrial Aspartate Aminotransferase, *J. Biol Chem.* 268: 3925-3937.

Mattingly, J.R.,Jr., Iriarte, A. and Martinez-Carrion, M. (1993b) Structural Features Which Control Folding of Homologous Proteins in Cell-free Translation Systems: The Effect of a Mitochondrial Targeting Presequence on the Aspartate Aminotransferase Isozymes. *J. Biol. Chem.* 268: 26320-26327.

Reyes, A., Iriarte, A. and Martinez-Carrion, M. (1993) Refolding of the Precursor and Mature Forms of Mitochondrial Aspartate Aminotransferase after Guanidine Hydrochloride Denaturation. *J. Biol Chem.* 268: 22281-2291.

Mitochondrial protein import: role of certain domains of mitochondrial aspartate aminotransferase

S. Giannattasio, A. Azzariti, R. A. Vacca, P. Lattanzio, R. S. Merafina and E. Marra

Centro di Studio sui Mitocondri e Metabolismo Energetico - C.N.R., Via Amendola 165/A, 70126, Bari and Sezione di Trani, Via Corato 17, 70059, Trani, Italy

Correct targeting of nuclear-encoded mitochondrial proteins is a complex process which has been intensively studied over the past fifteen years. Essential features have been identified in the structure of imported polypeptides which recognize specific receptors at the mitochondrial surface. Moreover, several cytosolic factors have been shown to be involved in the translocation and import of cytoplasmically synthesised mitochondrial proteins (Glover and Lindsay, 1992).

Most nuclear-encoded mitochondrial proteins are synthesized as higher molecular weight precursors with amino-terminal peptide extensions, which are proteolytically removed upon translocation into mitochondria, and proved to contain information for intramitochondrial localization. Others are synthesised as mature sized proteins and contain all mitochondrial targeting information within their own structure.

Mitochondrial aspartate aminotransferase (mAspAT) is encoded by the nuclear genome and synthesised on free cytoplasmic ribosomes as a precursor with an N-terminal extrasequence (pmAspAT) cleaved upon translocation into mitochondria, yielding the mature form. Our initial experimental evidence showed that mitochondrial aspartate aminotransferase can enter isolated mitochondria as a purified protein, whereas its cytosolic isoenzyme cannot; many features of the process have been comprehensively investigated (for ref. see Doonan et al., 1984). Further experiments were also carried out with chemically modified purified mAspAT from which inference of the involvement of the N-terminal region and of a cysteine residue of mature mAspAT was also made (O'Donovan et al., 1985; Barile et al., 1990; Marra et al., 1979). Thus, experimental evidence obtained strongly suggested that information for the correct mitochondrial localization of mAspAT must reside in the structure of the mature protein, with presequence of pmAspAT not strictly required for the translocation process.

So as to carry out investigations on the protein domains of mitochondrial aspartate aminotransferase involved in the mitochondrial import process, use was made of recombinant

DNA technology to construct recombinant expression plasmids, which contain DNA sequences encoding for precursor and mature forms of mAspAT as well as for mutant and chimeric proteins (fig.1), thus allowing for studying their import into isolated mitochondria.

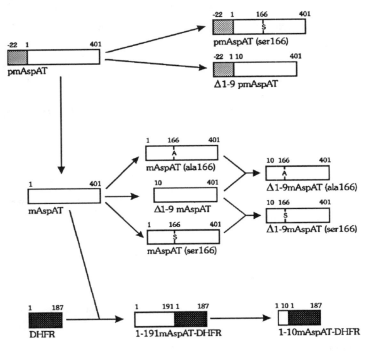

Figure 1. Schematic representation of the procedure to construct mutant and fused DNA sequences encoding for mutant and chimeric proteins, starting from pmAspAT coding sequence. Coding sequence for mature mAspAT or part of it is indicated with white box, that for presequence of pmAspAT with grey box and that for DHFR with black box.

A comparative study of import into isolated mitochondria of <u>in vitro</u> synthesised precursor and mature mAspAT showed that both proteins were incorporated into isolated mitochondria with the same efficiency (Table I) with the precursor correctly processed to its mature form. In addition, competitive inhibition of the import rate of pmAspAT into mitochondria by externally added purified mAspAT was shown, thus demonstrating that pmAspAT and mAspAT share the same import pathway in isolated mitochondria (Giannattasio et al., 1991).

To ascertain the role of specific protein domains in mAspAT targeting to mitochondrial matrix, mutations were produced in the polypeptide chain of mature mAspAT, cysteine 166 was changed into either serine or alanine (mAspAT(ser166) and mAspAT(ala166)) and the nine N-terminal amino acids were deleted (Δ1-9 mAspAT).

Table I. Import into mitochondria of mutant and chimeric proteins. Mitochondrial import of in vitro synthesised proteins was studied, and radioactivity associated with the protein bands measured as described in Giannattasio et al. 1991. In each case import was measured as a percentage of added radioactivity recovered in the mitochondrial pellet. Percent of import is expressed as the ratio between import and import measured after completion for pmAspAT, to which a value of 100 was given. Experimental values are means of different experiments, with the relative standard deviations. +, synthesis or import assay carried out; n.s., not studied; n.d., not determined; S.D., standard deviation

PROTEIN	IN VITRO SYNTHESIS	MITOCHONDRIAL IMPORT	PERCENT OF IMPORT MEAN VALUE±S.D.
pmAspAT	+	+	100
mAspAT	+	+	93±8.3
Δ1-9 mAspAT	+	+	42±2.8
mAspAT (ala166)	+	+	53±7.2
mAspAT (ser166)	+	+	53±3.5
Δ1-9 mAspAT (ala166)	+	n.s.	n.d.
Δ1-9 mAspAT (ser166)	+	n.s.	n.d.
Δ1-9 pmAspAT	+	n.s.	n.d.
pmAspAT (ser166)	+	n.s.	n.d.
1-10 mAspAT-DHFR	+	+	280±38,4
1-191 mAspAT-DHFR	+	+	50±5,5
DHFR	+	+	0

In vitro synthesised mutant and wild type mature mAspAT were incubated with isolated mitochondria to study their import process. In the case of point mutations involving cysteine 166, the amount of imported mAspAT(ser166) and mAspAT(ala166) was found to be about 50% lower than in the case of mAspAT, whereas in the case Δ1-9 mAspAT the percentage of import was about 40% of that of the wild type protein (Table I) (Giannattasio et al., 1992). The involvement of these protein domains is substantiated by the observation that cysteine 166 is conserved in mitochondrial aspartate aminotransferases from differrent species, the amino-terminal region of mAspAT is more conserved than the corresponding region of the cytosolic isoform. In addition, the degree of interspecies identity at the N-terminal segment between two mitochondrial enzymes exceeds the average degree of identity of the two polypetide chains, whereas the degree of interspecies identity between two cytosolic AspATs is lower than the average of the polypeptide chain (Graf-Hausner et al., 1983). mAspAT receptor binding (Marra et al., 1985) and subsequent import is thus seen as dependent on a variety of chemical interactions between at least the N-terminal region and cysteine 166 and the mitochondrial membrane.

Delineation of the exact regions in precursor proteins which are responsible for mitochondrial targeting has been demonstrated in several cases by gene fusion experiments in which parts of a mitochondrial precursor protein can be attached to a non-mitochondrial "passenger" protein (Hurt and van Loon, 1986). Similarly, so as to investigate further the mitochondrial targeting information of the N-terminus of mature mAspAT, import of the chimeric proteins 1-10mAspAT-DHFR and 1-191mAspAT-DHFR as well as DHFR was studied and compared with that of mAspAT and pmAspAT. Mitochondria were found to be impermeable to DHFR whereas both chimeric proteins were internalized by the organelles. The percent of uptake of the in vitro synthesised 1-191mAspAT-DHFR was found to be lower than that of authentic pmAspAT, whereas that of 1-10mAspAT-DHFR is three times higher (Table I), thus indicating that the 10 N-terminal amino acids of the mature moiety of pmAspAT contain sufficient information to direct a cytosolic protein into mitochondria (Giannattasio et al., 1994).

It has now been well established that one requirement for the import of proteins into mitochondria is a partially folded or flexible conformation. This import competent conformation is maintained by 70-kDa heat shock proteins while 60-kDa heat shock proteins assist imported mitochondrial proteins in their intramitochondrial folding and assembly (Neupert et al., 1990; Baker and Schatz, 1991). Recent experimental evidence has shown that the primary sequence of the mature part of pmAspAT seems to dictate whether or how molecular chaperones regulate folding events (Mattingly et al., 1993), thus leading to speculation that the N-terminal region of mature mAspAT binds a chaperone interfering with adjacent domains, thereby creating additional sites for chaperone binding within cytosolic DHFR structure, which do not normally bind molecular chaperones involved in mitochondrial import process.

The finding that the presequence of a nuclear-encoded mitochondrial protein is not strictly required for its mitochondrial localization is not unique: similar experimental evidence has been gathered for the import into mitochondria of mitochondrial malate dehydrogenase (mMDH) both as a purified protein (for ref. see Doonan et al., 1984) and as a protein synthesized in yeast, where the presequence of the mMDH precursor was not found to be essential for efficient mitochondrial localization or function (Thompson and Mc Allister-Henn, 1989). Furthermore deletion of the presequence and 40 residues from the N-terminus of mature 5-aminolevulinate synthase from yeast does not prevent import of the enzyme into mitochondria in vivo (Volland and Urban-Grimal, 1988).

The fact that mature mAspAT contain structural information for interaction with mitochondrial membrane is also substantiated by the change of its protease sensitivity on binding with mitochondrial membranes (Marra et al., 1980). Consistently, it has been shown that the mature form of different imported mitochondrial proteins, including mAspAT, undergoes conformational changes upon binding to isolated mitochondria (Hartmann et al., 1993).

In order to investigate further how the two domains of mAspAT involved in import into mitocondria influence each other it seems worthwhile to study mitochondrial import of multiple mutant forms of mature mAspAT, which involve both deletion of the first nine amino acids and mutation of cysteine 166 in serine or alanine. Other mutations that allow for clarification of the interrelation between presequence and mature moiety of pmAspAT are deletion of the nine N-terminal amino acids of the mature part and mutation of cysteine 166 of pmAspAT (Fig. 1).

Sequences encoding for these new mutant proteins were cloned into pBluescript expression vector in order to study mitochondrial import of their _in vitro_ synthesised expression products.

Acknowledgements
This work was financed by a grant of C.N.R Target Project BTBS.

References

Baker, K. P., and Schatz, G. (1991) Mitochondrial proteins essential for viability mediate protein import into yest mitochondria. *Nature* (London) 349: 205-208.

Barile, M., Giannattasio, S., Marra, E., Passarella, S., Pucci, P., Sannia, G. and Quagliariello, E. (1990) Certain N-terminal peptides inhibit uptake of mature aspartate aminotransferase by isolated mitochondria. *Biochem. Biophys. Res. Commun.* 170: 609-615.

Doonan, S., Marra, E., Passarella, S., Saccone, C. and Quagliariello, E. (1984) Transport of proteins into mitochondria. *Int. Rev. Cytol.* 91: 141-186.

Giannattasio, S., Marra, E., Abruzzese, M.F., Greco, M. and Quagliariello, E. (1991) The _in vitro_-synthesised precursor and mature mitochondrial aspartate aminotransferase share the same import pathway in isolated mitochondria. *Arch. Biochem. Biophys.* 290: 528-534.

Giannattasio, S., Marra, E., Vacca, R.A., Iannace, G. and Quagliariello, E. (1992) Import of mutant forms of mitochondrial aspartate aminotransferase into isolated mitochondria. *Arch. Biochem. Biophys.* 298: 532-538.

Giannattasio, S., Azzariti, A., Marra, E. and Quagliariello, E. (1994) The N-terminal region of mature aspartate aminotransferase can direct cytosolic dihydrofolate reductase into mitochondria _in vitro_. *Biochem. Biophys. Res. Commun.* (in press).

Glover, L.A. and Lindsay, J.G. (1992) Targeting proteins to mitochondria: a corrent overview. *Biochem. J.* 284: 609-620.

Graf-Hausner, U., Wilson, K.J. and Christen, P. (1983) The covalent structure of mitochondrial aspartate aminotrnsferase from chicken. *J. Biol. Chem.* 258: 8813-8826.

Hartmann, C. M., Gehring, H., and Christen, P. (1993) The mature form of imported mitochondrial proteins undergoes conformational changes upon binding to isolated mitochondria. *Eur. J. Biochem.* 218: 905-910.

Hurt, E. C. and van Loon, A. P. G. M. (1986) How proteins find mitochondria and intramitochondria compartments. *Trends Biochem. Sci.* 11: 204-207.

Marra, E., Passarella, S., Doonan, S., Saccone, C. and Quagliariello, E. (1979) The effect of sulphydryl group reagents on the permeation of mitochondrial aspartate aminotransferase into mitochondria _in vitro_. *Arch. Biochem. Biophys.* 195: 269-279.

Marra, E., Passarella, S., Doonan, S., Quagliariello, E. and Saccone, C. (1980) Protease resistance of aspartate aminotransferase imported in mitochondria. *FEBS Lett.* 122: 33-36.

Marra, E., Passarella, S., Casamassima, E., Perlino, E., Doonan, S. and Quagliarielli, E. (1985) Kinetic studies of the uptake of asparate aminotransferase and malate dehydrogenase into mitochondria _in vitro_. *Biochem. J.* 228: 493-503.

Mattingly, J. R., Jr., Iriarte, A., and Martinez-Carrion, M. (1993) Structural features which control folding of homologous proteins in cell-free translation systems. The effect of a mitochondrial-targeting presequence on aspartate aminotransferase isozymes. *J. Biol. Chem.* 268: 26320-26327.

Neupert, W., Hartl, F.-U., Craig, E. A., and Pfanner, N. (1990) How do polypeptides cross the mitochondrial membranes? *Cell* 63: 447-450.

O'Donovan, K.M.C., Doonan, S., Marra, E., Passarella, S. and Quagliariello, E. (1985) Removal of an N-terminal peptide from mitochondrial aspartate aminotransferase abolishes its interactions with mitochondria _in vitro_. *Biochem. J.* 228: 609-614.

Thompson, L. M., and McAllister-Henn, L. (1989) Disposable presequence for cellular localization and function of mitochondrial malate dehydrogenase from Saccharomyces cerevisiae. *J. Biol. Chem.* 264: 12091-12096.

Volland, C., and Urban-Grimal, D. (1988) The presequence of yeast 5-aminolevulinate synthase is not required for targeting to mitochondria. *J. Biol. Chem.* 263: 8294-8299.

Biochemistry of Vitamin B$_6$ and PQQ
G. Marino, G. Sannia and F. Bossa (eds.)
© 1994 Birkhäuser Verlag Basel/Switzerland

Cytosolic aspartate aminotransferase : tissue-specific hormonal regulation of a housekeeping gene promoter

R. Barouki, M. Garlatti, S. Feilleux-Duché, C. Toussaint, M. Aggerbeck and J. Hanoune

INSERM Unité 99, Hôpital Henri Mondor, 94010 Créteil, France

Summary

The cytosolic aspartate aminotransferase gene is an unusual housekeeping gene that is hormonally regulated in a highly tissue-specific manner. The cAspAT enzyme is involved in several cellular metabolic pathways. In the liver and hepatoma cells, the enzyme participates in gluconeogenesis and is transcriptionally regulated by glucocorticoids, cAMP and insulin. Glucocorticoids induce cAspAT in the liver and in the kidney but not in other tissues. Using in situ hybridization, we have shown that the effect of glucocorticoids on the cAspAT mRNAs in the kidney is restricted to the distal tubule of the nephron. In the liver, the induction is restricted to the periportal hepatocytes. In both organs, the basal expression is uniformly distributed. Thus, the hormonal regulation but not the basal expression of cAspAT displays a stringent tissue specificity.

We carried out functional and structural studies on the cAspAT gene promoter. Using transient and stable transfections in the Fao hepatoma cells, we have shown that two distinct regions were responsible for the hormonal regulation of the promoter. Both regions were necessary for maximal glucocorticoid effect. The inhibitory insulin effect and the stimulatory cAMP effect could be separated and were mediated by the distal and proximal regions respectively.

DNA-protein interactions were studied using in vitro DNase I footprinting and gel retardation assays. In the liver, heat resistant C/EBP-related proteins bind to the promoter at three sites. In the other organs, two of these sites are bound by heat sensitive C/EBP-related proteins and one of them is bound by NF1 or CP1 related proteins. We conclude that the nuclear proteins bound to this housekeeping gene promoter are different in different tissues. Some of these proteins display a tissue specific expression. These surprising results could account for the tissue specific regulation of an otherwise ubiquitously expressed gene.

Introduction

Cytosolic Aspartate Aminotransferase (cAspAT) is a metabolic enzyme that participates in both constitutive metabolic pathways and tissue-specific regulated pathways. Together with the mitochondrial isoenzyme (mAspAT) and the cytosolic and mitochondrial isoenzymes of malate dehydrogenase, it constitutes the widely distributed malate aspartate shuttle (Cooper and Meister, 1985). In the liver, cAspAT also participates in gluconeogenesis, a highly regulated tissue-specific pathway (Ferré and Williamson, 1978 ; Horio et al., 1978). In agreement with its metabolic functions, the cAspAT gene exhibits a ubiquitous basal expression and a hormonal regulation that is restricted to the liver and the kidney (Pavé-Preux et al., 1988). In the liver, cAspAT is regulated under several physiological and pathological conditions. It is induced by glucocorticoids, glucagon, high-protein diet, starvation, and diabetes (Katunuma et al., 1966). In the Fao hepatoma cell line, the cAspAT mRNAs as well as the transcription of the cAspAT gene are increased by glucocorticoids and cAMP, and decreased by insulin (Barouki et al., 1989 ; Aggerbeck et al., 1993). Recently, the cloning of the proximal 5' end of the gene coding for the rat cAspAT allowed us to analyze its promoter. Although it has the classical characteristics expected for a housekeeping gene promoter (the absence of a TATA box, a high G + C content, the presence of Sp1 sites and multiple initiation sites), the cAspAT promoter also contains CCAAT boxes and glucocorticoid responsive elements (GREs) (Pavé-Preux et al., 1990), which is unusual for this type of promoter. Two putative GREs are found at positions -585/-571 and -462/-442, and a hemipalindrome can also be detected at position -382. These dual properties of the cAspAT promoter correlate well with the metabolic pathways in which the enzyme participates. Some pathways are constitutive with ubiquitous expression of the enzyme (Cooper and Meister, 1985), whereas other pathways are metabolically and hormonally regulated in a tissue-specific manner (Pavé-Preux et al., 1988). During the last few years, we have conducted a cellular and molecular analysis of the basal expression and hormonal regulation of cAspAT.

Results and Discussion

Cell specific regulation of cAspAT

We have previously shown that cAspAT activity and mRNAs are induced by glucocorticoids in the liver and the kidney but not in the brain and the heart (Pavé-Preux et al., 1988). We next asked in which cells of both organs cAspAT regulation occurs. Using in situ hybridization of tissue sections, we found that glucocorticoids induced cAspAT mRNAs specifically in the periportal but not in the perivenous hepatocytes, while basal expression was uniformly distributed (Feilleux-Duché et al., 1994). Interestingly, gluconeogenesis is localized in the periportal hepatocytes. In the kidney, cAspAT mRNAs were also uniformly distributed except in the papilla where their expression was very weak. Again, glucocorticoids induced these mRNAs only in a subset of kidney cells, namely in the thick ascending limb and in the distal convoluted tubule (Feilleux-Duché et al., 1993). Glucocorticoids are known to increase energy metabolism specifically in these cells. Surprisingly, there was no increase in cAspAT mRNAs in the proximal tubules where renal gluconeogenesis is localized.

We next asked whether the induction of cAspAT by other treatments displayed the same cellular specificity. Streptozotocin-induced diabetes increased cAspAT activity and mRNAs in the liver but not in the kidney. This induction occurred, within the liver acinus, in the periportal zone as well as in the intermediate zone but not in the perivenous zone. Thus, the regulation of cAspAT in this case occurred in a larger zone than in the case of glucocorticoid treatment.

We conclude from these studies that, while basal expression of cAspAT is widely distributed, its regulation displays a strong cell specificity which depends on the inducing agent.

Table I. Expression and regulation of cAspAT

	Basal expression	Glucocorticoid regulation
Liver		
• periport hepatocytes	+	++
• perivenous hepatocytes	+	-
Kidney cortex		
• glomerulus..	+	-
• distal tubule	+	++
• proximal tubule..	+	-

Molecular determinants of basal expression

As previously mentioned, the cAspAT gene promoter displays some characteristics of housekeeping gene promoters. We have shown that the basal promoter activity was carried by a fragment of 260 bp (-286, -26 from the translation initiation site). We have studied the DNA-protein interactions at this fragment by DNase I footprinting and electrophoretic mobility shift assay (Garlatti et al., 1993). Using liver nuclear extracts, we found three regions that were protected from nuclease digestions : P2, P3, P4. All three regions bound heat resistant C/EBP-related proteins, probably C/EBP α and β. This result was surprising since those transcription factors have a limited tissue distribution and could not account for the widespread expression of the gene. When nuclear extracts from other tissues were used, the binding of C/EBP-related proteins was observed (Garlatti et al., 1993 ; Toussaint et al., 1994). However, these proteins were heat sensitive and correspond to different members of this family of proteins than the ones present in the liver. Furthermore, in the kidney, CP1/NF1 proteins were found to bind to the P1 site which overlaps with the P2 site, thus preventing C/EBP from binding. We conclude from this study that the cAspAT housekeeping gene promoter is recognized by nuclear proteins in all tissues tested ; however these proteins are different in different tissues. This could possibly contribute to the tissue-specific regulation of this unusual housekeeping gene.

Table II. Binding of nuclear proteins to the cAspAT gene promoter in different tissues

	Footprint	Liver	Kidney	Brain	Testis
P1	-126, -155	-	CP1/NF1	CP1/NF1	-
P2	-147, -170	C/EBP(R)	-	C/EBP(S)	C/EBP
P3	-192, -218	C/EBP(R)	C/EBP	C/EBP(S)	C/EBP(RS)
P4	-234, -255	C/EBP(R)	C/EBP(RS)	C/EBP(S)	C/EBP(RS)

CP1 :	CCAAT protein 1.
NF1 :	Nuclear Factor 1
C/EBP :	CCAAT/Enhancer Binding Protein.
C/EBP(R) :	Heat Resistant C/EBP.
C/EBP(S) :	Heat Sensitive C/EBP.
C/EBP (RS) :	Partially Heat Resistant C/EBP.

Hormonal regulation of the cAspAT gene promoter

The rat cAspAT gene promoter was cloned upstream of the chloramphenicol acetyltransferase (CAT) gene and transfected into either the Fao or the HepG2 cells. When a CAT construct including a 2.4 kb promoter fragment was stably transfected into the Fao cells, CAT activity was induced by glucocorticoids and cAMP and inhibited by insulin exactly like the endogenous gene. Deletion analysis was then performed which allowed us to localize promoter fragments that were critical for hormonal regulation (Aggerbeck et al., 1993). The cAMP regulation was at least partially localized in the proximal fragment bearing basal promoter activity (-286, -26). Glucocorticoids act at two distinct sites : a distal one (-1983, -1718) and a proximal one (-553, -398).

The distal fragment carrying the glucocorticoid effect is also responsible for the inhibitory insulin effect. Several putative glucocorticoid responsive elements are present in this fragment as well as several binding sites for liver nuclear proteins. We are now conducting site directed mutagenesis to determine which site is responsible for the insulin effect.

The proximal fragment contains a sequence called GRE A that mediates the glucocorticoid effect. GRE A is also active in the context of a heterologous promoter (ΔMMTV CAT). Binding studies with the purified glucocorticoid receptor as well as transfection studies of mutated sites revealed that GRE A has a very unusual structure. It is, in fact, constituted of two overlapping glucocorticoid responsive elements (GRE). Each element can bind a glucocorticoid receptor dimer. The resulting (GRE A) site binds two receptor dimers in a highly cooperative manner.

Our model predicts that each dimer binds on a different side of the DNA helix. This is the first demonstration that such an unusual structure can mediate glucocorticoid regulation of genes.

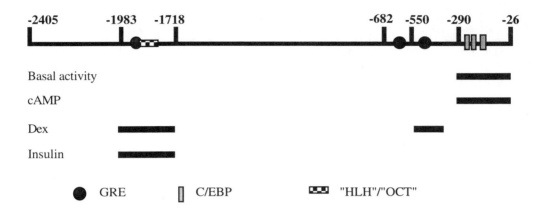

Figure 1. Localization of the DNA sites mediating hormonal effects within the cAspAT gene promoter.

Conclusion

Using in situ hybridization, we have shown that the regulation of the cAspAT housekeeping gene is highly cell specific. We then addressed the molecular mechanisms of basal expression and hormonal regulation. Despite the widespread activity of the cAspAT promoter, it is recognized by tissue-specific transcription factors which may partially account for the specificity of its regulation. The DNA sites responsible for the hormonal regulation have been mapped and are currently beeing characterized further.

References

Aggerbeck, M., Garlatti, M., Feilleux-Duché, S., Veyssier, C., Daheshia, M., Hanoune, J., and Barouki, R. (1993) Regulation of the cytosolic aspartate aminotransferase housekeeping gene promoter by glucocorticoids, cAMP and insulin. *Biochemistry* 32: 9065-9072.

Barouki, R., Pavé-Preux, M., Bousquet-Lemercier, B., Pol, S., Bouguet, J., and Hanoune, J. (1989) Regulation of cytosolic aspartate aminotransferase mRNAs in the Fao rat hepatoma cell line by dexamethasone, insulin and cyclic AMP. *Eur. J. Biochem.* 186: 79-85.

Cooper, A.J.L., and Meister, A. Metabolic significance of transamination (1985) In: P. Christen, and Metzler, D.E. (eds.): *Transaminases*, Wiley, New York, PP. 534-563.

Feilleux-Duché, S., Garlatti, M., Aggerbeck, M., Poyard, M., Bouguet, J., Hanoune, J., and Barouki, R. (1993) Cell specific regulation of cytosolic aspartate aminotransferase by glucocorticoids in the rat kidney. *Am. J. Physiol* 265: C1298-C1305.

92

Feilleux-Duché, S., Garlatti, M., Burcelin, R., Aggerbeck, M., Bouguet, J., Girard, J., Hanoune, J., and Barouki, R. (1994) Acinar zonation of the hormonal regulation of the housekeeping cytosolic aspartate aminotransferase gene in the liver. *Amer. J. Physiol.* 266: C911-C918.

Ferré, P., and Williamson, H. (1978) Evidence for the participation of aspartate aminotransferase in hepatic glucose synthesis in the suckling newborn rat. *Biochem. J.* 176: 335-338.

Garlatti, M., Tchesnokov, V., Daheshia, M., Feilleux-Duché, S., Hanoune, J., Aggerbeck, M., Barouki, R. (1993) C/EBP-related proteins bind to the unusual promoter of the aspartate aminotransferase housekeeping gene. *J. Biol. Chem.* 268: 6567-6574.

Horio, Y., Tanaka, T., Taketoshi, M., Uno, T., and Wada, H. (1988) Rat cytosolic aspartate aminotransferase: regulation of its mRNA and contribution to gluconeogenesis. *J. Biochem.* 103: 805-808.

Katunuma, N., Okada, M., and Nishii, Y. (1966) Regulation of the urea cycle and TCA cycle by ammonia. *Adv. Enzyme Regul.* 4: 317-335.

Pavé-Preux, M., Aggerbeck, M., Veyssier, C., Bousquet-Lemercier, B., Hanoune, J., and Barouki, R. (1990) Hormonal discrimination among transcription start sites of aspartate aminotransferase. *J. Biol. Chem.* 265: 4444-4448.

Pavé-Preux, M., Ferry, N., Bouguet, J., Hanoune, J., and Barouki, R. Nucleotide sequence and glucocorticoid regulation of the mRNAs for the isoenzymes of rat aspartate aminotransferase. *J. Biol. Chem.* 263: 17459-17466.

Toussaint, C., Bousquet-Lemercier, B., Garlatti, M., Hanoune, J., and Barouki, R. (1994) Testis-specific transcription start site in the aspartate aminotransferase housekeeping gene promoter. *J. Biol. Chem.* in press.

Biochemistry of Vitamin B$_6$ and PQQ
G. Marino, G. Sannia and F. Bossa (eds.)
© 1994 Birkhäuser Verlag Basel/Switzerland

Regulation by glucagon of serine:pyruvate/alanine:glyoxylate aminotransferase gene expression in cultured hepatocytes

C. Uchida, T. Funai, K. Ohbayashi, T. Oda and A. Ichiyama

Dept. of Biochemistry, Hamamatsu University School of Medicine, 3600 Handa-cho, Hamamatsu, Shizuoka, 431-31, Japan

Summary

In rat liver, serine:pyruvate/alanine:glyoxylate aminotransferase (SPT/AGT) locates in both mitochondria and peroxisomes, and only the mitochondrial enzyme is markedly induced by glucagon. In the rat, a single SPT/AGT gene locates on chromosome 9q34-q36, and there are two transcription initiation sites in the first exon. Transcription from the upstream and downstream start sites generate mRNAs for the precursor of mitochondrial SPT/AGT (mitochondrial SPT/AGT-mRNA) and peroxisomal SPT/AGT-mRNA, respectively. In the present study, the effect of glucagon on SPT/AGT gene expression were studied in primary cultured rat hepatocytes. Hepatocytes were first precultured for 16-18 h under serum- and hormone-free conditions. Glucagon and/or other effectors were then added, and the culture was continued as required. Under these conditions, the addition of glucagon caused a remarkable increase in the cellular level of mitochondrial SPT/AGT-mRNA via the cAMP-protein kinase A signaling pathway. A run-on transcription assay revealed that activation of transcription is responsible for the increase in mitochondrial SPT/AGT-mRNA. Notable features of the activation of SPT/AGT gene transcription by glucagon or cAMP are inhibition by cycloheximide and a slow response taking as long as 90 min for the maximum rate of transcription, suggesting that a protein synthesis is involved in this process. It appears that the rat SPT/AGT gene is a dual promoter gene. In this case, a remarkable feature of this gene is that the alternative usage of the two promoters eventually determines the alternative organelle localization of the expression product.

Introduction

Serine:pyruvate aminotransferase (SPT) has been studied in the 1970's mainly from a viewpoint of gluconeogenesis from serine, because the SPT activity in rat liver was shown to be induced by glucagon (Rowsell *et al.*, 1973). Now we know that SPT/AGT also acts on glyoxylate as alanine:glyoxylate aminotransferase (AGT) (Noguchi *et al.*, 1978) and that the AGT activity has an important role in the liver. In this paper, this enzyme is referred to as SPT/AGT.

One of the most interesting characteristics of SPT/AGT is that its organelle distribution differs with animal species. In carnivores, SPT/AGT locates mostly in mitochondria, while in herbivores, it is entirely peroxisomal (Takada and Noguchi, 1982; Danpure *et al.*, 1990). Peroxisomes are the major intracellular compartment where glyoxylate, an immediate precursor of oxalate, is synthesized. Therefore, peroxisomal localization of SPT/AGT is essential, especially for herbivores, to remove glyoxylate by transamination to glycine and to keep animals from harmful overproduction of oxalate (Yanagisawa *et al.*, 1983; Noguchi, 1987). In fact, primary hyperoxaluria type 1, a congenital metabolic disease characterized by increased production of oxalate and precipitation of calcium oxalate crystals in many tissues, is caused by a defect in peroxisomal SPT/AGT (Danpure and Jennings, 1986). In rat liver, SPT/AGT locates in both mitochondria and peroxisomes, and only the mitochondrial enzyme is markedly induced by glucagon (Noguchi *et al.*, 1978; Oda *et al.*, 1982). We have been interested in how the same enzyme locates in two different organelles and how the synthesis of only the mitochondrial SPT/AGT is enhanced by glucagon.

In the rat, the SPT/AGT gene is single and locates on chromosome 9q34-q36 (Oda *et al.*, 1990; Mori *et al.*, 1992), but there are two transcription initiation sites in exon 1. Transcription from the upstream and downstream sites generates mitochondrial SPT/AGT-mRNA and peroxisomal SPT/AGT-mRNA, respectively. Mitochondrial SPT/AGT-mRNA is translated from the first ATG codon to produce a precursor containing a mitochondria-targeting N-terminal extension peptide. The product is translocated into mitochondria and converted to the mature form with processing of the targeting peptide. On the other hand, translation of peroxisomal SPT/AGT-mRNA begins from the ATG codon which corresponds to Met at the N-terminal of mature mitochondrial SPT/AGT (Fig. 1). Without the mitochondria-targeting signal, the product is translocated into peroxisomes, being directed by an intramolecular peroxisome-targeting sequence (Oda *et al.*, 1990; Yokota *et al.*, 1991). When glucagon is injected into rat, mitochondrial SPT/AGT-mRNA is markedly induced, while peroxisomal mRNA is not affected (Oda *et al.*, 1990). In this paper,

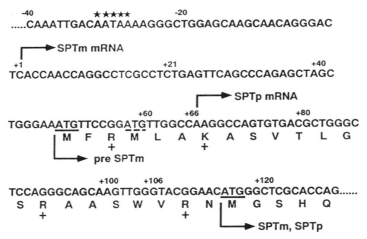

Figure 1. Transcription start sites of rat SPT/AGT gene. The upstream start site is numbered +1. Mitochondrial and peroxisomal SPT/AGTs are abbreviated to SPTm, SPTp, respectively. Translation initiation ATG codones are underlined. Amino acid sequence was represented by one-letter abbreviations and basic amino acid residues are marked with +. Asterisk indicates a TATA-like sequence.

we describe the mechanism of the specific induction of mitochondrial SPT/AGT-mRNA by glucagon in primary cultured rat hepatocytes.

Materials and Methods

Hepatocytes were precultured in the absence of serum and hormones for 16-18 h (or for 2 h where indicated), and then incubated with 5-500 nM glucagon, 0.1 mM 8-Br-cAMP or other effectors. The methods for northern blot analysis, run-on transcription assay and RNase protection analysis have been described previously (Uchida *et al.*, 1994).

Results and Discussion

We decided to use primary cultured rat hepatocytes for analysis of the induction by glucagon of mitochondrial SPT/AGT-mRNA, because complexities seen *in vivo* such as contribution of other hormones or metabolites are eliminated in this system. We were able to reproduce in the cultured hepatocyte system the glucagon-induced increase in the level of SPT/AGT-mRNA. This increase occurred after an apparent lag of 2 h, reaching a plateau by 4-6 h. The concentration of glucagon for half-maximal induction was 20 nM. We also confirmed by RNase protection analysis that hepatocytes contain both the mitochondrial and peroxisomal SPT/AGT-mRNAs and that the mRNA induced by glucagon is the one for mitochondrial SPT/AGT. With regard to the second messenger system, the ability of glucagon to increase SPT/AGT-mRNA was reproduced, at least qualitatively, by 8-Br-cAMP and forskolin, but neither TPA, nor calcium ionophore A23187, nor their combination was effective in place of glucagon. In addition, effects of both glucagon and 8-Br-cAMP were inhibited by H89, a selective inhibitor of protein kinase A, indicating that cAMP and protein kinase A are involved in the signaling pathway.

We then performed run-on transcription experiments with isolated nuclei in order to examine whether or not the increase in SPT/AGT-mRNA by glucagon is due to activation of the SPT/AGT gene transcription. Addition of glucagon to hepatocytes resulted in a clear-cut enhancement of the SPT/AGT gene transcription, but the activation was a slow process, taking 90 min for the maximum rate of transcription.

One of notable features of the glucagon-activation of the SPT/AGT gene transcription is the effect of dexamethasone. In general, effects of glucocorticoids are cooperative with glucagon, especially when gluconeogenesis and glycogenolysis are concerned, but in this case, no transcription of the SPT/AGT gene was detected, when hepatocytes were exposed to 0.1 µM dexamethasone for 30 min either prior to or after 90 min incubation with glucagon. It appears that dexamethasone interferes with the SPT/AGT gene transcription that has been activated by glucagon.

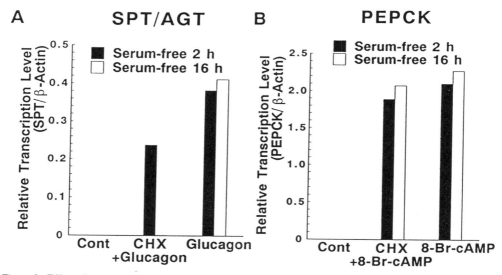

Figure 2. Effect of cycloheximide on activation of transcription by glucagon or 8-Br-cAMP. Hepatocytes were precultured without serum and hormones for 2 h or 16 h, followed by a 0.5 h culture under the same conditions, except that 1 µM cycloheximide was included in the culture medium where indicated. Then 90 min incubation was carried out in the absence (control) or presence of 0.5 µM glucagon or 0.1 mM 8-Br-cAMP. Transcription rate was determined by run-on transcription assay and expressed as the ratio to transcription rate of the β-actin gene.

Another feature of the glucagon-activation of the SPT/AGT gene transcription is the effect of cycloheximide. It is well documented that a cAMP-responsive element (CRE) and CRE-biding protein (CREB) play key roles in the activation of transcription by cAMP (Montminy *et al.*, 1990). It is also generally accepted that most of the CRE- and CREB-mediated activation of transcription by cAMP occurs rapidly reaching a maximum within 30 min and is independent of new protein synthesis. In contrast, the activation of the SPT/AGT gene transcription by cAMP or glucagon took 90 min and was strongly inhibited by 1 µM cycloheximide, when hepatocytes had been precultured for 16 h under serum- and hormone-free conditions (Fig. 2, panel A). When the preculture was shortened to 2 h, the activation by glucagon occurred a little more rapidly and was less sensitive to the cycloheximide inhibition. On the other hand, activation of the PEPCK gene transcription by 8-Br-cAMP examined as a typical example of the CRE- and CREB-mediated response was not affected by cycloheximide, irrespective of the preculture time of 2 h or 16 h, as shown in panel B, Fig. 2. It is possible that a new type of CRE-CREB system mediates the activation of SPT/AGT gene transcription by glucagon.

We think that the rat SPT/AGT gene is a dual promoter gene. Recently we found that the +21 to +106 region promotes transcription from the downstream start site (Ohbayashi *et al.*, submitted for publication) (cf. Fig. 1). Transcription from the upstream start site may also occur in the presence of its own promoter which interacts with a putative cAMP-responsive enhancer complex. In this case, a remarkable feature of this gene is that the alternative usage of the two promoters eventually determines the alternative organelle localization of the expression products. It is well known that in eukaryotic cells each organelle plays different roles in cellular functions, and proteins are synthesized being destined to be localized in a relevant subcellular compartment. Therefore, the food habit-dependent mitochondrial or peroxisomal localization of SPT/AGT in carnivores or herbivores suggests that each class of animals has gained, according to metabolic needs and as a result of natural selection, a mechanism to supply the enzyme to a proper organelle. Whether or not the peroxisome-targeting and mitochondria-targeting signals seen in rat SPT/AGT or its precursor are also used by other animal species is of great interest.

Acknowledgments
We thank Drs. Y. Tomita and A. Ichihara, University of Tokushima, for teaching us the hepatocyte primary culture technique, Dr. H. Hidaka, University of Nagoya, for generous supply of H89, and Drs. C. Caldwell and D.K. Granner, University of Vanderbilt, for kind supply of a cDNA for rat PEPCK, pPC116.

References
Danpure, C.J., and Jennings, P.R. (1986) Peroxisomal alanine:glyoxylate aminotransferase deficiency in primary hyperoxaluria type 1. FEBS Lett. 201: 20-25

Danpure, C.J., Guttrige, K.M., Fryer, P., Jennings, P.R., Allsop, J., and Purdue, P.E. (1990) Subcellular distribution of hepatic alanine:glyoxylate aminotransferase in various mammalian species. J. Cell Sci. 97: 669-678

Montminy, M.R., Gonzalez, G.A., and Yamamoto, K.K. (1990) Regulation of cAMP-inducible genes by CREB. TINS. 13: 184-188

Mori, M., Oda, T., Nishiyama, K., Serikawa, T., Yamada, J., and Ichiyama, A. (1992) A single serine:pyruvate aminotransferase gene on rat chromosome 9q34-q36. Genomics 13: 686-689

Noguchi, T. (1987) Amino acid metabolism in animal peroxisomes. In: Fahimi, H.D. and Sies, H. (eds.): Peroxisomes in Biology and Medicine, Springer-Verlag, Berlin, Heidelberg, pp. 234-243

Noguchi, T., Okuno, E., Takada, Y., Minatogawa, Y., Okai, K., and Kido, R. (1978) Characteristics of hepatic alanine-glyoxylate aminotransferase activity in different mammalian species. Biochem. J. 169: 113-122

Oda, T., Yanagisawa, M., and Ichiyama, A. (1982) Induction of serine:pyruvate aminotransferase in rat liver organelles by glucagon and a high protein diet. J. Biochem. 91: 219-232

Oda, T., Funai, T., and Ichiyama, A. (1990) Generation from a single gene of two mRNAs that encode the mitochondrial and peroxisomal serine:pyruvate aminotransferase of rat liver. J. Biol. Chem. 265: 7513-7519

Rowsell, E.V., Al-Tai, A.H., Carnie, J.A., and Rowsell, K.V. (1973) Increased liver L-serine-pyruvate aminotransferase activity under gluconeogenic conditions. Biochem. J. 134: 349-351

Takada, Y., and Noguchi, T. (1982) Subcellular distribution, and physical and immunological properties of hepatic alanine:glyoxylate aminotransferase isoenzymes in different mammalian species. Comp. Biochem. Physiol. 72B: 597-604

Uchida, C., Funai, T., Oda, T., Ohbayashi, K., and Ichiyama, A. (1994) Regulation by glucagon of serine:pyruvate/alanine:glyoxylate aminotransferase gene expression in cultured rat hepatocytes. J. Biol. Chem. 269: 8849-8859

Yanagisawa, M., Higashi, S., Oda, T., and Ichiyama, A. (1983) Properties and possible physiological role of rat liver serine:pyruvate aminotransferase. In: Lennon, D.L.F., Stratman, F.W., and Zahlten, R.N. (eds.): Biochemistry of Metabolic Processes, Elsevier Biomedical, New York, Amsterdam, Oxford, pp. 413-426

Yokota, S., Funai, T., and Ichiyama, A. (1991) Organelle localization of rat liver serine:pyruvate aminotransferase expressed in transfected Cos-1 cells. Biomed. Res. 12: 53-59

Biochemistry of Vitamin B$_6$ and PQQ
G. Marino, G. Sannia and F. Bossa (eds.)
© 1994 Birkhäuser Verlag Basel/Switzerland

Glutamate 1-semialdehyde aminotransferase, a unique enzyme in chlorophyll biosynthesis

Bernhard Grimm

Institut für Pflanzengenetik und Kulturpflanzenforschung, Corrensstr. 3, 06466 Gatersleben, Germany

Glutamate 1-semialdehyde aminotransferase (GSA-AT) has been first described in barley. Gough and Kannangara [1] found an enzyme in the chloroplast stromal preparation of greening barley that catalyses the transamination of glutamate 1-semialdehyde (GSA) to δ-aminolevulinate (ALA). This is the final step of the C5 pathway which in three enzymatic reactions converts glutamate into ALA, the precursor for all tetrapyrroles [2, 3]. The primary structure of GSA-AT from barley has been obtained by partial amino acid sequence determination and nucleotide sequencing of a cDNA clone [4]. Subsequently, a number of bacterial and plant genes for GSA-AT have been sequenced [5-11].

All deduced amino acid sequences of GSA-AT known to date show a high overall sequence identity, indicating a common structural organization and a common catalytic mechanism. Purified recombinant Synechococcus GSA-AT has been the primary model enzyme to study the reaction mechanism of ALA synthesis [12-15]. The enzyme is active as a homodimer and catalyses the net intramolecular transfer of an amino group from the C2 to C1 position of GSA. The vitamin B6 derivatives PMP and PLP are integral parts of the active site of GSA-AT functioning as amino group acceptor and donor. Both coenzyme forms exhibit spectral changes upon addition of GSA and its analogues. It is noteworthy, that GSA contains carbonyl and amino functional groups and reacts with the enzyme in both coenzyme forms. Resulting products are dioxo- (DOVA) and diamino valerate (DAVA) which are considered as putative intermediates in the transfer of the amino group. Several lines of evidence show that DAVA is the active intermediate in the conversion of GSA to ALA, and DOVA is a pseudo intermediate [12-15]. By analogy with other aminotransferases ALA forms an abortive complex with the PLP form and a reactive complex with the PMP form of GSA-AT [13]. According to kinetic data of GSA-AT the formation of ALA proceeds in two half reactions by a Ping Pong Bi Bi mechanism [13,14], similar to other transaminases, e.g. aspartate aminotransferase [16]. The PMP form initiates the synthesis of ALA. The intermediate formed in the first half-reaction of transamination, DAVA, is converted to ALA by the donation of the C4 amino group of DAVA to the PLP form of GSA-AT. DAVA dissociates from the enzyme and is released by transaldimination giving the corresponding internal aldimine with the active site lysine side chain. For the second half reaction the process is reversed via an external aldimine yielding ALA. (S)GSA is the natural substrate for GSA-AT and is immediately converted to ALA, while the R-enantiomer is a substrate only for the first half reaction. [17]. No back reaction of ALA to GSA was observed, suggesting a thermodynamic preference of the amino transfer from the C4 position. However, experiments with the active site mutant Lys272Arg of Synechococcus GSA-AT indicate that the C5 amino group of DAVA was preferentially transferred, while the C4 amino group seems to be inaccessible for transamination by the cofactor in this mutant enzyme [18].

GSA-AT is particularly susceptible to an inhibitory mechanism known as mechanism based inhibition. The high specificity of these inhibitors based on the fact, that they are recognized as normal substrates, but the intermediates reacts covalently or irreversibly with the enzyme. It is intended to test GSA-AT as target for new designed herbicidal compounds with potentials of mechanism based inhibitors. Structural and physiological prerequisites for the use of new designed herbicides of GSA-AT were initially determined in two different approaches. Both experiments provided information either on active site residues, which are responsible for the high sensitivity towards suicide inhibitors, or if GSA-AT is essential for tetrapyrrole synthesis in higher plants.

A compound, which has been tested to affect chlorophyll biosynthesis negatively is gabaculine. It is a neurotoxin and inhibits chlorophyll synthesis by inactivation of GSA-AT. It was considered as a derivative of γ-aminobutyrate and inhibits γ-aminobutyrate transaminase. Gabaculine reacts only with the PLP form of the enzyme. Enzyme inactivation is associated with an immediate spectral shift upon addition of gabaculine from 418nm to 338 nm indicating the formation of m-carboxyphenyl-PMP.

Dr. Arnold Smith, Aberystwyth, presented a gabaculine tolerant mutant of Synechococcus [19]. The gene coding for GSA-AT of this mutant strain showed two changes in the nucleotide sequence. A deletion of 9 bases resulted in the elimination of amino acid No 5-7 and a nucleotide substitution causes the exchange from Met 248 to Ile

[12]. Recombinant GSA-AT containing only one of the two mutations were tested for their tolerance to gabaculine. The sensitivity towards gabaculine was indicated in the ability to synthesize ALA in the presence of the increasing amounts of the inhibitor (Fig.1). The wild-type (WT) enzyme and the deletion mutant (DEL 5-7) were inactivated with the same low concentration, while 100-300 times higher concentration of gabaculine are required to inactivate the primary mutant (GR6) and the point mutant (M248I). Although Met248 was identified to be part of the active site of GSA-AT, reasons for the decrease in substrate specificity of gabaculine are still speculative.

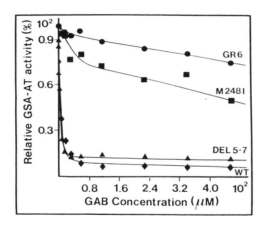

Figure 1. Gabaculine resistance of recombinant wild-type (WT) and three mutant GSA-AT (GR6, M248I, DEL5-7). Initial rates of ALA synthesis were determined in the presence of various fixed concentrations of GAB and expressed in terms of the percent of the uninhibited reaction rate.

In light of the important function of GSA-AT providing ALA for tetrapyrroles we asked for the indispensability of the enzyme for the pathway. Antisense genes for GSA-AT were introduced into tobacco plants using the leaf disk transformation technique [20]. Antisense RNA was expected to inactivate the endogenous transcripts most likely by RNA-RNA-hybrid formation [21]. As result of the eliminated RNA, plants suffer from lack of gene products. Inactivation of GSA-AT expression by antisense RNA synthesis simulates

102

herbicidal effects on the enzyme and, in addition, enables studies on regulatory effects on the chlorophyll pathway and other plastid functions.

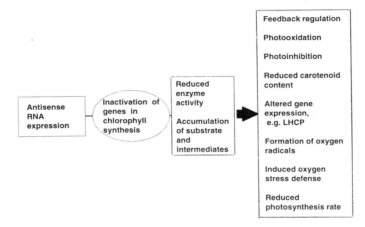

Figure 2. Flow diagram illustrating effects of antisense gene expression in chlorophyll biosynthesis

Transformants with one or more antisense genes for GSA-AT were selected by the phenotypical changes in pigment content [11]. The plants showed different degrees of chlorophyll reduction and variegation pattern. The leaves of some transformants were uniform pale, others patchy with sectors of different pigmentation. The chlorophyll concentration was reduced to less than 10% and correlated with reduced GSA-AT activity. Lower activities were consequences of the inhibited gene expression of GSA-AT indicated by Northern and Western Blot analysis. Since GSA accumulation could not be observed, it is assumed that the activity, stability or synthesis of the initial enzymes in the ALA-pathway were affected. Interestingly, the levels of carotinoids and chlorophyll binding proteins were reduced compared to wild-type levels. These findings indicate that chlorophyll and carotinoids are required to stabilize certain pigment protein complexes and that the deficient amount of one of the components limits the amount of the others which are degraded or hardly synthesized. Furthermore, lack of pigments affects stronger the accumulation of light harvesting components rather than of core proteins. Again, the reduced light harvesting protein and carotinoid levels cause severe impairments in the primary protection against phototoxic reactions and oxygen stress.

The visible phenotypical changes of the transformants with GSA-AT antisense genes mirror inhibition of chlorophyll synthesis and give good evidence for the actual activity of GSA-AT. The inactivation of GSA-AT synthesis elicits a series of dramatic processes in transgenic plants. It influences the regulation of the ALA synthesizing pathway. Chlorophyll deficiency impairs subsequently energy absorption and the photosynthesis rate. These effects become more intense since the transgenic plants are sensitized to light and oxygen radicals (Fig.2)

Acknowledgements
This work was partially supported by a grant from the EC network programme for Human Capital and Mobility "The Design of Vitamin B6-Dependent Enzymes with Catalytic Properties and Altered Susceptibilities to Mechanism-Based Inhibitors"

References
[1]   Kannangara, C.G. and Gough, S.P. (1978) Carlsberg Res. Commun. 43, 185-194
[2]   Beale, S.I. and Weinstein, J.D. (1990) in: *Biosynthesis of Heme and Chlorophyll* (Dailey, H.A., ed.) pp. 287-391, McGraw-Hill Publishing Co., New York
[3]   Smith, A. and Griffith, T.G. (1993) In *Methods in Plant Biochemistry* (Lea, P.J. ed.), Vol.9, pp. 299-343, Academic Press ltd., London
[4]   Grimm, B. (1990) Proc. Natl. Acad. Sci. USA 87, 4169-4173
[5]   Elliott, T., Avissar, Y.J., Rhie, G.E. and Beale, S.I. (1990) J. Bacteriol. 172, 7071-7084
[6]   Grimm, B., Bull, A. and Breu, V. (1991) Mol. Gen. Genet. 225, 1-10
[7]   Hansson, M., Rutberg, L., Schröder, I. and Hederstedt, L. (1991) J. Bacteriol. 173, 2590-2599
[8]   Sangwan, I. and O'Brian, M.R. (1993) Plant Physiol. 102, 829-836
[9]   Ilag, L.L., Kumar, A.M. and Söll, D. (1994) Plant Cell 6, 265-275
[10]   Matters G.L. and Beale, S.I. (1994) Plant Mol.Biol. 24, 617-629
[11]   Höfgen, R., Axelsen, K.B., Kannangara, C.G., Schüttke I., Pohlenz, H.D., Willmitzer L., Grimm, B. and von Wettstein, D. (1994) Proc.Natl.Acad.Sci. 91, 1726-1730
[12]   Grimm, B., Smith, A.J., Kannangara, C.G. and Smith, M.A. (1991) J. Biol. Chem. 12495-12501
[13]   Smith, M.A., Kannangara, C.G., Grimm, B. and von Wettstein, D. (1991) Eur. J. Biochem. 202, 749-757
[14]   Smith, M.A., Grimm, B., Kannangara, C.G. and von Wettstein, D. (1991) Proc. Natl. Acad. Sci. USA 88, 9775-9779
[15]   Pugh, C.E., Harwood, J.L. and John, R.A. (1992) J. Biol. Chem. 267, 1584-1588
[16]   Velick, S.F. and Vavra, J. (1962) J. Biol. Chem. 237, 2109-2122
[17]   Smith, M.A., Kannangara, C.G. and Grimm, B. (1992) Biochemistry, 31 11249-11254
[18]   Grimm, B. Smith, M.A. and von Wettstein, D. (1992) Eur. J. Biochem. 206, 579-585 (1992)
[19]   Bull, A., Breu, V., Kannangara, C.G., Rogers, L.J. and Smith, A.J. (1990) Arch. Mircobiol. 154, 56-59
[20]   Horsch, R.B., Fry, J.E., Hoffmann, N.L., Eichholtz, D., Rogers S.G. and Fraley, R.T. (1985) Science 227, 1229-1231
[21]   Murray, J.A.H. and Crockett, N. (1992) in *Modern Cell Biology: Antisense RNA and DNA*, ed. Murray, J.A.H. (Wiley-Liss, New York), Vol.11, pp 1-49

Biochemistry of Vitamin B$_6$ and PQQ
G. Marino, G. Sannia and F. Bossa (eds.)
© 1994 Birkhäuser Verlag Basel/Switzerland

Mechanism of glutamate semialdehyde aminotransferase probed with substrate analogues

Robin Tyacke, Bernhard Grimm[1], John L. Harwood and Robert A. John

Department of Biochemistry, University of Wales, Cardiff CF1 1ST, Wales, U.K.
[1]*Institut für Pflanzengenetik und Kulturpflanzenforschung, D-06466 Gatersleben, Germany*

Summary

Stopped-flow diode-array spectrophotometry is used to investigate the mechanism of action of glutamate semialdehyde amiunotransferase on close analogues of the intermediate diaminovalerate namely 4-aminohex-5-enoate and 4-aminohex-5-ynoate as well as on diaminovalerate itself.

Introduction

In all forms of life the basic component from which tetrapyrroles are derived appears to be δ-aminolaevulinate. However, whereas in animals this compound is synthesised from succinyl coenzyme A and glycine (Jordan & Shemin, 1972) in plants and bacteria it arises from glutamate 1-semialdehydeyde (GSA, Kannangara *et al.*, 1988). The conversion of GSA to aminolaevulinate, an isomerisation in which the positions of amino and oxo groups on the same molecule are exchanged, is catalysed by glutamate semialdehyde aminotransferase (GSAT). The reaction proceeds by initial combination of the enzyme in its pyridoxamine form (E$_M$) with the aldehyde group of GSA. Diaminovalerate is an intermediate in the reaction and dissociates to an extent determined by the concentration of the enzyme. Because of this dissociation the enzyme is left partially in the free 420nm-absorbing internal pyridoxaldimine form (E$_L$) at the end of an reaction with GSA *in vitro* (Smith *et al.*, 1991, Pugh *et al.*, 1992, Tyacke *et al.*, 1993) and this form of the enzyme forms a significant part of preparations obtained from plants (Pugh *et al.*, 1992). E$_L$ reacts only very slowly with GSA but rapidly with diaminovalerate. Here we report the results of experiments in which we have used structural analogues of the enzyme's substrate to investigate the enzyme's mechanism.

Materials and Methods

R and S enantiomers of 4-aminohex-5-enoate, and racemic 4-aminohex-5-ynoate were generously provided by Marion Merrell-Dow International Research Centre, Strasbourg France. (S)-Glutamate 1- semialdehyde was synthesised from (S)-4-aminohex-5-enoate as described previously (Pugh et al. 1991).

The enzyme was prepared either from pea leaves as described earlier (Pugh et al. 1992) or from *Escherichia coli* overexpressing the gene encoding the enzyme from the photosynthetic bacterium *Synechococcus* and purified as described earlier (Grimm et al.,1991). The enzyme prepared from either source had virtually the same properties. The activity of the enzyme was assayed by the method of Pugh et al., (1991) and its concentration was determined using ε_{280} $=35,000M^{-1}cm^{-1}$ (Smith et al, 1991). At the end of the preparation, the enzyme is obtained as a mixture of E_L and E_M forms with E_M predominating. Conversion to E_L was achieved using succinic semialdehyde. To ensure virtually complete conversion, the equilibrium was displaced by gel filtration using the method of Dixon & Severin (1968).

A stopped-flow diode-array spectrophotometer (Hi-Tech, Salisbury, UK) was used to obtain absorption spectra within 2ms of mixing. Absorption spectra, each consisting of 366 data points collected from 290nm to 580nm were recorded at intervals and the data stored on floppy discs. The observed absorbance changes at individual wavelengths were analysed using the IS-2 kinetics software suite provided with the instrument. Goodness of fit was judged on the basis of an even distribution of residuals between experimental results and theoretically predicted curve. Absorption spectra of intermediates, or more correctly of mixtures of chromophores which behaved as single intermediates in terms of a particular kinetic scheme, were determined using the multivariate data analysis package SPECFIT (Hi-Tech Salisbury, UK).

Results and Discussion

Fig. 1 (a) shows the spectral changes occurring when the enzyme (E_L) was mixed with diaminovalerate. No chromophore having λ_{max} greater than 430nm is discernible indicating that any quinonoid intermediate on the reaction pathway does not accumulate significantly. Most of the reaction is ascribable to conversion of E_L to E_M and follows a single exponential characterised by $k_{app} = 2s^{-1}$. However analysis of the spectra obtained over shorter time intervals revealed a more rapid process Fig 1 (b). The amplitude of this process varied with wavelength and changed direction at 400nm. This behaviour is consistent with the interconversion of two forms of the enzyme having slightly different λ_{max} values but both being close to 420nm.

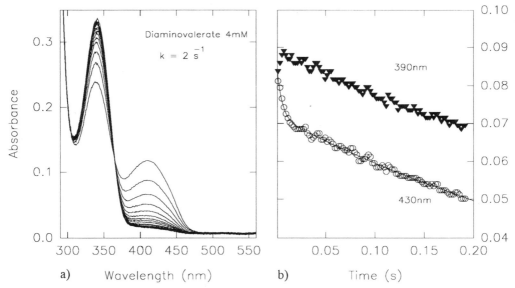

Figure 1. Absorbance changes associated with the reaction of diaminovalerate with E_L. The enzyme 0.2mM was mixed in equal volume with diaminovalerate (4mM) and spectra were recorded at intervals. (a) Spectra taken at 17ms intervals over 4s. (b) Course of absorbance change at single wavelengths indicated.

The most likely interpretation of these results is that one protonated aldimine is being rapidly converted to another. At present it is not clear whether the conversion observed is from the external aldimine to one of the two possible internal aldimines or from one external aldimine to the other.

Fig. 2 shows the reaction occurring with 4-aminohex-5-enoate a close structural analogue of diaminovalerate and of glutamate semialdehyde. In this case a small transient increase in absorbance at about 490nm is observed.

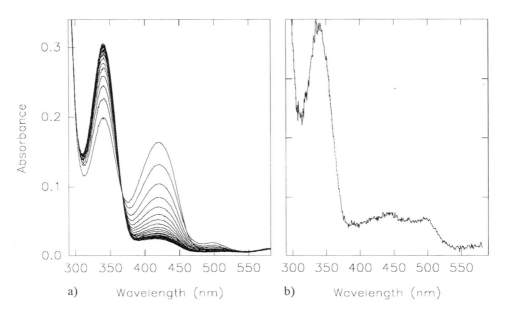

Figure 2. Absorbance changes associated with the reaction of aminohexenoate with E_L. The enzyme (E_L 0.2mM) was mixed with aminohexenoate (4mM). (a) The spectra shown are taken at 40ms intervals over 1s. (b) The spectrum found by SPECFIT for the transient "intermediate".

The data at 490nm (Fig 2c) fit well to a scheme consisting of two steps in which k1 = 7s-1 characterises the first step and k2 = 160s-1 characterises the second. Analysis of the spectra by SPECFIT gave a spectrum (Fig 2b). which indicates the presence of chromophores absorbing maximally at 500nm, 440nm and 330nm. We suggest that these are respectively the quinonoid, a second external aldimine formed by shift of the double bond, and the ketimine formed by completion of the transamination cycle. Aminohexenoate must combine through its single 4-amino group. This is structurally analogous to the 4-amino group of diaminovalerate and to the amino group of glutamate semialdehyde itself. It is therefore curious that the first two compounds undergo rapid transamination with the EL form of the enzyme while glutamate semialdehyde itself which is sterically almost identical with aminohexenoate reacts only very slowly. The explanation must lie in the different chemical reactivities of -CH=CH2 versus CH=O and a possible explanation is that GSA forms a non-productive complex between its aldehyde and the lysine that forms the internal aldimine.

Acknowledgements

We thank the Marion Merrell Dow International Research Institute, Strasbourg, for their generous gifts of aminohexenoate and aminohexynoate. This work was supported by the EC Human Capital and Mobility programme Contract Number CHRX-CT93-0179 (DG DSCS).

References

Dixon, H. B. F. and Severin (1968) Dissociation of the Prosthetic Group of Aspartate Aminotransferase. *Biochem J.* 110, 18P

Grimm, B., Smith, A. J., Kannangara, G. C. & Smith, M. (1991) Gabaculine Resistant Glutamate semialdehyde Aminotransferase of *Synechococcus*. *J. Biol. Chem.* 266, 12495 - 12501

Jordan, P. M. & Shemin, D. (1972) Aminolaevulinate Synthase In: Boyer, G (ed) *The Enzymes*, Third Edition volVII, pp.339-356

Kannangara, G., Gough, S. P., Bryant, P., Hoober, J.K., Kahn, A. and von Wettstein, D. (1988) tRNAglu as a cofactor in aminolaevulinate synthesis. *Trends Biochem. Sci.* 13, 139 - 143.

Pugh, C. E., Nair, S. P., Harwood, J. L. & John, R. A. (1991) Conditions for the Assay of Glutamate Semialdehyde Aminotransferase that overcome the Problem of Substrate Instability. *Anal Biochem.* 198: 43 - 46

Pugh, C. E., Nair, S. P., Harwood, J. L. & John, R. A. (1992) Mechanism of Glutamate Semialdehyde Aminotransferase. *J. Biol. Chem.* 267: 1584 - 1588

Smith, M. A., Kannangara, C. G., Grimm, B. & Von Wettstein, D. (1991) Characterisation of Glutamate Semiialdehyde Aminotransferase of *Synechococcus* . *Eur. J. Biochem.* 202, 749 - 747

TRYPTOPHAN-SYNTHASE AND DECARBOXYLASES

Crystallographic and kinetic studies of the tryptophan synthase $\alpha_2\beta_2$ complex with a mutation in β subunit lysine-87 that binds pyridoxal phosphate

E.W. Miles, U. Banik, Z. Lu, S.A. Ahmed, K.D. Parris, C.C. Hyde and D.R. Davies

National Institutes of Health, Building 8 Room 2A09, Bethesda, MD 20892, U.S.A.

Summary

To probe the mechanism of reactions catalyzed by the tryptophan synthase $\alpha_2\beta_2$ complex, we have substituted threonine for β subunit lysine-87 that forms an internal aldimine with pyridoxal phosphate. Our finding that the mutant $\alpha_2\beta_2$ complex (K87T) is inactive, but forms external aldimine complexes of pyridoxal phosphate with L-serine and L-tryptophan, provides evidence that lysine-87 serves critical roles in transimination, catalysis and product release. Kinetic studies demonstrate that formation of a stable aminoacrylate intermediate at the β site of the K87T $\alpha_2\beta_2$ complex results in activation of the α subunit. Crystallographic analyses at ~2 Å resolution of the L-serine and L-tryptophan intermediates with the K87T $\alpha_2\beta_2$ complex localize the substrate and product binding sites of the β subunit.

Introduction

The bacterial tryptophan synthase $\alpha_2\beta_2$ complex catalyzes the last two reactions in L-tryptophan biosynthesis. The first reaction, cleavage of indole-3-glycerol phosphate to D-glyceraldehyde 3-phosphate and indole, is catalyzed by the α subunit. The second reaction, condensation of indole and L-serine, proceeds through a series of pyridoxal phosphate (PLP) intermediates at the active site of the β subunit (Scheme IA). To probe the functional roles of β subunit lysine-87 that forms an internal aldimine with PLP, we have used site-directed mutagenesis to change lysine-87 to threonine (Lu *et al.*, 1993). The purified K87T $\alpha_2\beta_2$ complex binds pyridoxal phosphate as the free aldehyde (E in Scheme IB). Thus, lysine-87 is not essential for PLP binding.

Scheme I: Reactions of the Wild Type (A) and K87T (B) Tryptophan Synthase $\alpha_2\beta_2$ Complexes

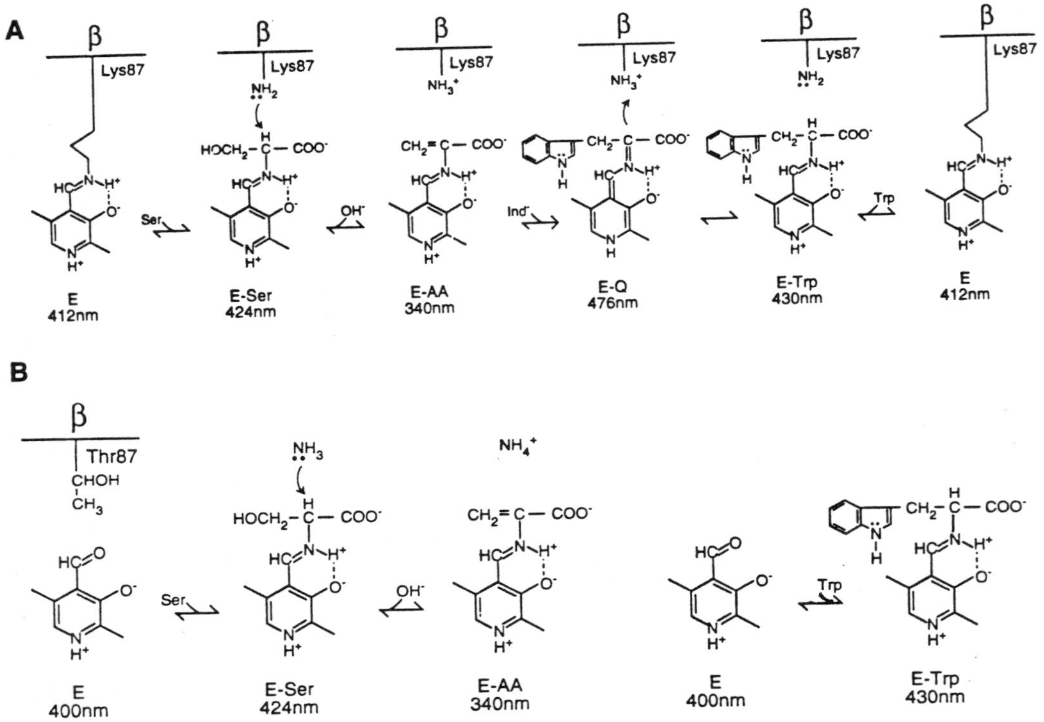
A
β
Lys87
Ser
OH⁻
Ind⁻
Trp
E
412nm
E-Ser
424nm
E-AA
340nm
E-Q
476nm
E-Trp
430nm
E
412nm
B
Thr87
CHOH
CH₃
NH₃
NH₄⁺
E
400nm
E-Ser
424nm
E-AA
340nm
E
400nm
E-Trp
430nm

Results and Discussion

Reactions of the K87T $\alpha_2\beta_2$ Complex

The K87T $\alpha_2\beta_2$ complex forms external aldimines with several amino acids including L-serine (Fig. 1) and L-tryptophan (Lu *et al.*, 1993). The K87T L-serine complex (E-Ser) is not converted enzymatically to the E-AA intermediate or to L-tryptophan in the presence of indole. These results provide evidence that lysine-87 serves a catalytic role as the acceptor of the α-proton of L-serine and as the donor of a proton in the conversion of E-Q to E-Trp in the formation of L-tryptophan (Scheme IB). Lysine-87 is important for substrate and product release since L-serine and L-tryptophan dissociate extremely slowly from the K87T $\alpha_2\beta_2$ complex.

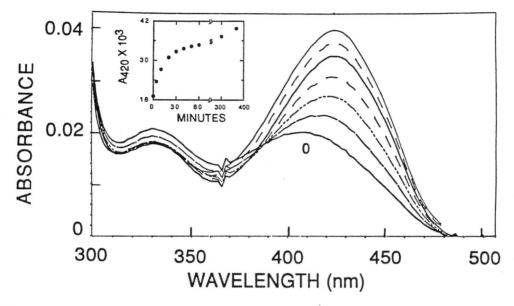

Fig. 1. Reaction of the K87T $\alpha_2\beta_2$ complex with L-serine. Absorption spectra of 10 μM enzyme at times up to 300 min after addition of 1 mM L-serine (Lu *et al.*, 1993).

Addition of 1 M ammonium chloride to the isolated K87T-L-serine complex at pH 7.5, results in a slow decrease in the absorbance at 424 nm (E-Ser) with a concomitant increase in the absorbance at 340 nm, which is assigned to E-AA (Fig. 2A). The pH dependence of the observed pseudo-first order rate constants for this reaction (Fig. 2B) implies that NH₃ serves as the acceptor of the α-proton of L-serine as shown in Scheme IB).

Steady-state Kinetic Studies

The K87T $\alpha_2\beta_2$ complex exhibits normal α site activity but does not convert L-serine and indole to tryptophan at the β site (Lu *et al.*, 1993). Previous kinetic studies suggest that conversion of L-serine to an aminoacrylate intermediate (E-AA) at the β site activates indole-3-glycerol phosphate (IGP) cleavage at the α site (Anderson *et al.*, 1991). We have tested this hypothesis by comparing steady-state kinetic values for the wild type and K87T $\alpha_2\beta_2$ complexes in the cleavage of IGP. The results show that k_{cat}/K_m for IGP cleavage in the absence of L-serine is ~7-fold higher for the K87T-AA derivative than for the wild type enzyme or K87T-

116

Ser derivative. Our results are a direct demonstration of the postulated mechanism of allosteric activation by the aminoacrylate intermediate in the absence of turnover.

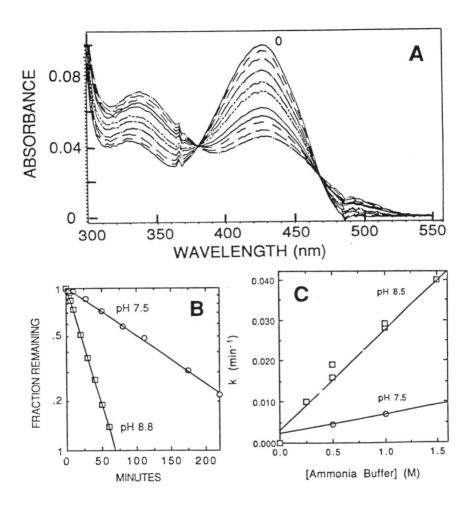

Fig. 2. Reactions of the K87T-L-serine complex that had been isolated by gel filtration. A, absorption spectra of the K87T-L-serine complex (19 μM) at times up to 325 min after addition of 1 M NH4Cl at pH 7.5. B, plot of fraction of unreacted enzyme versus time at pH 7.5 or pH 8.5. C, effect of NH4Cl concentration on the rate of reaction at pH 8.5 (Lu *et al.*, 1993).

X-Ray Crystallography

The three-dimensional structure of the wild type $\alpha_2\beta_2$ complex has been determined at 2.5 Å (Hyde *et al.*, 1988). Crystallographic analyses at ~2 Å resolution of the external aldimine derivatives of the K87T $\alpha_2\beta_2$ complex with L-serine and L-tryptophan (E-Ser and E-Trp in Scheme IB) localize the substrate and product binding sites of the β subunit. A comparison between the structures of the K87T L-tryptophan and L-serine complexes and that of the unliganded wild type $\alpha_2\beta_2$ complex (Hyde *et al.*, 1988) reveals that the β subunit has different conformational states in each of the structures. Examination of the L-tryptophan complex reveals a large movement (~4 Å) of helix 6 and smaller movements of neighboring regions in the N-terminal domain of the β subunit. The conformation of the β subunit in the L-serine complex is intermediate between that in the L-tryptophan complex and in the unliganded wild type $\alpha_2\beta_2$ complex. The conformational changes in the L-tryptophan and L-serine complexes result in the closure of the indole tunnel in the β subunit. Alterations in the tunnel may play roles in intersubunit communication.

Conclusions

The use of a mutant form of the tryptophan synthase $\alpha_2\beta_2$ complex (K87T) has allowed us to obtain stable enzyme-substrate intermediates. These intermediates have provided useful materials for crystallographic studies and for kinetic studies that probe the allosteric mechanism. Future crystallographic studies of the K87T-AA may elucidate the conformational changes responsible for this allosteric activation.

References

Anderson, K. S., Miles, E. W. , and Johnson, K. A. (1991) Serine modulates substrate channeling in tryptophan synthase: a novel intersubunit triggering mechanism. *J. Biol. Chem.* 266: 8020-8033.

Hyde, C. C., Ahmed, S. A., Padlan, E. A., Miles, E. W. , and Davies, D. R. (1988) Three-dimensional structure of the tryptophan synthase $\alpha_2\beta_2$ multienzyme complex from *Salmonella typhimurium. J. Biol. Chem.* 263: 17857-17871.

Lu, Z., Nagata, S., Mc Phie, P. , and Miles, E. W. (1993) Lysine-87 in the β subunit of tryptophan synthase that forms an internal aldimine with pyridoxal phosphate serves critical roles in transimination, catalysis, and product release. *J. Biol. Chem.* 268: 8727-8734.

Biochemistry of Vitamin B_6 and PQQ
G. Marino, G. Sannia and F. Bossa (eds.)
© 1994 Birkhäuser Verlag Basel/Switzerland

The Roles of Chemical Transformation, Loop Closure, Tunnel Function and Metal Ion Activation in the Tryptophan Synthase Mechanism

Michael F. Dunn, Peter S. Brzovic, Catherine A. Leja, Peng Pan and Eilika U. Woehl

Department of Biochemistry, University of California, Riverside, California, 92521, USA

Summary

An overview of the recent results derived from X-ray crystallography, physical biochemical methods, rapid kinetic techniques and site-directed mutagenesis that have shaped current understanding of tryptophan synthase structure-function relationships is presented. An integrated mechanism relating the chemical transformations and metal ion activation to tunnel function and allosteric regulation is proposed.

Introduction

The bacterial tryptophan synthase bienzyme complex is an important example for the study of the subtle interplay between structure and function (Drewe and Dunn, 1985; 1986; Kawasaki et al., 1987; Hyde et al., 1988; Houben and Dunn, 1990; Dunn et al., 1990; Miles, 1991; Lane and Kirschner, 1991; Kirschner et al., 1991; Anderson et al., 1991; Brzovic et al., 1992a, b; 1993; Yang et al., 1993). The catalytic transformations at the α- and β-sites are rich in chemical variety, involving C-C, C-H, C-N, C-O, N-H and O-H scission/synthesis. The 2.5 Å resolution X-ray structures of the *S. typhimurium* enzyme (Hyde et al., 1988) revealed a 25 Å-long tunnel connecting the α- and β-subunit sites. Kinetic studies have demonstrated that the transfer of indole between the two active sites occurs via this tunnel (Dunn et al., 1990; Lane and Kirschner, 1991; Anderson et al., 1991). Ligand-mediated heterotropic allosteric interactions between the α- and β-sites that involve both physical binding and covalent transformations regulate transitions between conformationally "open" and "closed" states of the protein (Houben and Dunn, 1990; Kirschner et al., 1991; Brzovic et al., 1992a,b; 1993). In the α-subunit, this transition involves loop structures that close down over the catalytic site, both preventing the escape of indole and activating α-catalysis by > 26-fold (Kirschner et al., 1991; Brzovic et al., 1992a,b; 1993). Catalysis at the β-site is strongly stimulated by the binding of Na^+ or K^+.

Materials and Methods

S. typhimurium tryptophan synthase (wildtype) was prepared as previously described (Nagata et al., 1989). Mutant enzyme species were kindly provided by Edith W. Miles. Studies of metal ion effects were carried out in buffers containing no monovalent metal ions. α-Glycerolphosphate (GP) and indole glycerolphosphate (IGP) were prepared as the triethanol ammonium salts free of all monovalent cations and ammonium ion. Single-wavelength and rapid-scanning stopped-flow (SWSF and RSSF) kinetic studies, steady-state kinetic studies and equilibrium binding measurements were performed as previously described (Drewe and Dunn, 1985; 1986; Dunn et al., 1990; Brzovic et al., 1992a.b; 1993).

Results and Conclusions

The Mechanism of Indole Reaction with the α- Aminoacrylate, E(A-A). The nucleophilic attack of indole on the E(A-A) to give E(Q) is the key chemical transformation that provides the allosteric signal to deactivate catalysis at the α-site. Even though indole is an extremely weak nucleophile (pKa = - 3.5), this Michael addition occurs very fast. We have used transient kinetic studies to investigate α-secondary deuterium kinetic isotope effects to further characterize this process. Comparison of the effects of ^2H substitution for ^1H at the β-C of E(A-A) on the rate of E(Q) formation via SWSF, show that the saturated value of $1/\tau_1$ increased from 390 ± 15 s^{-1} (^1H) to 500 ± 15 s^{-1}(^2H). This α-secondary kinetic isotope effect (apparent $k_H/k_D = 0.78$) is consistent with the formation of an sp^3-like transition state from the E(A-A) ground state. The concentration dependence of $1/\tau_1$ implies a two step process (Bernasconi, 1976):

$$E \text{ (A-A)} + Nu \underset{}{\overset{K_1}{\rightleftharpoons}} E \text{ (A-A)(Nu)} \underset{k_{-2}}{\overset{k_2}{\rightleftharpoons}} E \text{ (Q), with } 1/\tau_1 = \{(k_2 K_1[Nu])/(1 + K_1[Nu]_0)\} + k_{-2}$$

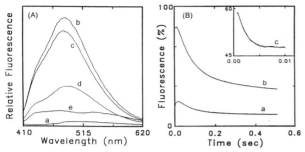

Figure 1: (A) Fluorescence spectra of (a) ANS; (b) $\alpha_2\beta_2$ + ANS; (c) $\alpha_2\beta_2$ +ANS + L-Trp; (d) $\alpha_2\beta_2$ + ANS + GP; (e) $\alpha_2\beta_2$ + ANS + L-Ser. (B) Time courses for the reactions of the $\alpha_2\beta_2$-ANS complex with (b) L-Ser; (c) GP. Trace (a), $\alpha_2\beta_2$ + L-Ser in the absence of ANS measured as in trace (b). Concentrations: [$\alpha_2\beta_2$] = 10 µM; [ANS] = 12 µM; [GP] = 20 mM; [L-Trp] 12.5 mM; [L-Ser] = 20 mM; 50 mM triethanolamine buffer, pH = 7.8 at 25 ° C.

The concentration dependence of k_H/k_D indicates that the major effect is on k_2 (not k_{-2}), suggesting the transition state is well along toward C-C bond formation. Since the attack of indole on E(A-A) provides the allosteric trigger that deactivates the α-site and shifts equilibrium in favor of an open conformation (Brzovic et al., 1992a,b; 1993), the change from sp^2 to sp^3 hybridization must provide the weak bonding interactions that switch the enzyme between active (closed) and inactive (open) conformations.

Activation of Indole Likely Involves the Carboxylate of βE109. The mutant βE109D exhibits altered kinetics in the reaction of indole with E(A-A) (Brzovic et al., 1992c). Compared to wildtype enzyme, the affinity for indole is decreased, the steady-state rate of the β-reaction is decreased 27-fold, and the transient formation of E(Q) can no longer be detected, findings consistent with a charge stabilization/acid-base catalytic role for βE109 in the activation of indole (Phillips et al., 1984).

Dynamics of the Interconversion of "Open" and "Closed" Conformations. We have used fluorogenic dyes to examine ligand-mediated changes between open and closed conformations of the enzyme. Our studies show that 8-anilino-1-naphthalenesulfonate (ANS) binds selectively to the open conformation, and exhibits enhanced fluorescence. ANS is displaced both by the reaction of L-Ser with the β-site to form E(A-A), and by the binding of GP to the α-site (Fig.1).

However, ANS is not displaced by the reactions of L-Trp, L-His or Gly. Hence, ANS displacement by L-Ser likely is due to a conformational transition. We propose that the binding of GP to the α-site and the formation of E(A-A) at the β-site trigger the change in conformation to a closed structure, while amino acids that are incapable of forming E(A-A) do not trigger the conformational transition (Brzovic et al., 1992a). Since L-Trp does not displace ANS, conversion of E(A-A) to E(Q) must convert the protein back to the open conformation.

Effects of Monovalent Metal Ions on Catalytic and Regulatory Functions. Monovalent metal ions such as Na^+, K^+ or Li^+ bind to the tryptophan synthase bienzyme complex with apparent dissociation constants in the mM range. The physiological $\alpha\beta$-reaction therefore occurs under saturating amounts of monovalent metal ions. Monovalent metal ion binding effects turnover rates, distribution of intermediates at the β-active site and the individual rates of steps in the α- and β-reaction. In the absence of metal ions, the turnover rates (k_{cat}) for the α-reaction alone and the $\alpha\beta$-reaction are the same (0.3 s^{-1}). In the presence of metal ions, k_{cat} of the α-reaction (absence of L-Ser) is decreased to 30% of its value in absence of metal ions (0.09 s^{-1}). However, the $\alpha\beta$-reaction k_{cat}, is stimulated 10-fold (3 s^{-1}). The 30-fold stimulation of the α-reaction upon formation of E(A-A) requires the presence of monovalent metal ions. Therefore, monovalent metal ions are essential for intersubunit communication. Monovalent metal ions severely alter the distribution of intermediates at the β-active site both in the transient- and the steady-state. In the reaction of E(A-A) with indole or IGP, E(Q) does not accumulate to significant amounts in the absence of monovalent metal ions, but forms a strong transient peak in their presence. The transient formation of E(Q) is thought to be the signal for the release of G3P at the α-site. Accumulation of E(Q) could therefore be an essential role for metal ions in the intersubunit signaling. In the reaction of $\alpha_2\beta_2$ with L-Ser ($\pm$IGP or $\pm$ indole) (Fig.2), E(Aex) accumulates to a much higher degree in the presence of metal ions, while decay rates are not significantly changed in presence of IGP or indole. Consequently, the metal ion induced accumulation of E(Aex) appears to result from lowering of the ground-state energy of that species. In absence of IGP or indole, the rate of formation of E(A-A) is reduced in the presence of monovalent metal ions. Metal ions could therefore also play a role in transmitting the allosteric signals between the α- and β-sites such that increased formation of E(A-A) occurs only in the presence of indole.

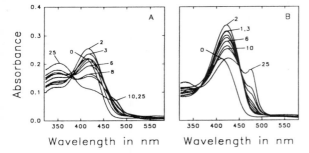

Figure 2: RSSF spectra for the reaction of $\alpha_2\beta_2$ with L-Ser and IGP in absence (A) and presence (B) of 100 mM NaCl. Final concentrations: $[\alpha_2\beta_2]$ = 17.5 μM; [L-Ser] = 40 mM and [IGP] = 0.5 mM. The total acquisition time is 0.34 seconds (spectrum 25) and the spectrum of $\alpha_2\beta_2$ alone is spectrum 0. Only a subset of the 25 collected scans is shown. The time between the first 5 scans is the same and continuously increases after that.

These studies establish the following: (a) The reaction of indole with E(A-A) is a chemically limited Michael addition. α-Secondary kinetic isotope effects indicate the transition state lies well along the reaction coordinate toward C-C bond formation with sp³ hybridization at C-β. (b) Studies with the dye ANS lend new support to the hypothesis that reaction to form E(A-A) at the β-site triggers a change in the conformation of $\alpha_2\beta_2$ to a closed conformation. This change is reversed by conversion of E(A-A) to E(Q). (c) Na^+ or K^+ binding is essential for activation of the bienzyme complex. This activation is accompanied by activation of the α-site in the physiological reaction, a redistribution of the covalent intermediates at the β-site and stimulation of the β-reaction alone. The redistribution of β-site intermediates strongly favors accumulation of E(Q), possibly providing the allosteric trigger for G3P release.

Acknowledgements

Supported by NSF grant DMB 9107808.

124

References

Anderson, K. S., Miles, E. W. and Johnson, K A. (1991) Serine modulates substrate channeling in tryptophan synthase. A novel intersubunit triggering mechanism. *J. Biol. Chem. 266*: 8020-8033.

Bernasconi, C. (1976) *Relaxation Kinetics,* Academic Press, New York, Chapter 3.

Brzovic, P. S., Ngo, K., and Dunn, M. F. (1992a) Allosteric interactions coordinate catalytic activity between successive metabolic enzymes in the tryptophan synthase bienzyme complex. *Biochemistry 31*: 3831-3839.

Brzovic, P. S., Sawa, Y., Miles, E. W. and Dunn, M. F. (1992b) Evidence that mutations in a loop region of the α–subunit inhibit the transition from an open to a closed conformation in the tryptophan synthase bienzyme complex. *J. Biol. Chem. 267*: 13028-13038.

Brzovic, P. S., Kayastha, A. M., Miles, E. W. and Dunn, M. F. (1922c) Substitution of glutamic acid 109 by aspartic acid alters the substrate specificity and catalytic activity of the β–subunit in the tryptophan synthase bienzyme complex from *Salmonella typhimurium. Biochemistry 31*: 1180-1190.

Brzovic, P. S., Hyde, C. C., Miles, E. W. and Dunn, M. F. (1993) Characterization of the functional role of a flexible loop in the the α–subunit of tryptophan synthase by rapid-scanning stopped-flow spectroscopy and site-directed mutagenesis. *Biochemistry 32*: 10404-10413.

Drewe, Jr., W. F. and Dunn, M. F. (1985) Detection and identification of intermediates in the reaction of L-serine with *E. coli* tryptophan synthase via rapid-scanning UV-visible spectroscopy. *Biochemistry 24*: 3977-3987.

Drewe, Jr., W. F. and Dunn, M. F. (1986) Characterization of the reaction of L-serine and indole with tryptophan synthase via rapid-scanning UV-visible spectroscopy. *Biochemistry 25*: 2494-2501.

Dunn, M. F., Aguilar, V., Brzovic, P. S., Drewe, W. F., Houben, K. F., Leja, C. A. and Roy, M. (1990) The tryptophan synthase bienzyme complex transfers indole between the α– and β–sites via a 25-30 A-long tunnel. *Biochemistry 29*: 8598-8607.

Houben, K. F. and Dunn, M. F. (1990) Allosteric effects acting over a distance of 20-25 A in the *E. coli* tryptophan synthase bienzyme complex increase ligand affinity and cause redistribution of covalent intermediates. *Biochemistry 29*: 2421-2429. βE109

Hyde, C. C., Ahmed, S. A., Padlan, E. A., Miles, E. W., and Davies, D. R. (1988) Three-dimensional structure of the tryptophan synthase $\alpha_2\beta_2$ multienzyme complex from *Salmonella typhimurium. J. Biol. Chem. 263*: 17857-17871.

Kawasaki, H., Baurle, R., Zon, G. , Ahmed, S., and Miles, E. W. (1987) Site-specific mutagenesis of the α–subunit of tryptophan synthase from *Salmonella typhimurium.* Changing arginine 179 to leucine alters the reciprocal transmission of substrate-induced conformational changes between the α and β_2 subunits. *J. Biol. Chem. 262*: 10678-10683.

Kirschner, K., Lane, A. N. and Strasser, A. W. N. (1991) Reciprocal communication between the lyase and synthase active sites of the tryptophan synthase bienzyme complex. *Biochemistry 30*: 472-478.

Lane, A. N. and Kirschner, K. (1991) Mechanism of the physiological reaction catalyzed by tryptophan synthase from *E. coli. Biochemistry 30*: 479-484.

Miles, E. W. (1991) Structural basis for catalysis by tryptophan synthase. *Adv. Enzymol. Relat. Areas Mol. Biol. 64*: 93-172.

Nagata, S., Hyde, C. C. and Miles, E. W. (1989) The α–subunit of tryptophan synthase. Evidence that aspartic acid 60 is a catalytic residue and that the double alteration of residues 175 and 211 in a second-site revertant restores the proper geometry of the substrate binding site. *J. Biol. Chem. 264*: 6288-6296.

Yang, X-J. and Miles, E. W. (1993) A novel intersubunit repair mechanism in the tryptophan synthase $\alpha_2\beta_2$ complex, -critical role of the β–subunit lysine-167 in intersubunit communication. *J. Biol. Chem. 286*: 22269-22272.

Effects of Monovalent Cations on Functional Properties of the Tryptophan Synthase $\alpha_2\beta_2$ Complex in Solution and in the Crystal

A. Peracchi, A. Mozzarelli and G. L. Rossi

Istituto di Scienze Biochimiche, Università di Parma, 43100 Parma, Italy

Summary

Synthesis of L-tryptophan, catalyzed by tryptophan synthase from *Salmonella typhimurium*, at 10°C is activated by monovalent cations in the order Cs$^+$ > Rb$^+$ > Li$^+$ > K$^+$ > Na$^+$. The most efficient cations increase V$_{max}$ and decrease K$_M$ for indole. Na$^+$ only affects K$_M$. In the absence of indole, the equilibrium distribution of the external aldimine and the α-aminoacrylate Schiff base depends on monovalent cations both in solution and in the crystalline state. The least activating ions, Na$^+$ and K$^+$, stabilize the external aldimine, whereas Cs$^+$, Rb$^+$ and Li$^+$ favor the accumulation of a species absorbing at 470 nm, tentatively identified as a tautomer of α-aminoacrylate. Activation of the enzyme might be associated with the stabilization of this more reactive intermediate.

Introduction

Several pyridoxal 5'-phosphate (PLP)-dependent enzymes, catalyzing β-elimination or β-replacement reactions, are known to be regulated by monovalent cations. Tryptophan synthase from enterobacteria is an $\alpha_2\beta_2$ complex that catalyzes the final two steps in the biosynthesis of L-tryptophan. First, α-subunits cleave indole-3-glycerol phosphate to form indole and glyceraldehyde-3-phosphate. Then, indole, channeled to the ß-active site, is condensed with the α-aminoacrylate resulting from the elimination of the β-hydroxyl group of L-serine (Yanofsky and Crawford, 1972; Miles, 1979; 1991). The effects of monovalent cations on the catalytic properties of isolated ß$_2$ dimers have been extensively investigated (Hatanaka et al., 1962; Crawford and Ito, 1964; Goldberg et al., 1968; York, 1972; Miles and Kumagai, 1974; Yang and Miles, 1992), while the effects on the catalytic properties of the $\alpha_2\beta_2$ complex have not been thoroughly explored. It was reported that, at 37°C, K$^+$ increases the catalytic activity, Na$^+$ has almost no effect and NH$_4^+$ inhibits it (Hatanaka et al., 1962; Schwartz and Bonner, 1964).

Suelter (1970) pointed out that β-replacement and β-elimination reactions involving different PLP-enzymes proceed via a structurally similar key intermediate, the α-aminoacrylate, and suggested that monovalent cations specifically interact with this intermediate. In the present work we report the effects of cations on the catalytic properties of the $\alpha_2\beta_2$ complex from *Salmonella typhimurium* in solution, as well as the effects on the equilibrium distribution between the external aldimine and the α-aminoacrylate Schiff base both in solution and in the crystalline state.

Materials and Methods

The tryptophan synthase $\alpha_2\beta_2$ complex from *Salmonella typhimurium* was obtained according to Kawasaki et al. (1987). Crystals of the enzyme were grown from polyethylene glycol solutions as previously described (Ahmed et al., 1985; Mozzarelli et al., 1989). All reagents were of the best commercially available quality and were used without further purification. Experiments were carried out using 25 mM Bis-Tris propane buffer. This buffer is particularly useful for studying cations effects since pH adjustement does not require the addition of external bases. pH measurements were performed using a pHM 83 Radiometer equipped with a U402-M3 Ingold microelectrode.

Activity of the $\alpha_2\beta_2$ complex was assayed spectrophotometrically by incubating the enzyme in a solution containing 50 mM L-serine, 10 µM PLP, 25 mM Bis-Tris propane pH 7.9, at 10° C, in the presence of different concentrations of cations and indole.

Absorption spectra of a solution containing the $\alpha_2\beta_2$ complex, and 50 mM L-serine in 25 mM Bis-Tris propane buffer were recorded in the presence of different cations, at pH 7.9 and 10 °C.

Enzyme crystals were suspended in a medium containing 20% (w/v) PEG M_r 8000, 25 mM Bis-Tris propane, at a defined cation concentration, pH 7.6, 20°C. Single crystal polarized absorption spectra were recorded by a Zeiss u.v. MPM03 microspectrophotometer. Handling of tryptophan synthase crystals and microspectrophotometric measurements have been previously described (Mozzarelli et al., 1989; Rossi et al., 1992).

Results and Discussion

The activities of tryptophan synthase in the absence and in the presence of increasing concentrations of different cations at pH 7.9 and 10°C are reported in Figure 1. Monovalent cations activate the reaction to a different extent, Cs^+ being the most efficient and Na^+ the least efficient effector. The bulky tetramethylammonium cation (TMA) as well as Ca^{2+} and Mg^{2+} do not significantly stimulate the reaction, indicating that the effect of monovalent cations is specific and not due to an ionic strength increase. The activation constant for each monovalent cation (i.e. the cation concentration that leads to half of the maximal activity) is in the millimolar range and increases with the ionic radius (Table I). Note that the metal ion effects are temperature-dependent. At 25° also Na^+ and K^+ become activating (data not shown).The affinity of L-serine for the $\alpha_2\beta_2$ complex is increased by cations. The calculated dissociation constant is 91 µM in the absence of monovalent cations, and 61 µM and 22 µM, respectively, in the presence of 20 mM NaCl and 20 mM CsCl. Experiments carried out at saturating concentrations of L-serine and cations and at different sub-saturating concentrations of indole allow to determine the kinetic parameters of the catalytic reaction. All monovalent cations decrease the apparent K_M of indole. Li^+, K^+, Rb^+ and Cs^+ also increase V_{max} (Table I).

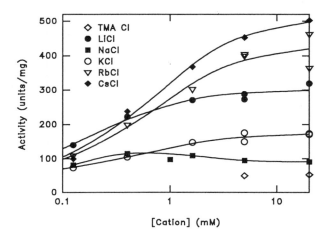

Figure 1: Effect of cations on the rate of L-tryptophan synthesis. Enzyme activity was assayed in a solution containing 50 mM L-serine, 0.2 mM indole, 10 μM PLP, 25 mM Bis-Tris propane pH 7.9, in the presence of increasing concentrations of various cations, at 10°C. Tryptophan was monitored at 290 nm.

Table I. The activation constants and catalytic parameters for L-tryptophan synthesis in the presence of monovalent cations. The rate of reaction was determined in an assay solution that contains 20 mM of a defined cation and indole concentrations varying between 0.01 and 1 mM, at 10°C. The catalytic parameters were obtained by fitting the data to the Michaelis-Menten equation

Cation	Ionic radius (Å)	$E_{Hydration}$ (Kcal/mol)	$K_{activation}$ (mM)	K_{M} indole (mM)	V_{max} (U/mg)
---	---	---	---	0.145	114
TMA	---	---	---	0.054	112
Li+	0.60	-98	0.22	0.024	455
Na+	0.95	-72	---	0.007	122
K+	1.33	-55	0.53	0.015	237
Rb+	1.48	-51	0.69	0.014	410
Cs+	1.69	-47	0.70	0.023	603

According to Suelter's hypothesis the activation effect should be paralleled by an increase in the concentration or in the reactivity of the key intermediate α-aminoacrylate. We have therefore investigated the effect of cations on the first part of the catalytic reaction, i.e. the formation of α-aminoacrylate in the reaction of L-serine with the $\alpha_2\beta_2$ complex, in the absence of indole.

The predominant PLP-derivatives in the presence of L-serine are the external aldimine (λ_{max}= 422 nm) and the α-aminoacrylate Schiff base (λ_{max}= 350 nm) (Miles, 1979; Drewe and Dunn, 1985). This distribution is affected by pH, temperature and allosteric effectors (Mozzarelli et al., 1991). We have now found that it is also dependent on monovalent cations (figure 2a). Binding of Na$^+$ or K$^+$ favors the accumulation of the external aldimine, whereas binding of Li$^+$, Rb$^+$, or Cs$^+$ leads to the formation of a new band absorbing at about 470 nm. This species is tentatively identified as a more reactive tautomer of the α-aminoacrylate, as observed in θ-acetylserine sulfhydrylase (Cook et al., 1992). If this is true, our findings are in agreement with Suelter's hypothesis.

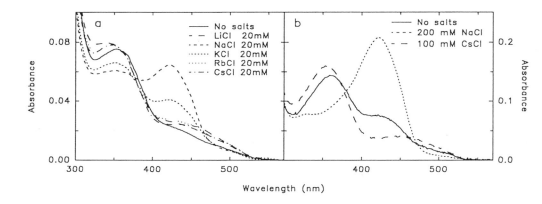

Figure 2. Absorption spectra of L-serine-$\alpha_2\beta_2$-complexes in the presence and in the absence of monovalent cations in solution and in the crystalline state.
a) Absorption spectra were recorded for a solution containing the $\alpha_2\beta_2$ complex (0.5 mg/ml), 50 mM L-serine, 25 mM Bis-Tris propane, 1 mM EDTA, pH 8, at 10 °C, in the absence and in the presence of Li$^+$, Na$^+$, K$^+$, Rb$^+$ or Cs$^+$.
b) Single crystal polarized absorption spectra were recorded with the electric vector of the linearly polarized light parallel to the x optical axis (Mozzarelli et al., 1989). The crystal was suspended in a solution containing 25 mM Bis-Tris propane, 20% PEG 8000 M$_r$, 1 mM EDTA, 50 mM L-serine, pH 7.6, at 20 °C, both in the absence and in the presence of Na$^+$ and Cs$^+$.

In order to verify whether the cation binding site(s) are maintained in the crystalline state of the enzyme, we carried out single crystal polarized absorption measurements (Mozzarelli et al., 1989; Rossi et al., 1992). The three dimensional structure of the enzyme has been determined (Hyde et al., 1988) and the catalytic competence of the enzyme in the crystalline state has been demonstrated (Ahmed et al., 1987; Mozzarelli et al., 1989). Single crystal polarized absorption spectra of the L-serine-enzyme complexes, both in the presence and in the absence of saturating concentrations of sodium and cesium ions (figure 2b), indicate that the effect of cations on the equilibrium distribution of intermediates in the crystal is similar to that observed for the soluble state of the enzyme. These findings indicate that it will eventually be possible to localize the cation binding sites by x-ray crystallography and to identify the structural changes associated with monovalent cation binding that are responsible for catalytic regulation.

Acknowledgements
This work was supported by funds from M.U.R.S.T. and from C.N.R. Target Project on Biotechnology and Bioinstrumentation.

References
Ahmed, S. A., Miles, E. W. and Davies, D. R. (1985) Crystallization and Preliminary X-ray Crystallographic Data of the Tryptophan Synthase $\alpha_2\beta_2$ Complex from *Salmonella typhimurium*. J. Biol. Chem. 260, 3716-3718

Ahmed, S. A., Hyde, C. C., Thomas, G., and Miles, E. W. (1987) Microcrystals of Tryptophan Synthase $\alpha_2\beta_2$ Complex from *Salmonella typhimurium* are Catalytically Active. Biochemistry 26, 5492-5498

Cook, P. F., Hara, S., Nalabolu, S. and Schnackerz, K. D. (1992) pH Dependence of the Absorbance and ^{31}P NMR Spectra of *O*-Acetylserine Sulfhydrylase in the Absence and in the Presence of *O*-Acetyl-L-serine. Biochemistry 31, 2298-2303

Crawford, I. P. and Ito, J (1964) Serine Deamination by the B Protein of *Escherichia coli* Tryptophan Synthetase. Proc. Natl. Acad. Sci. USA 51, 390-397

Drewe, W. F., and Dunn, M. F. (1985) Detection and Identification of Intermediates in the Reaction of L-serine with *Escherichia coli* Tryptophan Synthase via Rapid-Scanning Ultraviolet-Visible Spectroscopy. Biochemistry 24, 3977-3987

Goldberg, M. E., York, S. S. and Stryer, L. (1968) Fluorescent Studies of Substrate and Subunit Interactions of the β_2 Protein of *Escherichia coli* Tryptophan Synthase. Biochemistry 7, 3662-3667

Hatanaka, M., White, E. A., Horibata, K and Crawford, I. P. (1962) A Study of the Catalytic Properties of *Escherichia coli* Tryptophan Synthase, a Two-Component Enzyme. Arch. Biochem. Biophys. 97, 596-606

Hyde, C. C., Ahmed, S. A., Padlan, E. A., Miles, E. W. and Davies, D. R. (1988) Three-dimensional Structure of the Tryptophan Synthase $\alpha_2\beta_2$ Complex from *Salmonella typhimurium*. J. Biol. Chem. 263, 17857-17871

Kawasaki, H., Bauerle, R., Zon, G., Ahmed, S. A., and Miles E. W. (1987) Site-specific Mutagenesis of the α subunit of Tryptophan Synthase from *Salmonella typhimurium*. J. Biol. Chem. 262, 10678-10683

Miles, E. W. (1979) Tryptophan Synthase: Structure, Function, and Subunit Interaction. Adv. Enzymology 49, 127-186

Miles, E. W. (1991) Structural Basis for Catalysis by Tryptophan Synthase. Adv. Enzymology, 64, 83-172

Miles, E. W. and Kumagai, H. (1974) Modification of Essential Histidyl Residues of the β_2 Subunit of Tryptophan Synthetase by Photo-oxidation in the Presence of Pyridoxal 5'-Phosphate and L-serine and Diethylpyrocarbonate. J. Biol. Chem. 249, 2843-2851

Mozzarelli, A., Peracchi, A., Rossi, G. L., Ahmed, S. A., and Miles, E. W. (1989) Microspectrophotometric Studies on Single Crystals of the Tryptophan Synthase $\alpha_2\beta_2$ Complex Demonstrate Formation of Enzyme-Substrate Intermediates. J. Biol. Chem. 264, 15774-15780

Mozzarelli, A., Peracchi, A., Bettati, S. and Rossi, G.L. (1991) Allosteric Regulation of Tryptophan Synthase: A pKa Change at β-active site Induced by α-Subunit Ligands. In "Enzyme Dependent on Pyridoxal Phosphate and Other Carbonyl Compounds as Cofactors" (eds. Fukui, T., Kagamiyama, H., Soda, K. and Wada, H.) 273-275

Rossi, G. L., Mozzarelli, A., Peracchi, A. and Rivetti, C. (1992) Time Course of Chemical and Structural Events in Protein Crystals Measured by Microspectrophotometry. Phyl. Trans. Royal. Soc. Lond. 340, 191-207

Schwartz, A. K. and Bonner, D. M. (1964) Tryptophan Synthetase in *Bacillus subtilis*: Effects of High Potassium Ion Concentration on a Two Component Enzyme. Biochim. Biophys. Acta 89, 337-347

Suelter, C. H. (1970) Enzyme Activated by Monovalent Cations. Science 168, 789-795

Yanofsky, C. and Crawford I. P. (1972) Tryptophan Synthetase. In The Enzymes, 3rd Ed. (Boyer, P. D. ed.) vol VII, pp.1-31, Academic Press, New York

Yang, X-J. and Miles, E. W. (1992) Threonine 183 and Adjacent Flexible Loop Residues in the Tryptophan Synthase α Subunit Have Critical Roles in Modulating the Enzymatic Activities of the β subunit in the $\alpha_2\beta_2$ complex. J. Biol. Chem. 267, 7520-7528

York, S. S. (1972) Kinetic Spectroscopic Studies of Substrate and Subunit Interactions of Tryptophan Synthase. Biochemistry 11, 2733-2740

Biochemistry of Vitamin B$_6$ and PQQ
G. Marino, G. Sannia and F. Bossa (eds.)
© 1994 Birkhäuser Verlag Basel/Switzerland

The long-range effect on the mutual activation of the α and β subunits in the α₂β₂ complex of tryptophan synthase

Kaori Hiraga and Katsuhide Yutani

Institute for Protein Research, Osaka University, Yamadaoka 3-2, Suita City, Osaka 565, Japan

Summary

In this paper, we discuss the mutual activation mechanism of the tryptophan synthase α₂β₂ complex, especially focusing on the long-range effect of the interaction between the α and β₂ subunits, due to the residue which is situated far from the α/β subunit interface. We found that mutant α subunit from *E. coli* substituted at the residue (Pro261), located far from the subunit interface, strongly affected the mutual activation. Additionally, the disadvantages of Pro261 mutant are compensated by double mutations at the residue (Lys109), located at the α/β interface. To elucidate the mechanism of the long-range effect from position-261 and compensation by position-109, the heterologous interactions of five α subunits (from *S. typhimurium*, *E. coli* and the three mutants of *E. coli*; P261A, K109N and K109N/P261A), with β₂ subunit (from *E. coli*), were investigated using a titration calorimeter (OMEGA).

Introduction

Bacterial tryptophan synthase is a multi-enzyme, α₂β₂ complex composed of non-identical and dissociable α and β₂ subunits. The isolated α and β₂ subunits catalyze the final two reactions in the biosynthesis of L-tryptophan, termed α and β reaction, respectively. When α and β₂ subunits associate to form α₂β₂ complex, the rates of α and β reactions are stimulated by 1-2 orders of magnitude (Miles, 1991). In order to analyze the mutual activation mechanism of the tryptophan synthase complex, we studied the interaction between α and β₂ subunits by a titration calorimetry (Ogasahara et al., 1992).

In this study, we investigated the mutants of α subunit from *E. coli* at two positions. The position-261 is far from subunit interface, whereas the position-109 is located at the interface. These positions are Lys109 and Pro261 in the α subunit from *E. coli*, and Asn109 and Ala261 in the α subunit from *S. typhimurium*. For the α subunit from *E. coli*, we made the Salmonella type mutations at these positions and measured the effect on the mutual activation and subunit interaction by measurement of activities and by titration calorimetry.

Materials and Methods

Materials---Two single mutant α subunits (P261A and K109N) and one double mutant (K109N/P261A) from *E. coli* were constructed by site-directed mutagenesis, and purified.

Measurement of activities---The activities of the forward α and β reactions for five α subunits were measured spectrophotometrically at pH8.0, 37℃.

Measurement of binding constants by isothermal titration calorimetry---The binding constants and enthalpies of five α subunits with two β_2 subunits were determined at 40℃ using the OMEGA titration calorimeter (Ogasahara et al., 1992; Wiseman et al., 1989).

Results and Discussion

Catalytic activities of five α subunits in the α and β reactions---In the presence of excess β_2 subunit, the values in the both reactions of P261A were much lower than those of the other proteins (62-67%; Table I). However, the inherent activity of P261A was comparable (95%), to that of the wild type measured in the absence of β_2 subunit. This result indicates that the substitution at position-261 interrupts stimulation of the activities, but does not affect the inherent activity. On the other hand, the activities of K109N/P261A were similar to those of the wild type. Since K109N has little effect on these activities, this result means that the additional substitution of Lys-109 by Asn can compensate for the disadvantages of P261A on the stimulation effects.

Binding constant measurements by titration calorimetry---The results obtained by calorimetric measurements(Figure 1) showed that the binding constant of the P261A with β_2 subunit was 1-order lower than that of the other α subunits(Table I). This suggests that the position 261 of α subunit plays an important role in the formation of the complex with β_2 subunit, although the position is far from the binding interface. The Ala replacement for Pro at position 261, has a long-range effect on the structure of interface and decreases the interaction between α and β_2 subunits. The binding constant of the double mutant, K109N/P261A was restored, to approximately that of the wild type. These results agreed with those obtained from activity measurements.

Conclusion

We conclude that the position-261 of the α subunit which is far from subunit interface, plays an important role in the interaction with β_2 subunit. The substitution at position-109, located on interface, can recover the disadvantage resulting from the substitution of position-261.

References

Miles, E.W. (1991) Structural basis for catalysis by tryptophan synthase. Adv. Emzymol. Relat. Areas Mol. Biol. 64: 93-172

Ogasahara, K., Hiraga, K., Ito, W., Miles, E. W. and Yutani, K. (1992) Origin of the mutual activation of the α and β$_2$ subunits in the α$_2$β$_2$ complex of tryptophan synthase. J. Biol. Chem. 267: 5222-5228

Wiseman, T., Williston, S., Brandts, J. F. and Lin, L.-N. (1989) Rapid measurement of binding constants and heats of binding using a new titration calorimeter. Anal. Biochem. 179: 131-137

Table I. Stimulation effects on the activities and binding constants with β$_2$ subunit for the various α subunits. The values for the stimulation activities are represented as a percentage of activities of the wild type α subunit from E. coli. The activities were measured in the presence of 3-fold molar excess of β chain from E. coli, except for the value in the parenthesis. The value in the parenthesis for P261A represents the inherent activity in α reaction measured in the absence of the β$_2$ subunit.

The values for the binding constants represent the molar concentration of β chain at 40 ℃, obtained from titration calorimetry.

α subunits	Stimulation activity		Binding constant (10^6/M)
	forward α reaction	β reaction	
from E. coli			
wild type	100% (100%)	100%	5.32
K109N	87%	99%	3.48
P261A	67% (95%)	62%	0.74
K109N/P261A	109%	105%	2.74
from S.typhimurium			
wild type	92%	98%	9.61

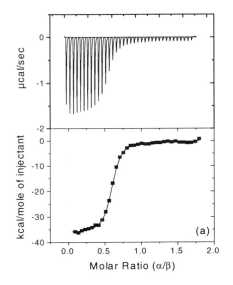
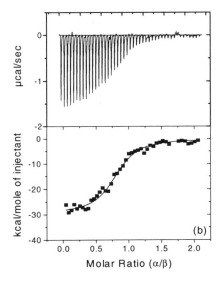

Figure 1. Binding heat obtained by calorimetric titration of the β$_2$ subunit from E. coli, with (a)the wild type and (b)P261A α subunits from E. coli, at pH7, 40 ℃.

Biochemistry of Vitamin B_6 and PQQ
G. Marino, G. Sannia and F. Bossa (eds.)
© 1994 Birkhäuser Verlag Basel/Switzerland

X-ray Structure, Sequence and Solution Properties of Ornithine Decarboxylase from *Lactobacillus 30a*

Marvin L. HACKERT, Don CARROLL, Ratna GHOSH, Andrew KERN, Cory MOMANY, Marcos OLIVEIRA and Liwen ZHANG

Department of Chemistry and Biochemistry, University of Texas at Austin, Austin, TX, USA 78712

Summary

The polyamines, putrescine, spermidine and spermine, are essential for all cells and their concentrations within cells are highly regulated. The synthesis of polyamines begins with the conversion of ornithine into putrescine which is also the starting material for the synthesis of spermidine and spermine. In mammalian cells, fungi, and most protozoa the only route available to synthesize putrescine is via the enzyme ornithine decarboxylase, a pyridoxal phosphate-dependent enzyme. We have determined the gene sequence and X-ray structure of ornithine decarboxylase (ODC) from *Lactobacillus 30a*. This ODC is a dodecamer of ~1MDa that crystallizes in space group P6, $\mathbf{a} = \mathbf{b} = 195.6$Å, $\mathbf{c} = 97.6$Å with two 730 a.a. residue monomers/ asymmetric unit.

The structure of the PLP-dependent decarboxylase is markedly different from what we found for pyruvoyl-dependent histidine decarboxylase. In the latter case the functional unit is a trimer of $\alpha\beta$ subunits, while in the PLP-dependent decarboxylases the functional unit is a dimer. Each dimer consists of a tightly packed "core" involving monomer/monomer contacts plus protruding "wing" domains that interlock with adjacent dimers to form the ring-like dodecamer. Each monomer may be further broken down into five folding domains: the N-terminal 107 residues form the 5-stranded β-sheet "wing" domain, residues 108-161 form a linker domain, residues 162-415 make up the PLP-binding scaffold which is reminiscent of the 7-stranded β-sheet observed in aspartate aminotransferase, and the final two domains (residues 416-571 and 572-730) help create a cleft that leads to the active site at the subunit interface deep within the dimeric "core."

Using the ODC structure as a guide, we have identified amino acid sequence motifs common to decarboxylases, transaminases, and other PLP-dependent enzymes. In particular, the conserved residues Asp316, Ala318, and Lys355 of ODC assume identical functional roles as in the aminotransferases. We have also identified a GTP effector site which has the effect of broadening the pH range over which the enzyme is active. The GTP site lies on the surface of the protein at the interface between the two subunits, but approximately 27Å from the PLP binding site. Kinetic studies show that the effector maintains enzyme activity by shifting the sharp rise in Km from pH 7 to pH 9, but that Vmax remains nearly constant over the pH range of 4 to 9. Preparation of inhibitor complexes and site-directed mutants to explore the functional role of individual residues are in progress.

Introduction

Many bacteria contain two types of amino acid decarboxylases, a biosynthetic enzyme which is constitutively expressed and an inducible or biodegradative form which can be induced in rich medium at low pH. Biodegradative ornithine decarboxylase (ODC) purified from *Lactobacillus 30a* is induced by low pH and the presence of ornithine and histidine in the growth medium (Guirard & Snell, 1980). The ornithine decarboxylase (ODC) from *Lactobacillus 30a* is representative of the large bacterial, PLP-dependent decarboxylases. This ODC exists as a dodecamer composed of six dimers with 730 amino acid residues per subunit (Hackert, et al., 1994). Biosynthetic and biodegradative ODC from *E. coli* have been shown to be actively stimulated by a number of positive effectors including nucleotides with guanosine triphosphate (GTP) being one of the most effective (Holtta et al., 1972).

We have determined the nucleotide sequence, GTP effector site characteristics (Carroll et al., 1994), and x-ray structure of ODC from *L30a* (Momany et al., 1994). GTP binding affinity was analyzed by Scatchard analysis and kinetics were used to study the changes of K_M and Vmax as a function of pH. The GTP binding site was located using low resolution, electron density difference maps. In addition, amino acid sequence alignments based on the structure of ODC and the AATs have been used to demonstrate the relatedness of many PLP-dependent decarboxylases.

Methods

The gene encoding this ornithine decarboxylase from *Lactobacillus* 30a was isolated from a genomic DNA library and sequenced by standard techniques. The x-ray structure was solved by the methods of Multiple Isomorphous Replacement. The binding of $(8, 5'-{}^3H)$-guanosine 5'-triphosphate (tetrasodium salt, 33 Ci/mmol) was performed in a 5-cell equilibrium dialyzer. The K_M for ornithine was determined at pHs 4.0, 5.8, 7.4, 8.0 and 9.4 in the presence of 0.1 mM GTP and at pH 4.0, 5.8 and 7.4 in the absence of GTP.

Results and Discussion

Kinetic analyses at pHs 4.0, 5.8, 7.4, 8.0, and 9.4 show that the Vmax remains essentially constant over this pH range. Thus the variation of specific activity with pH under normal assay conditions is primarily the result of changes in K_M. In the absence of GTP, the K_M is 1.6 mM at the pH optima but is 30 fold higher at pH 4.0 and 7.4. In the presence of 0.1 mM GTP, the observed variation in K_M as a function of pH goes through a much broader minimum with K_M reduced to 0.31 mM at pH 8.0, consistent with the pH profile of specific activity.

The slope of the line for the Scatchard plot at pH 5.8 corresponds to a microscropic dissociation constant of 0.11 µM. The GTP dissociation constant at pH 8.0 was estimated to be about 1.6 µM, but this value should be viewed only as an indication of weaker binding at the higher pH because the presence of multiple oligomeric forms of ODC at pH 8.0 make analysis of the binding data more difficult to interpret.

Sequence analysis showed a 2190 nucleotide open reading frame which encodes a 730 amino acid protein. The calculated molecular size of this enzyme is 82,551 daltons which agrees well with the subunit size of 85,000 Da determined by SDS PAGE. The deduced protein sequence of the *L*30a ODC was compared to sequences of several *E. coli* decarboxylase enzymes: the induced and constitutive forms of the ODC (Kashiwagi et al., 1991; Barroso et al., 1990), the induced arginine decarboxylase (Stim & Bennett, 1993) and the lysine decarboxylase (Meng & Bennett, 1992). It was also compared to sequences of *Hafnia alvei* LDC (Fecker et al.,1986). There are 107 residues (~ 15%) that are identically conserved in all six decarboxylase sequences, including the **FDxAW** sequence containing the Asp316 that pairs with the N1 of the cofactor and Lys355 in **SxHK** that forms the internal aldimine.

```
  0  MSSSLKIASTQEARQYFDTDRVVVDAVGSDFTDVGAVIAMDYETDVIDAADATKFGIPVF
 60  AVTKDAQAISADELKKIFHIIDLENKFDATVNAREIETAVNNYEDSILPPFFKSLKEYVS
120  RGLIQFDCPGHQGGQYYRKHPAGREFYDFFGETVFRADLCNADVALGDLLIHEGPAVAAE
180  KHAARVYNADKTYFVLGGSSNANNTVTSALVSNGDLVLFDRNNHKSVYNSALAMAGGRPV
240  YLQTNRNPYGFIGGIYDSDFDEKKIRELAAKVDPERAKWKRPFRLAVIQLGTYDGTIYNA
300  HEVVKRIGHLCDYIEFDSAWVGYEQFIPMMRNSSPLLIDDLGPEDPGIIVVQSVHKQQAG
360  FSQTSQIHKKDSHIKGQLRYCDHKHFNNSFNLFMSTSPFYPMYAALDVNAAMQEGEAGRK
420  LWHDLLITTIEARKKLIKAGSMFRPFVPPVVNGKKWEDGDTEDMANNIDYWRFEKGAKWH
480  AYEGYGDNQYYVDPNKFMLTTPGINPETGDYEDFGVPATIVANYLRDHGIIPEKSDLNSI
540  LFLMTPAETPAKMNNLITQLLQLQRLIEEDAPLKQVLPSIYAANEERYNGYTIRELCQEL
600  HDFYKNNNTFTYQKRLFLREFFPEQGMLPYEARQEFIRNHNKLVPLNKIEGEIALEGALP
660  YPPGVFCVAPGEKWSETAVKYFTILQDGINNFPGFAPEIQGVYFKQEGDKVVAYGEVYDA
720  EVAKNDDRYNN
```

Figure 1. Deduced amino acid sequence of ODC from L. 30a. Residues in **bold** are conserved in six, large basic amino acid decarboxylases. Underlined residues are discussed below.

Early in our crystallographic analysis we recognized that one of ODC's five major domains was structurally similar to the PLP-binding domain of aspartate aminotransferase (Figure 2).

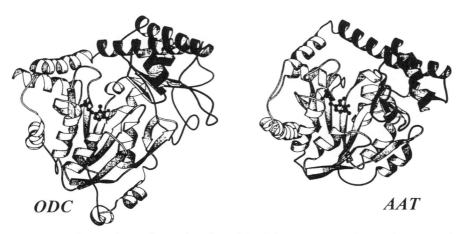

Figure 2. Comparison of PLP domains of ODC from *L. 30a* and AAT from *E. coli* .

In addition to having a similar fold (a seven-stranded β-sheet with flanking helices), several clusters of residues that interact with the PLP are conserved in both the decarboxylases and aminotransferases. Using these active site residues as a guide, a sequence alignment with other decarboxylases was generated (Figure 3). In addition, other PLP-dependent enzymes also have these conserved, active site residues, implying that they have a similar PLP binding site (Toney et al., 1993; Antson et al., 1993). Like in the AATs, two monomers are necessary to define the PLP-binding pocket in ODC. This feature will probably be common to all of the related PLP-dependent enzymes.

```
L30aODC    311DYIEFDSAWVGYEQFIPMMRNSSPLLIDDLGPEDPGIIVVQSVHKQQ357
HumHisDC   268LWLHIDAAYAGTAFLCPEFR------GFLKGIEYADSFTF-NPSKWM307
HumDopaDC  266IWLHVDAAYAGSAFICPEFR------HLLNGVEFADSFNF-NPHKWL305
HumGluDC   359IWMHVDAAWGGGLLMSRKHK------WKLSGVERANSVTW-NPHKMM398
ChkAAT     215LFPFFDSAYQGFASGSLD-KD--AWAVRYFVSEGFELFCAQSFSKNF258
```

Figure 3. Sequence alignment of active site residues of several decarboxylases around the PLP-lysine illustrating the conserved -**D-A**- $(x)_{30-40}$ -**K**- motif.

Functional roles can be assigned to amino acid residues found in these conserved clusters. The *Lactobacillus* ODC sequence ^{315}FDSAW^{319}, forming part of a β-sheet immediately behind the cofactor, is conserved among the decarboxylases as well as aminotransferases (Mehta et al., 1993). Asp316, which forms an ion-pair with the N1 of the pyridinium ring of PLP, is absolutely conserved in aminotransferases and decarboxylases. The methyl side chain of Ala 318 lies directly behind the ring of the cofactor. The phosphate of the PLP is bound by a cluster of hydroxyls from serine and threonine residues (Ser 198, 199, 352, 394, 396, and Thr 395), as well as main chain amide nitrogens, frequently from glycines (Gly 197). Charge stabilization of the pyridoxal-5'-phosphate is provided by the dipole moment arising from helices as noted in the AATs, plus the presence of His 354 in the classic decarboxylase fingerprint sequence, Ser-X-His-Lys. His354 may provide the charge neutralization role similar to that of Arg266 in the AATs rather than act as a potential proton donor during catalysis.

Another significant difference between ODC and AAT is the replacement of a tryptophan (Trp140, AAT) lying over the cofactor in AATs with a histidine (His223, ODC) in the decarboxylases. Sequence alignment algorithms readily associate the His in ^{220}RNNHKSVYNSA^{230} in the *Lactobacillus* ODC with the conserved His in ^{140}WPNHKSVFNSA^{150} in *E. coli* AAT. However, the X-ray crystal structure of ODC reveals that a rotation of the helix occurs to bring this histidine into an equivalent position over the PLP cofactor held by Trp140 in AATs.

The lack of overall sequence identity, but the presence of a common PLP-binding motif consisting of clusters of conserved residues, suggests that the decarboxylases and aminotransferases have a common, but very distant ancestor. A surprising result of our sequence analysis is that this motif is not recognizable in eukaryotic ODCs, *E. coli* bADC, or diaminopimelate decarboxylases, but that the sequences of these enzymes align well with each other. This supports the idea of a second class of PLP-dependent decarboxylases The recognition that the PLP-dependent decarboxylases can be divided into two distinct structural classes suggests that care should be taken in extrapolating results from one class to the other. We are now focusing our efforts on the structure determination of the biosynthetic arginine decarboxylase from *E. coli* and mouse ODC. These results should clarify how significant the structural differences are between the two classes of decarboxylases.

Acknowledgments

We gratefully acknowledge the encouragement of Prof. Esmond Snell who introduced us to B6 enzymes and support provided by grants from the NIH (GM 30105) and the Foundation for Res..

References

Antson, A., Demidkina, T., Gollnick, P., Dauter, Z., Von Tersch, R., Long, J., Berezhnoy, S., Phillips, R., Harutyunyan, E., and Wilson, K. (1993) "Three-Dimensional Structure of Tyrosine Phenol-Lyase" Biochem. 32, 4195-4206.

Barroso, L., Moore, R., Wright, J., Patel, T. and Boyle, S. M. (1990) GenBank, accession #M33766.

Fecker, L.F., Beier, H. and Berlin, J. (1986) "Cloning and Characterization of a Lysine Decarboxylase Gene from *Hafnia alvei*." Mol.Gen. Genet. 203, 177-184.

Guirard, B. M. and Snell, E. E. (1980) Purification and Properties of Ornithine Decarboxylase from *Lactobacillus* 30a." J. Biol Chem. 255, 5960-5964.

Holtta, E., Janne, J. and Pispa J. (1972) "Ornithine Decarboxylase from *E. coli*: Stimulation of the Enzyme Activity by Nucleotides." Bioch. Biophs. Res. Comm. 47, 1165-1171.

Kashiwagi, K., Suzuke, T., Suzuki, F., Furuchi, T., Kobayashi, H. and Igarashi, K. (1991) "Coexistence of Genes for Putrescine Transport Protein and Ornithine Decarboxylase at 16min on *E. coli* Chromosome." J. Biol. Chem. 266, 20922-20927.

Mehta, P. K., Hale, T. I. and Christen, P. (1993) "Aminotransferases: Demonstration of Homology and Division into Evolutionary Subgroups." Eur. J. Biochem. 214, 549-561.

Meng, S-Y. and Bennett, G. N. (1992) "Nucleotide Sequence of the *E. coli* cad Operon: a System for Neutralization of Low Extracellular pH." J. Bact. 174, 2659-2669.

Stim, K. P. and Bennett, G. N. (1993) "Nucleotide Sequence of the *adi* Gene which Encodes the Biodegradative, Acid-Induced Arginine Decarboxylase of *E. coli*." J. Bact. 175, 1221-1234.

Toney, M. D., Hohenester, E., Cowan, S. W. and Jansonius, J. N. (1993) "Dialkylglycine Decarboxylase Structure: Bifunctional Active Site and Alkali Metal Sites." Science, 261 756-759.

Hackert, M.L., Carroll, D.W., Davidson, L. Kim,S.-O., Momany, C. Vaaler, G.L. and Zhang, L., "Sequence, Analysis and Expression of Ornithine Decarboxylase from *Lactobacillus 30a*," J. Bact., submitted (1994).

Carroll, D.W., Momany, C., Davidson, L., Hackert, M.L., "Characterization of the GTP Effector Site and Effect of GTP on the Kinetics of Ornithine Decarboxylase from *Lactobacillus 30a*," Prot. Sci., in prep. (1994).

Momany, C., Ghosh, R., Hackert, M.L., "Two Structural Motifs For Pyridoxal-5'-Phosphate Binding In Decarboxylases: An Analysis Based on the Crystal Structure of the *Lactobacillus* 30A Ornithine Decarboxylase" Protein Science, in preparation (1994).

Biochemistry of Vitamin B₆ and PQQ
G. Marino, G. Sannia and F. Bossa (eds.)
© 1994 Birkhäuser Verlag Basel/Switzerland

Dialkylglycine decarboxylase structure: alkali metal binding sites and bifunctional active site

Michael D. Toney[1], Erhard Hohenester, John W. Keller[2] and Johan N. Jansonius

Abteilung Strukturbiologie, Biozentrum der Universität Basel, Klingelbergstrasse 70, CH-4056 Basel, Switzerland
[1]*Department of Chemistry, University of California, Berkeley, California 94720, U. S. A.*
[2]*Department of Chemistry, University of Alaska Fairbanks, Fairbanks, Alaska 99775, U. S. A.*

Summary

The structure of the pyridoxal phosphate dependent enzyme dialkylglycine decarboxylase (DGD) has been solved by X-ray crystallography. DGD catalyzes the oxidative decarboxylation of 2,2-dialkylglycines in the first half-reaction of its catalytic cycle, which is completed by a classical transamination half-reaction. The enzyme has two alkali metal ion binding sites, and two distinct structures differing in metal content were solved. One structure, DGD-K⁺, has a potassium ion bound at site 1, which is near the active site, and a sodium ion bound at site 2, which is at the surface of the molecule. The second structure, DGD-Na⁺, has sodium ions at both binding sites. The change in the active site structure due to the ion exchange at site 1 likely accounts for the dependence of DGD activity on K⁺ and the inhibitory effect of Na⁺. Models of the external aldimine intermediates with L-isovaline and L-alanine were built in order to provide insight into potential mechanisms of action. In both external aldimine models, the scissile bonds are held in an orientation perpendicular to the plane of the PLP ring plane, providing maximum stereoelectronic activation. In the L-isovaline model, the substrate carboxylate group makes hydrogen bonds with the side chain amide nitrogen of Gln52, the amino group of Lys272, and the guanidino group of Arg406. These interactions enable the enzyme to populate the productive conformation about Cα, in competition with a second, possibly more favorable but nonproductive one. This second conformation about Cα is found in our L-alanine model, where the substrate carboxylate group makes a double hydrogen bond-salt bridge interaction with Arg406. This conformation places the Cα-H bond perpendicular to the PLP ring plane, with the Lys272 amino group well positioned to provide general base catalysis of the transamination reaction.

Introduction

The mechanistic diversity of pyridoxal phosphate dependent enzymes fascinates many an enzymologist, and we found dialkylglycine decarboxylase (DGD) to be particularly intriguing due to its ability to catalyze two reactions, decarboxylation and transamination, in its normal catalytic cycle. Keller *et al.* (1990) reported the cloning, sequencing, and expression in *E. coli* of the DGD gene from the soil bacterium *Pseudomonas cepacia*. Their sequence alignments suggest that, evolutionarily, DGD is related not to classical decarboxylases rather to aminotransferases. Little is known about the physiological role of DGD. 2,2-Dialkylglycines are major constituents of fungal antibiotics, and it may be that the utilization of these as fixed nitrogen sources is its principal function.

We previously reported the structure determination of DGD (Toney *et al.*, 1993). Two different structures, differing in alkali metal content, have been solved and fully refined. DGD-K^+ is the active form of the enzyme in which a potassium ion is bound near the active site, and DGD-Na^+ is an inactive form of the enzyme in which a sodium ion has been exchanged for the potassium ion. The two structures provide insight into how the binding of different alkali metal ions can control protein structure and function.

The mechanistic questions posed by the bifunctional nature of the DGD active site are absorbing: Are there two spatially distinct subsites in the active site that catalyze the decarboxylation and transamination reactions? Assuming a single catalytic subsite, how does it catalyze the mechanistically dissimilar decarboxylation and transamination reactions? We are interested in answering these and other questions, and we approach them here using the hypothetical structures of L-isovaline and L-alanine external aldimine models obtained through model building.

Materials and Methods

Crystals of DGD (hexagonal rods, typically 1.0 x 0.5 x 0.5 mm in size; space group $P6_422$; $a=b=152.7$, $c=86.6$; $\alpha=\beta=90^o$, $\gamma=120^o$) were obtained as described previously (Toney *et al.*, 1991). All data sets were collected on an Enraf-Nonius FAST area detector diffactometer except for the high resolution DGD-Na^+ data, which were collected on an image plate using synchrotron radiation from DESY in Hamburg. The structure solution has been described (Toney *et al.*, 1993) and a detailed account is in preparation (Toney *et al.*, in preparation).

Results and Discussion

The DGD-K^+ and DGD-Na^+ models have been refined to crystallographic R values of 17.6% and 17.8% at 2.6 Å and 2.1 Å resolution, respectively. The fold of the monomer is very similar to that of ω-amino acid aminotransferase (Watanabe *et al.*, 1989) and somewhat less similar to those of aspartate aminotransferase (Jansonius & Vincent, 1986) and tyrosine phenol-lyase (Antson *et al.*, 1993). A superposition of the Cα traces of the large domains of DGD and

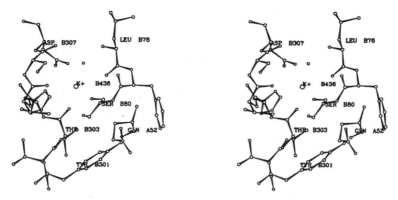

Figure 1. Structure of alkali metal ion binding site 1 with potassium bound.

aspartate aminotransferase can be made such that 140 atoms (52%) are aligned with an rms deviation of 2.1 Å.

Two alkali metal ion binding sites were found in the DGD structure. Metal binding site 2 was the first site found and is located at the C-terminus of helix 3 in a tight type II reverse turn preceding strand *a* of the central β-sheet of the large domain. This is on the surface of the molecule, opposite the active site. A sodium ion is found at this site in both the DGD-K+ and DGD-Na+ structures. The coordination geometry is octahedral with all ligands being oxygen atoms (Toney *et al.*, 1993). It appears from the specificity for sodium and the location distal from the active site that this ion preforms a structural role only.

Metal binding site 1 is located close to the active site at the dimer interface. This metal binding site is not specific for sodium as is site 2, and we have solved the structures of the enzyme with potassium (DGD-K+; Fig. 1) and sodium (DGD-Na+; Fig. 2) bound at this site. The potassium ion bound at site 1 has an octahedral coordination geometry with all ligands being oxygen atoms. The average metal-ligand distance is 2.73 ± 0.12 Å. The sodium ion bound at site

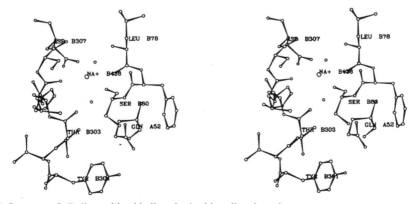

Figure 2. Structure of alkali metal ion binding site 1 with sodium bound.

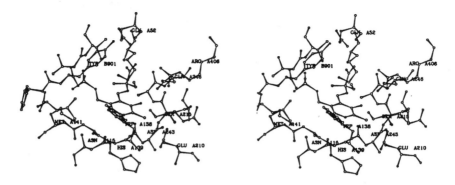

Figure 3. Hypothetical structure of the L-isovaline external aldimine intermediate.

1 has a trigonal bipyramidal coordination geometry instead of the octahedral geometry observed with potassium. The average metal-ligand distance for the sodium ion is 2.33 ± 0.16 Å.

The gross change in coordination geometry is not expected based on the geometric preferences of the metal ions (Glusker, 1991). Rather, our analyses indicate that it is easier for the protein structure to expand and allow a water molecule to replace the Ser80 and Thr303 interactions, since the necessary compaction of the protein structure in order to accomodate the shorter sodium-ligand vs. potassium-ligand distances in the six-coordinate geometry would lead to steric clashes between Ser80 and Thr302. Accompanying the change in coordination geometry to trigonal bipyramidal are conformational changes of Ser80 and Tyr301. The change in conformation of the latter residue places its phenolic side chain in the substrate binding site, and we propose that this may be the source of the inhibition of activity by sodium ions.

Models of the L-isovaline and L-alanine external aldimine intermediates were built in order to aid in the understanding of the catalytic mechanism. Our models use as a guideline the proposal of Dunathan (1966) that PLP dependent enzymes orient the scissile bond such that it is perpendicular to the plane of the pyridine ring plane so as to maximize stereoelectronic advantages. Fig. 3 shows the model of the L-isovaline external aldimine intermediate. It should be stressed that this is not an experimentally determined structure, but one based on computer modeling.

The labile substrate carboxylate group is held perpendicular to the coenzyme ring plane by three good hydrogen bonds in our model, which are donated by Lys272, Gln52, and Arg406. The latter two residues are likely to be positively charged and would thereby stabilize the ground state in the decarboxylation step. A similar situation is found in isocitrate dehydrogenase. Theoretical studies on this enzyme (Hurley & Remington, 1992) suggest that the ground state stabilization due to hydrogen bonds is more than offset in transition state stabilization since they help provide the interaction energy that draws the reactive metal-substrate complex into the catalytic environment of the active site. We suggest that in DGD the hydrogen bonds to the substrate carboxylate in the proposed L-isovaline external aldimine structure are necessary in order to significantly populate the conformation that is productive for decarboxylation.

The alternative, competing binding mode for the substrate carboxylate is that in which Arg406 makes a double hydrogen bond-salt bridge to this group. This corresponds to a 120° clockwise rotation about the substrate Cα-N bond in the view of Fig. 3. This external aldimine conformation is that which we propose for the L-alanine external aldimine model. In this model, the above mentioned interaction between the substrate carboxylate group and Arg406 orients the substrate methyl group toward Met141, and the Cα-H bond is then oriented perpendicular to the plane of the PLP ring. The Lys 272 amino group can be brought into close proximity of the α-hydrogen, and we propose that the 1,3-protropic shift that interconverts the external aldimine and ketimine intermediates is catalyzed by this group, in analogy to the mechanism of aspartate aminotransferase (Jansonius & Vincent, 1986).

References

Antson, A. A., Demidkina, T. V., Gollnick, P., Dauter, Z., Von Tersch, R. L., Long, J., Berezhnoy, S. N., Phillips, R. S., Harutyunyan, E. H., Wilson, K. S. (1993). Three-dimensional structure of tyrosine phenol-lyase. *Biochemistry* **32**, 4195-4206.

Dunathan, H. C. (1966). Conformation and reaction specificity in pyridoxal phosphate enzymes. *Proc. Nat. Acad. Sci. U. S. A.* **55**, 712-716.

Glusker, J. P. (1991). Structural aspects of metal liganding to functional groups in proteins. *Adv. Prot. Chem.* **42**, 1-76.

Hurley, J. H. & Remington, S. J. (1992). Contribution of charged side chains, Mg^{2+}, and solvent exclusion to enzymatic β-decarboxylation of α-keto acids. *J. Am. Chem. Soc.* **114**, 4769-4773.

Jansonius, J. N. & Vincent, M. G. (1987). Structural basis for catalysis by aspartate aminotransferase. In *Biological Macromolecules & Assemblies* (Jurnak, F. A., & McPherson, A., eds.) Vol. 3, Wiley & Sons, New York, pp. 187-288.

Keller, J. W., Baurick, K. B., Rutt, G. C., O'Malley, M. V., Sonafrank, N. L., Reynolds, R. A., Ebbesson, L. O. E., & Vajdos, F. F. (1990). *Pseudomonas cepacia* 2,2-dialkylglycine decarboxylase. Sequence and expression in *Escherichia coli* of structural and repressor genes. *J. Biol. Chem.* **265**, 5531-5539.

Toney, M. D., Hohenester, E., Cowan, S. W. & Jansonius, J. N. (1993). Dialkylglycine decarboxylase structure: bifunctional active site and alkali metal sites. *Science* **261**, 756-759.

Toney, M. D., Keller, J. W., Pauptit, R. A., Jaeger, J., Wise, M. K., Sauder, U., & Jansonius, J. N. (1991). Crystallization and preliminary X-ray diffraction studies of dialkylglycine decarboxylase, a decarboxylating transaminase. *J. Mol. Biol.* **222**, 873-875.

Watanabe, N., Sakabe, K., Sakabe, N., Higashi, T., Sasaki, K., Aibara, S., Morita, Y., Yonaha, K., Toyama, S. & Fukutani, H. (1989). Crystal structure analysis of ω-amino acid:pyruvate aminotransferase with a newly developed Weissenberg camera and an imaging plate using synchrotron radiation. *J. Biochem.* **105**, 1-3.

Biochemistry of Vitamin B$_6$ and PQQ
G. Marino, G. Sannia and F. Bossa (eds.)
© 1994 Birkhäuser Verlag Basel/Switzerland

The Location and Role of Active-Site Bases in PLP-Dependent Decarboxylase Enzymes as Deduced from Stereochemical and Kinetic Studies

David Gani , Mahmoud Akhtar, Janet E. Rose and Kevin Tilley

School of Chemistry, The Purdie Building, University of St. Andrews, St Andrews, Fife, Scotland, KY16 9ST, UK

Summary

Pyridoxal 5'-phosphate dependent *Escherichia coli* glutamic acid decarboxylase reprotonates the quinonoid intermediate derived from the coenzyme and its natural substrate, (2S)-glutamic acid on the 4'-*si*-face of the coenzyme during an abortive decarboxylation-transamination reaction. The enzyme introduces the 3-*pro-R* hydrogen of β-alanine with retention of configuration during the decarboxylation of (2S)-aspartic acid. Treatment of the inactive apoenzyme with $N^{4'}$-(2''-phosphoethyl)-pyridoxamine 5'-phosphate results in the formation of active holoenzyme *via* a mechanism in which the 1''-*pro-R* hydrogen and phosphate are eliminated from the phosphoethyl moiety. The results suggest that protonations and deprotonations at C$^\alpha$ of quinonoid intermediates derived from the coenzyme and the substrate occur from the 4'-*si*-face of the coenzyme and that the distal binding groups of the substrates and inhibitors occupy similar positions at the active site on the 3'-phenolic group side of the coenzyme. It is also demonstrated that the decarboxylase is inactivated by (2R)-serine *O*-sulphate, as well as by the (2S)-enantiomer of the suicide inhibitor, and that inactivation by the (2S)-enantiomer involves C$^\alpha$-H bond cleavage while inactivation by the (2R)-isomer involves C$^\alpha$-decarboxylation. Both processes occur on the 4'-*re*-face of the coenzyme, the opposite face to that utilised in the natural decarboxylation reaction.

Introduction

In view of their potential as targets for chemotherapeutic agents, suicide inhibitors have been designed and prepared for many pyridoxal 5'-phosphate (PLP) dependent decarboxylases (Gani, 1990). In several cases the mechanistic and stereochemical features of the suicide inactivation processes have been difficult to rationalise within the context of the known properties of pyridoxal dependent systems. In certain cases bonds connected to C$^\alpha$ were *apparently* cleaved on the wrong and unexpected 4'-*Re*-face of the coenzyme, for example, for acetylenic GABA [4-aminohex-5-ynoic acid **1**] (Bouclier et al., 1979; Danzin et al., 1984) and (2S)-serine *O*-sulfate (**2**) (Likos et al., 1982). In order to define the conformations of substrates and inhibitors and, hence, the positions of the distal binding groups at the active-site of GAD from *E. coli*, four stereochemical investigations were undertaken. The objectives were:

1) To determine the facial selectivity for protonation at the C-4' position of the coenzyme during an abortive decarboxylation-transamination reaction mediated by (2S)-glutamic acid (**3**).

2) To determine the stereochemical course and fidelity of the decarboxylation-reprotonation at C$^\alpha$ of the quinonoid intermediate derived from a 'loose' substrate, (2S)-aspartic acid (**4**).

3) To assess the ability of *E. coli* apoglutamic acid decarboxylase to reactivate itself in the presence of $N^{4'}$-(2"-phosphoethyl)-pyridoxamine 5'-phosphate (**5**) and to determine the stereochemical preference for the proton abstraction step. A parallel reaction had been reported for the mammalian brain enzyme (Choi & Churchich, 1986).

4) To gain further information on the mechanism of inactivation by serine *O*-sulphates (**2** and **7**).

Results and Discussion

The stereospecificity of the protonation of the quinonoid intermediate at C-4' during abortive decarboxylation-transamination was determined using the natural substrate, (2S)-glutamic acid (**3**). An earlier study had employed (2RS)-2-methylglutamic acid to perform a similar stereochemical correlation and had indicated that 4'-H_S of pyridoxamine 5'-phosphate was introduced during the transamination (Sukareva & Braunstein, 1971), but it could not be assumed that the same stereochemical course would have been followed in the much less frequent transamination reaction which occurs with the natural substrate. There was also some question as to whether the same or different proton-donating groups acted upon the quinonoid intermediates derived from (2S)-glutamic acid and its methyl homologue (Yamada & O'Leary, 1977).

[4'-^{3}H]-PLP was prepared as described previously (Stevenson et al., 1990) and was incubated with *E. coli* GAD at pH 6.0 in the presence of (2S)-glutamic acid. The purified tritiated PMP transamination product was treated with alkaline phosphatase and the resulting 4'-tritiated pyridoxamine was purified. The absolute configuration at C-4' in the sample was determined using apoaspartate aminotransferase which is known to exchange the 4'-*pro-S* hydrogen of pyridoxamine with solvent. None of the tritium was exchanged into the solvent in the sample derived from the decarboxylation incubation whereas 50% of the the tritium in a racemic synthetic sample was exchanged. This result indicates that a proton is transferred to the 4'-*si*-face of the coenzyme during the abortive transamination, in accord with the results obtained for methionine decarboxylase (Stevenson et al., 1990).

In order to determine the stereochemical course of the protonation at C^α in the quinonoid intermediate derived from a 'loose-fit' substrate, (2S)-[2-^{2}H]-aspartic acid and unlabelled aspartic acid were incubated with *E. coli* GAD in protium oxide and in deuterium oxide, respectively. When the decarboxylation reactions were complete the labelled β-alanine products were purified and were each converted to their N-(1S,4R)-camphanamide derivatives. Comparison of the NMR spectra of the samples with those obtained for synthetic C-3 chirally deuteriated samples (Gani & Young, 1985) indicated that the decarboxylation reaction occurred stereospecifically and with retention of configuration at C^α. These results, $i.e.$ high chiral integrity and retention of configuration, are analogous to those obtained for methionine decarboxylase (which has been probed with a wide range of substrates and at extreme pH's) (Stevenson et al., 1990; Akhtar et al., 1990) and suggest that the enzymes share common active-site structural features. Unfortunately $E. coli$ GAD is not stable above pH 6.0 (Fonda, 1972a; O'Leary et al., 1981) and, therefore, it has not been possible to test the stereospecificity for protonation at C^α at high pH as it was in the case of methionine decarboxylase.

The regeneration of active holoenzyme from apoenzyme and $N^{4'}$-(2"-phosphoethyl)-pyridoxamine 5'-phosphate (5) had not been reported for $E. coli$ GAD but was known for the porcine brain enzyme (Chio & Churchich, 1986) and a mechanism involving the elimination of phosphoric acid from the phosphoethyl moiety (to give PLP and ethylamine) had been proposed (Gani, 1986). Hence, compound (5) was prepared and was incubated with freshly prepared $E.$ $coli$ glutamic acid decarboxylase apoenzyme (Wang & Metzler, 1979). Aliquots of the enzyme solution were removed over a period of several hours and were assayed for activity using (2S)-[1-^{14}C]-glutamic acid (Fonda, 1972b). Active enzyme was slowly generated and in this respect the bacterial enzyme was similar to the mammalian enzyme.

In order to determine the stereochemical course of the elimination reaction, dideuteriated and chirally deuteriated samples of compound (5) were prepared (Tilley et al., 1992). Each of the four $N^{4'}$-(2"-phosphoethyl)-pyridoxamine 5'-phosphates (5, $H_A = H_B = H$; $H_A = {}^2H$, $H_B = H$; $H_A = H$, $H_B = {}^2H$, and; $H_A = H_B = {}^2H$) were incubated at a range of concentrations with apoGAD at 30 °C, and aliquots of the enzyme solutions were removed and were assayed for activity. The apparent rate constants for the reactivation were determined from the negative slopes of plots of $\log_e\{[E_{Apo}]-[E.PLP]\}$ versus time and from the increase in gradient ($-k^{App}$) with increasing activator concentration, the values for k_{cat} and K_{Act} were determined. For each compound the values of K_{Act} were similar (52 $\pm$5 μM) but the values of k_{cat} differed and were 1.6 x 10^{-5} s^{-1} for the unlabelled and (1"S)-monodeuteriated isotopomer and 0.9 x 10^{-5} s^{-1} for the dideuteriated and (1"R)-monodeuteriated isotopomer of compound (5). Thus, the enzyme removes the 1"-pro-R hydrogen from compound (5) during the reactivation process. Notably, this hydrogen atom is expected to occupy the spatially equivalent position to that occupied by the 4-pro-R hydrogen of γ-aminobutyric acid and the 3-pro-R proton of β-alanine, if all of the distal anionic binding groups occupy similar positions on the 3-OH side of the pyridine heterocycle. This result and those described above are in keeping with the two base/conjugate acid active site model proposed for methionine decarboxylase (Gani, 1991) in which an ε-ammoniun group from lysine operates at C-4' and an imidazolium group of histidine operates at C^α, both on the 4'-si-face of the coenzyme. Also, in accord with these ideas, for *E. coli* GAD it has been demonstrated that a His residue is important for catalysis but not for substrate binding (Mishin & Sukhareva, 1986).

Ongoing studies in our laboratory had indicated only (2S)-homocysteic acid [and not the (2R)-antipode] was a substrate and that (2R)-serine *O*-sulphate was a suicide inactivator of *E. coli* GAD. In order to further probe these findings and also Metzler's proposed mechanism (Likos et al., 1982) for suicide inactivation by (2S)-serine *O*-sulphate, α–deuteriated (2S)- and (2R)-serine were prepared (Rose et al., 1992a). Samples of the unlabelled and deuteriated serines were then converted to the corresponding *O*-sulphates (**2**, Y = O, H_A = H and ^{2}H, and; **7**, Y = O, H_A = H and ^{2}H) (Rose et al., 1992b) and the rates of GAD inactivation were measured for each of the isotopomers at a range of concentrations and the deuterium isotope effects for inactivation were determined for each enantiomer.

For the (2S)-enantiomer, the observed isotope effects were normal, ^DV [that is k_H/k_D] was 1.3 and $^D(V/K)$ [that is $(k_H/k_D)/(K_H/K_D)$] was 2.3, indicating that C^α-H bond cleavage does, indeed, occur. Thus, the inactivation of GAD by (2S)-serine *O*-sulphate involves the removal of an electrofuge from the 4'-*re*-face of the coenzyme. For (2R)-serine *O*-sulphate, ^DV was 0.13 (inverse) and $^D(V/K)$ was 1.0. The large apparent inverse isotope effect indicates that the substitution by deuterium increases the frequency of inactivation events. Presumably this arises because an alternative reaction pathway for the inhibitor which does not cause irreversible inactivation, but which involves C^α-H bond cleavage (probably transamination of the coenzyme [which does not cause inactivation if excess PLP is available]), expresses a large isotope effect of ~8.0. Nevertheless, the result indicates that for the (2R)-enantiomer C^α-H bond cleavage does not occur during the inactivation process and suggests that C^α- CO_2^- bond cleavage occurs.

In order to verify the unexpected conclusions that (2S)- and (2R)-serine *O*-sulphate lose a proton and a carboxyl group respectively in their inactivations of GAD, samples of (2S)-[U-^{14}C] and (2RS)-[U-^{14}C]serine *O*-sulphate were prepared from the appropriately labelled serines. The uniformity of the label in the (2S)-[U-^{14}C]serine was checked and verified by chemical decarboxylation (Gani & Young, 1985) and the racemic material was prepared from this sample. Each of the ^{14}C-serine *O*-sulphates were incubated with GAD and any liberated CO_2 was collected in barium hydroxide solution. The radioactivities of the incubation solutions and the barium hydroxide solutions were determined by scintillation counting before the start of the reactions and after the inactivations were complete. No $^{14}CO_2$ whatsoever was released during the inactivation of the enzyme by the (2S)-isomer but, the sample of (2RS)-[U-^{14}C]-serine *O*-sulphate gave some $^{14}CO_2$. The amount of radioactivity released was in accord with expectations given that a) most of the enzyme would have been processed through inactivation mediated by the (2S)-enantiomer (which possesses a larger value of V/K) and b) an alternative reaction pathway which involves C^α-H bond cleavage but which does not cause irreversible inactivation is available to the (2R)-enantiomer, *vide supra*.

In view of the strong evidence that the distal $-SO_3^-$ binding group in each of the external aldimines of the two suicide substrates should occupy the same position, *vide supra*, both inactivation events must involve the loss of electrofuges from the 4'-*re*-face of the coenzyme. In the light of the fact that the enzyme has evolved to decarboxylate and reprotonate substrates on the 4'-*si*-face, these are intriguing results.

Acknowledgement

We thank the Science and Engineering Research Council for Studentships for J.E.R and K.T.

References

Akhtar, M., Stevenson, D. E., & Gani, D. (1990) Fern L-methionine decarboxylase: kinetics and mechanism of decarboxylation and abortive transamination. *Biochemistry*, 29: 7648-7660.

Bouclier, M., Jung, M. J., & Lippert, B. (1979) Stereochemistry of reactions catalysed by mammalian-brain L-glutamate 1-carboxy-lyase and 4-aminobutyrate: 2-Oxoglutarate aminotransferase. *Eur. J. Biochem.*, 98: 363-368.

Chio, S. Y., & Churchich, J. E. (1986) Glutamate decarboxylase side reactions catalysed by the enzyme. *Eur. J. Biochem.*, 60: 515-520.

Danzin, C., Claverie, N., & Jung, M. J. (1984) Stereochemistry of the inactivation of 4-aminobutyrate: 2-Oxoglutarate aminotransferase and L-glutamate 1-carboxy-lyase by 4-aminohex-5-ynoic acid enantiomers. *Biochem. Pharmacol.*, 33: 1741-1746.

Fonda, M. L. (1972a) Glutamate decarboxylase: Substrate specificity and inhibition by carboxylic acids. *Biochemistry*, 11: 1304-1309.

Fonda, M. L. (1972b) Glutamate decarboxylase: Inhibition by monocarboxylic acids. *Arch. Biochem. Biophys.*, 153: 763-768.

Gani, D., & Young, D. W. (1985) Stereochemistry of catabolism of the RNA base uracil. *J. Chem. Soc. Perkin Trans. I*, 1355-1362.

Gani, D. (1986) Enzyme Chemistry. *Ann. Rep. prog. Chem.*, (B), 83: 303-330.

Gani, D. (1990) Pyridoxal dependent systems. *Section 6.5 in Comprehensive Medicinal Chemistry*, ed. Sammes, P.G., Pergamon Press, Oxford, vol. 2, pp. 213-254.

Gani, D. (1991) A structural and mechanistic comparison of pyridoxal 5'-phosphate dependent decarboxylase and transaminase enzymes. *Philosophical Trans. (B)* 332: 131-139.

Likos, J. J., Ueno, H., Feldhaus, R. W., & Metzler, D. E. (1982) A novel reaction of the coenzyme of glutamate decarboxylase with L-seine O-sulphate. *Biochemistry*, 21: 4377-4386.

Mishin, A. A., & Sukharaeva, B. S. (1986) Glutamate decarboxylase from *Escherichia coli*: Catalytic role of a histidine residue. *Dokl. Acad. Nauk SSSR*, 290: 1268-1271.

O'Leary, M. H., Yamada, H., & Yapp, C. J. (1981) Multiple isotope effect probes of glutamate decarboxylase. *Biochemistry*, 20: 1476-1481.

Rose, J. E., Leeson P. D., & Gani, D. (1992a) Regiospecific deuteriation of chiral 2,5-dimethoxy-3-isopropyl-3,6-dihydropyrazines in the stereospecific synthesis of α-deuteriated α-amino acids. *J. Chem. Soc. Perkin Trans. I*, 1563-1565.

Rose, J. E., Leeson P. D., & Gani, D. (1992b) Mechanism of the inactivation of *E. coli* glutamate decarboxylase by L- and D- serine O-sulphate. *J. Chem. Soc. Chem. Comm.*, 1784-1786.

Stevenson, D. E., Akhtar, M., & Gani, D. (1990) L-Methionine decarboxylase from *Dryopteris filix-mas*: purification, characterization, substrate specificity; abortive transamination of the coenzyme and the stereochemical courses of substrate decarboxylation and coenzyme transamination. *Biochemistry*, 29: 7631-7647.

Sukhareva, B. S., & Braunstein, A. E. (1971) Investigation of the nature of the interactions of glutamate decarboxylase from *Escherichia coli* with substrate and its analogues. *J. Mol. Biol. S.S.R*, 5: 302-317.

Tilley, K., Akhtar, M., & Gani, D. (1992) The stereochemical course of reactions catalysed by *E. coli* glutamate decarboxylase. *J. Chem. Soc. Chem. Comm.*, 68-70.

Wang, B. I-Y., & Metzler, D. E. (1979) Pyridoxal 5'-phosphate and analogues as probes of coenzyme-protein interaction. *Methods Enzymol.*, 62: 528-551.

Yamada H. & O'Leary, M. H. (1977) A solvent isotope effect probe for enzyme mediated proton transfers. *J. Am. Chem. Soc.*, 99: 1660-1661.

Biochemistry of Vitamin B$_6$ and PQQ
G. Marino, G. Sannia and F. Bossa (eds.)
© 1994 Birkhäuser Verlag Basel/Switzerland

GuCl-induced unfolding of pig kidney dopa decarboxylase: Evidence for a multi-state process

Paola Dominici, Patrick S. Moore and Carla Borri Voltattorni

Università di Verona, Istituto di Chimica Biologica, 37134 Verona, Italy

Summary

The guanidinium chloride (GuCl) induced unfolding of dopa decarboxylase (DDC) has been studied by monitoring its effects on enzymatic activity, hydrodynamic volume, far-uv cd, and intrinsic fluorescence. Due to its spectral properties, pyridoxal 5'-phosphate (PLP) was also used as a probe of structural changes occuring at the active site during the unfolding/refolding process. The combination of these studies revealed that the unfolding of DDC occurs as a multi-step process minimally composed of at least three steps that could be identified at equilibrium. The first step occurs at 0-1 M GuCl and gives rise to an inactive dimeric species which is devoid of coenzyme. At 1-2.2 M GuCl a second transition is observed, consisting in subunit dissociation and partial loss of tertiary and secondary structure accompanied by structural alterations of the coenzyme microenvironment leading to a "structured monomer". The third and final phase of the unfolding process is complete at about 4.5 M GuCl and is characterized by complete subunit unfolding. Further increasing the GuCl concentration failed to cause a change in any of the parameters followed. While enzymatic activity could never be regained starting from fully denatured protein, partial reactivation was seen starting from enzyme treated with GuCl concentrations less than 1.5 M. Together with an more in-depth investigation into the refolding, it is suggested that, at least under the experimental condition tested, the monomer-dimer transition is impaired during this process. These results are discussed in terms of a model for the unfolding/refolding of pig kidney dopa decarboxylase.

Introduction

Dopa decarboxylase (DDC) from pig kidney exists as a homodimer with a subunit molecular weight of about 54 kD (Borri Voltattorni et al., 1987). It contains 1 mol of PLP per dimer and the spectral properties of the coenzyme-bound apoenzyme and of the enzyme-substrate bound complexes have been determined (Borri Voltattorni et al., 1971; Borri Voltattorni et al., 1983; Fiori et al., 1975). The complete primary structure has also been elucidated which allowed for the localization of a number of structural features that are crucial for enzyme function (Maras et al., 1991). Crystals of the enzyme have recently been obtained and the determination of the three-dimensional structure is in progress (Malashkevich et al., 1992). However, as information correlating its spatial structure and activity are still lacking, a study of the unfolding/refolding process was undertaken in an attempt to gain insight in this regard.

Experimental Methods

<u>Enzyme denaturation.</u> Denaturation of DDC was performed by mixing stock solutions of enzyme and 6 M GuCl (both dissolved in 50 mM potassium phosphate, pH 7, 0.5 mM EDTA, and 1 mM DTT (buffer A)) to yield the desired concentration of protein and denaturant.

<u>Spectroscopy.</u> Cd spectra were recorded on a Cary model 60 at 20° at protein concentrations from 0.075-0.15 mg/ml for far uv and 1.5 mg/ml for near uv-vis experiments. Fluorescence measurements were carried out with a Kontron SFM 25 at 25°. Native protein fluorescence was monitored at 326 nm (excitation at 278 nm) while $NaBH_4$ reduced enzyme was also monitored at 385 nm (excitation at 325 nm).

<u>Gel-filtration chromatography.</u> All experiments were carried out at 4° with FPLC equipped with a Superose 12 column. A linear gradient of GuCl was formed by mixing 100 ml of buffer A containing 300 mM NaCl (buffer B) with 100 ml of buffer B containing 6 M GuCl. Successive 50 μl samples of native DDC were injected after each 0.1 M increment in GuCl concentration. The elution profile was monitored by absorbance at 280 nm.

Results and Discussion

Under equilibrium conditions, the effect of increasing concentrations of guanidinium chloride (GuCl) on the enzyme was followed by monitoring enzymatic activity, hydrodynamic volume, far-uv cd, and intrinsic fluorescence. PLP was also used as a probe to follow the local conformational changes occuring at the active site during GuCl denaturation of the enzyme. The combination of these studies have shown that the unfolding of DDC occurs in at least three phases with distinct intermediates. The first phase of the unfolding process occurs at GuCl concentrations from 0-1 M. In this range there was a progressive loss of activity with 50% remaining at 0.4 M GuCl and less than 10% remaining at 1 M GuCl (data not shown). This inactive species retains all of its secondary and tertiary structure (Fig. 1a) and is still in the dimeric form (data not shown). However, the enzyme has lost PLP as indicated by the following lines of evidence. 1) The absorption spectra of the holoenzyme displays two peaks at 335 and 420 nm, which are also seen in visible cd. The presence of increasing concentrations of GuCl causes the gradual decrease of these absorbing and dichroic bands and the concomitant appearance of a absorbing band at 388 nm, due to free PLP (data not shown). This process is complete at 1 M GuCl. 2) As shown in Fig. 1a, there is an increase in the quantum yield of the holoenzyme in this GuCl concentration range, while the fluorescence of the apoenzyme remains constant. This suggests that the intrinsic fluorescence is quenched by coenzyme and that when PLP is no longer associated with the enzyme, the exposure of previously buried tryptophan residues to solvent leads to an increased quantum yield. 3) PLP fluorescence was also measured using $NaBH_4$ reduced DDC to gain information on the coenzyme binding region. With increasing concentrations of denaturant, a maximum increase in fluorescence is reached at 1 M GuCl (data not shown) suggesting that slight local structural alterations have occurred which could be responsible for the release of PLP from the active site. 4) When intrinsic fluorescence of the reduced enzyme is measured, two emission peaks are observed at 326 and 385 nm, the latter being most likely due to energy transfer between a tryptophan residue(s) and the coenzyme (Fig. 1b). In the 0-1 M GuCl range a variation of the efficiency of this process is observed (Fig. 1b). Taken together, these data indicate that in this denaturant concentration range a slight disturbance of the correct spatial geometry of the functional groups in the active site responsible for catalysis occurs. This leads to the loss of enzymatic activity before any gross conformational changes have taken place.

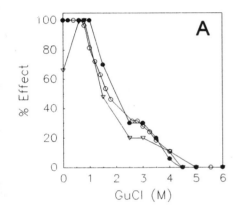 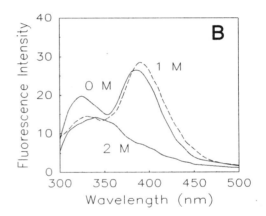

Figure 1. A) GuCl dependent unfolding as measured by fluorescence and far-uv cd spectroscopy. Protein fluorescence of native holo (∇) and apo (●) enzyme was measured as described in the experimental methods. Changes in ellipticity were measured at 222 nm at the indicated GuCl concentrations (O). B) The fluorescence spectra of $NaBH_4$ reduced enzyme were measured at the indicated GuCl concentrations as described in the experimental methods.

The second phase of the unfolding process which occurs in the denaturant range of 1-2.2 M involves dimer dissociation and partial loss of higher order structure. Measurements of intrinsic fluorescence showed a cooperative decrease in this range before reaching a plateau at about 2 M GuCl. This decrease was accompanied by a red-shift in the emission maximum from 326 to 341 nm. As in fluorescence, the far-uv cd decreases in this range and reaches a plateau at 2 M GuCl (Fig. 1a). The 385 nm fluorescence intensity of reduced PLP begins to decline and at 2 M GuCl the emission intensities of reduced PLP and free PMP coincide with one another (data not shown). Intrinsic fluorescence measurements of the reduced enzyme showed that the emission at

385 nm has fully disappeared at 2 M (Fig. 1b), indicating that the adequate requirements of distance and orientation are not met. Measurements of hydrodynamic volume demonstrated that the protein has dissociated into monomers by 2 M GuCl. In fact, while the native enzyme elutes with an apparent molecular mass of 104 kD, in good agreement with the true mass, at 2 M GuCl the retention volume increases and a species with an apparent molecular mass of 56 kD elutes. The second phase is therefore characterized by dimer dissociation, partial loss of secondary and tertiary structure (as seen by fluorescence and cd), and gross conformational changes at or near the active site leading to a complete exposure of the PLP binding site to solvent.

The third and final phase of the unfolding represents the complete unfolding of the protein. At GuCl concentrations from 2.2-4.5 M, a gradual loss of the intrinsic fluorescence and far-uv CD signals is seen. Hydrodynamic volume measurements also showed a gradual decrease of the elution volume as expected for complete unfolding of the monomeric species.. This phase is complete at about 4.5 M GuCl. Further increasing the denaturant concentration resulted in no further changes in any of the parameters followed.

With regards to the process of refolding of DDC, partial enzymatic activity can be recovered starting from material treated with denaturant concentrations of less than 1.5 M. Starting from protein treated with higher concentrations of GuCl, the enzyme is irreversibly inactivated. Numerous attempts under a wide variety of conditions proved to be unsuccessful, including those recommended by Jaenicke and Rudolph (1989), either by step-dilution or dialysis. However, when fully-denatured samples were quick-diluted to a GuCl concentration that would be expected to support native enzyme in the presence of 0.9 M sodium sulfate, a fluorescence spectrum almost coincident with that of the native enzyme was observed. This species, termed X, exhibits a 1 nm red shift in the emission maximum and a 15% increase in the emission intensity with respect to the native enzyme, while its hydrodymanic volume is between that of the native enzyme and the fully unfolded form (data not shown). Although this species is able to interact with coenzyme, it nonetheless does not display energy transfer. The unfolding of this species as monitored by intrinsic fluorescence showed that with increasing denaturant concentration there is a decrease of the emission intensity accompanied by a red-shift (data not shown). Unlike the native enzyme this species unfolds in a simple cooperative transition from the "refolded" to the fully unfolded form. Further investigation into the refolding process by step-dilution revealed that from 6-2 M GuCl the changes in the emission intensity and maximum parallel those of the unfolding pathway. Below 2 M GuCl, there were no further consistent or significant changes in fluorescence.

The unfolding process has been divided into three identifiable steps. The first step leads to the formation of a modified dimer (D'). The second step represents the dissociation of the dimeric protein into its subunits (D' ⇨ 2M): "M" is considered to be a "structured" monomer. The third step involves the complete unfolding of the structured monomer in to the unfolded monomer "U". The refolding process was reversible down to about 2 M GuCl, supporting the concept that the refolding process is reversible in the range of 2-6 M GuCl. Thus it would appear that the bimolecular reaction corresponding to the monomer-dimer transition is impaired, at least under the experimental conditions tested. The inactive abortive species, X, may represent a kinetically trapped conformer that limits the refolding process and has unfolding characteristics consistent with a two-state mechanism involving only X and the unfolded monomer, U. Based on the above we have proposed the following model for the unfolding/refolding of pig kidney DDC:

$$D \Leftrightarrow D' \leftrightarrow 2M \Leftrightarrow 2U$$
$$\Updownarrow$$
$$X$$

where D and D' represent "folded dimeric" forms of the enzyme which are fully active and partially reversible inactivated states, respectively; M indicates the "structured" monomer; U the unfolded monomer; and X the inactive abortive state. The solid arrows indicate an irreversible transition.

Acknowledgements

This research was supported by the Italian MURST and C.I.S.M.I. (Milan, Pavia, Verona).

References

Borri Voltattorni, C., Minelli, A., and Turano, C. (1971) Spectral properties of the coenzyme bound to dopa decarboxylase from pig kidney. *FEBS Lett.* 17: 231-235.

Borri Voltattorni, C., Minelli, A., and Dominici, P. (1983) Interaction of aromatic amino acids in D- and L- forms with 3,4-dihydroxyphenylalanine decarboxylase from pig kidney. *Biochemistry* 22: 2249-2254.

Borri Voltattorni, C., Giartosio, A., and Turano, C. (1987) Aromatic amino acid decarboxylase from pig kidney. *Methods Enzymol.* 142: 179-187.

Fiori, A., Borri Voltattorni, C., Minelli, A., and Turano C. (1975) Interaction of L-Dopa decarboxylase with substrates: A spectrophotometric study. *FEBS Lett.* 54: 122-125.

Jaenicke, R. & Rudolph R. (1989) in *Protein Folding* (Horecker, B., ed.). Academic Press, Orlando, FL, pp. 289-296.

Maras, B., Dominici, P., Barra, D., Bossa, F., and Borri Voltattorni, C. (1991) Dopa decarboxylase: The pig kidney enzyme. Primary structure and relationship to other amino acid decarboxylases. *Eur. J. Biochem.* 201: 385-391.

Malashkevich, V.N., Fillipponi, P., Sauder, U., Dominici, P., Jansonius, J.N., and Borri Voltattorni, C. (1992) Crystallization and preliminary X-ray analysis of pig kidney dopa decarboxylase. *J. Mol. Biol.* 224: 1167-1170.

PHOSPHORYLASES

Biochemistry of Vitamin B_6 and PQQ
G. Marino, G. Sannia and F. Bossa (eds.)
© 1994 Birkhäuser Verlag Basel/Switzerland

The transition state complex in the phosphorylase catalyzed reaction

Dieter Palm, Stefan Becker and Reinhard Schinzel

Department of Physiological Chemistry, Theodor-Boveri-Institut für Biowissenschaften, Universität Würzburg
Am Hubland, D-97074 Würzburg, F.R.G

Summary
            A glucosylcarbonium ion is the central intermediate on the reaction pathway of the reversible phosphorylase catalyzed reaction. The contribution of pyridoxal-5′-phosphate to improve on the enzyme complementarity to the transition state by a tightly coordinated phosphate anion and two essential basic amino acid residues might be essential for the transition state complex.

Phosphorylases catalyze the phosphorolysis of polysaccharides by a mechanism which involves protonation of the glycosidic oxygen of the nonreducing terminal glucose residue, cleavage of the C1-O bond, and attack of the remaining glucosyl residue by a phosphate anion (Palm et al., 1990). The reaction (**I**) is fully reversible *in vitro* with glucose-1-P and a *primer*, $(\text{glucose})_{n=4}$, serving as substrates:

$$(\text{glucose})_n + H_2PO_4^- \;\; \rightleftharpoons \;\; (\text{glucose})_{n-1} + \text{glucose-1-P} \quad (\mathbf{I})$$

The existence of a carbonium ion-like transition state was anticipated from similarities with other glycosyltransferases, retaining the same anomeric configuration of substrate and products.

Complementarity to the transition state is a common feature of the active site structure of a large number of enzymes. This has given rise to the hypothesis catalysis, might be crucially dependent on the potential of the active site to assume conformations that are complementary to the transition state configurations of the reactants. Consequently, to gain more informations and to describe in more details the *transition state complex of the phosphorylase reaction*, it would be necessary to combine informations on the chemical and structural nature of the transition state or a transition state-like intermediate, and about the complementary protein conformations, responsible for either ground or transition state binding.

The common conception concerning the reaction pathway leading to products with retention of configuration is based on successive displacements each occurring with inversions, most

162

commonly two, but any even number of displacements will lead to the same result (Fersht, 1985).

Starting with an α-glycosidic substrate, solution chemistry would suggest a ß-glycosidic intermediate (first *inversion*), which on attack by the second substrate will yield a product with α-configuration (second *inversion*). Transferring this mechanism to an enzyme, this condition would be best satisfied by a covalent enzyme intermediate. On the other hand, formation of a carbonium ion intermediate by an S_N1 mechanism in solution would lead to loss of stereospecifity, but a carbonium ion stabilized in the active site of an enzyme can be expected to react stereospecificically on the enzyme. Thus stereochemical evidence can not proof the mechanism but can serve to discern alternative pathways if some of the requirements for interactions with the substrate are not met. In the case of phosphorylases, two situations are imaginable: direct participation of the enzyme forming a covalent, *inverted* glucosyl intermediate, which will be subsequently displaced by the second substrate with inversion of configuration at the glucosyl residue - or - stabilization of the transition state-like glucosylcarbonium ion by electrostatic forces. The shortened chain diffuses away from the enzyme; the carbonium ion intermediate then reacts with fixed chirality with the second substrate, or a nucleophile from the solvent. Examples of both types can be found among glycosyltransferases: The first case is represented by ß-galactosidase or, more prone to the present problem, by sucrose phosphorylase (Voet & Abeles, 1970), where a covalent glucosyl-intermediate could be demonstrated, and the second case is represented by lysozyme, where the intermediate was stabilized by an essential aspartate anion in a polar environment, which makes it likely that the intermediate forms a glycosylcarbonium ion (Phillips, 1966; Fersht, 1985).

Both cases appeared not to be applicable to glycogen phosphorylases for structural reasons (Johnson et al., 1990), since in the former cases an essential carboxyl residue on the opposite side of the sugar ring was provided by the enzyme, but there is no equivalent in the active site structure of phosphorylase. Therefore, an alternative solution had to be looked for.

With respect to the forementioned principles, a search was made for possible catalytic groups close to the cleavable glycosidic bond. By analogy to the lysozyme mechanism, likely candidates are groups that can serve as proton donors and acceptors. Although pyridoxal phosphate was suspected (for review see Helmreich & Klein, 1980) the increasingly refined X-ray structure made it clear that any involvement of pyridoxal-P must be indirect (Klein et al., 1984;

McLaughlin et al., 1984). Recent Fourier-transform infrared spectroscopic (FTIR) studies on phosphate hydrogen bonds of free and phosphorylase-bound pyridoxal-P demonstrate the exceptional capabilities of the cofactor phosphate to promote proton transfer (cf. Zundel & Eckert, 1989; F. Bartl, G. Zundel, D. Palm, R. Schinzel, unpublished results). This, together with the observation that the phosphorylase catalyzed reaction is essentially dependent on a *catalytic* phosphate anion, as demonstrated with glycosylic substrate analogs like D-glucal (Klein et al., 1982) let us suggest that pyridoxal-P together with a mobile phosphate provide the proton donor and the electrostatic stabilization for the proposed carbonium ion intermediate (Klein et al., 1982; Klein et al., 1984; Klein et al., 1986; Palm et al., 1990).

Moreover, the products of the D-glucal utilization met all stereochemical criteria required for phosphorylase catalyzed reactions and thus intermediates found in this pathway might give a clue to the natural substrates. If the reaction with D-glucal was performed in the presence of ^2H_2O, a 2-deoxy-α-D-[2(e)-^{2}H]glucopyranosyl-residue was found in all products (Klein et al., 1982). To conceive a reaction pathway which complies to these conditions the most simple and straightforward proposal would be to attach the proton to the electron rich double bond leading to a 2-deoxyglucosylcarbonium ion. The deoxyglucosylcarbonium ion consequently is subject to attack by nucleophiles in accordance with the specificity of the substrate binding site. Therefore, the product depends also on the chiral presentation of the nucleophile. Depending on substrate concentrations and substrate availibity two products were found (Fig. 1A): (α-1,4-)-2-deoxy-glucosyl-glucose$_n$ and α-D-deoxyglucose-1-phosphate as suggested by (**IIa** and **IIb**):

D-glucal + glucose$_n$ ⟶ [P$_i$] ⟶ 2-deoxyglucosyl-glucose$_n$ (**IIa**)
D-glucal + P$_i$ ⟶ [glucose$_n$] ⟶ 2-deoxyglucose-1-P (**IIb**)

However, the, at the first sight, unconventional reaction, left the faint suspicion, that the reaction might not be a part of the common phosphorylase reaction pathway and therefore could not provide valid proof of a glucosylcarbonium ion intermediate as part of the reaction mechanism.

In the course of a more detailed inspection of the properties of the deoxyglucosyl-primer derivative we studied the phosphorolysis of 2-deoxyglucosyl-glucose$_n$ and the reversible reaction of 2-deoxyglucose-1-P with a glucose$_4$-primer. Unlike the product pattern expected from the natural substrates in reaction (**I**) one additional product showed up if the 2-deoxyglucosyl-analogs were chosen for substrates (Fig. 1B and 1C). The new product can be easily identified

164

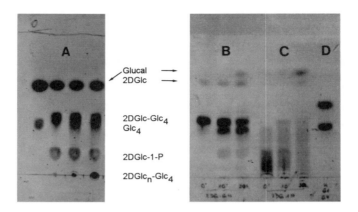

Fig. 1. **Products formed from (A) D-glucal (B) 2-deoxyglycosyl-glucose$_4$ and (C) 2-deoxyglucose-1-P in the phosphorylase catalyzed reaction.** E.coli maltodextrin phosphorylase was incubated with (A) D-glucal, maltotetraose and phosphate; (B) 2-deoxyglycosyl-glucose$_4$ and phosphate; (C) 2-deoxyglucose-1-P and maltotetraose, and aliquots were applied on TLC at intervals between zero time and 20 hours; (D) Controls: Glc and Glc$_4$. The primary products of reaction (A) were isolated and subsequently used as substrates in reaction (B) and (C). Note that the substrate in reaction (C) contains a trace amount of 2-deoxyglucose, which increased during the incubation due to the hydrolytic error (see text).

if we compare the pattern with the D-glucal reaction (Fig.1A). The product pattern can be rationalized if we assume that the products are formed by

$$\text{2-deoxyglucosyl-glucose}_n + P_i \longrightarrow \text{glucose}_n + \text{2-deoxyglucose-1-P} + \text{D-glucal} \quad (\textbf{IIIa})$$

$$\text{2-deoxyglucosyl-1-P} + \text{glucose}_n \xrightarrow{\lfloor P_i \rfloor} \text{2-deoxyglucosyl-glucose}_n + \text{D-glucal} \quad (\textbf{IIIb})$$

Formation of D-glucal in any of the former reactions is feasible by deprotonation of a 2-deoxyglucosyl intermediate, most probably a deoxyglucosylcarbonium ion. It must therefore be concluded that the deoxyglucosylcarbonium ion is on the reaction pathway. By common criteria this can be considered as proof for the existence of an glucosyloxocarbonium ion intermediate (Fersht, 1985).

These findings repudiate arguments about a separate mechanism of D-glucal turnover by phosphorylases. In our mind the reversibility of the D-glucal/2-deoxyglucosyloligosaccharide reaction suggests two points:

1) The transition state like intermediate can be attacked by a nucleophile, e.g. a phosphate anion or the hydroxyl of the terminal glucose of a growing chain, or it can be stabilized by deprotonation. This is exactly the reversal of the protonation reaction. The 2-deoxyglycosylcarbonium ion intermediate is the only conceivable intermediate which can stabilize itself by deprotonation and thus provides the hitherto best proof for the existence of such an intermediate.

2) The simultaneous formation of 2-deoxyglucose-1-P or 2-deoxyglucosyl-glucose$_n$ with D-glucal require similar activation energies and small differences in Gibbs free energy. The reversibility makes it probable that catalysis by phosphorylase in the phosphorolytic or synthetic mode proceeds by a similar sequence of steps.

Since for the phosphorolysis of 2-deoxyglucosyl-glucose$_4$ the substrate is activated by protonation of the glycosidic oxygen and cleavage of the C1-O bond similar to catalysis of the natural substrates it can be concluded that the transition state-like intermediate resulting from the cleavage of the natural maltooligosachcharides will be a glucosylcarbonium ion. The latter can be attacked by nucleophiles but cannot stabilize itself by deprotonation.

It might be noted that accidentally water might replace phosphate serving as a nucleophilic agent in the active site. To the extent that the specificity pocket of the substrate binding site fits closely to the O2-hydroxyl of the terminal glucose residue or glucose-1-P, the hydrolytic error will increase in the presence of substrates like 2-deoxyglucosyl derivatives which are sterically less demanding than the natural substrates. This can be observed in Fig. 1.

Concluding remarks

The proposed transition state complex and the basic phosphorylase mechanism did not turn out as a violation of classical glycosyl transferase mechanisms. We find all elements like protonation of the glycosidic bond, stabilization of the transition state by electrostatic forces and chiral nucleophilic attack.

What than make up special features in the mechanism of phosphorylases?

Electrostatic stabilization of the glucosylcarbonium ion is obtained by a *mobile* phosphate anion, which unlike a specific amino acid residue, is more flexible to adjust to the sterical requirements on the reaction pathway in both directions. The disposition and orientation of the phosphate anion is crucially dependent on pyridoxal-P and on two basic amino acid residues forming a charge network in the active site: Arg534 and Lys539 (Schinzel & Drueckes, 1991; R. Schinzel, this Symposium). Phosphate-phosphate interactions like those formed between the cofactor phosphate and the mobile phosphate allow easy exchange of protons and equilibration of charge without changes of net charge. The unique combination of pyridoxal-P and a phosphate anion thus constitutes an optimal agent to achieve enzyme - transition state complementarity.

Acknowledgements The studies on the mechanism of phosphorylases have been supported by grants from the Deutsche Forschungsgemeinschaft.

References

Fersht, A. (1985). Enzyme Structure and Mechanism (2nd ed.). San Francisco: Freeman.

Helmreich, E., & Klein, H. W. (1980). The role of pyridoxal phosphate in the catalysis of glycogen phosphorylases. Angew. Chem. Int. Ed. Engl., 19, 441-5.

Johnson, L. N., Acharya, K. R., Jordan, M. D., & McLaughlin, P. J. (1990). Refined crystal structure of the phosphorylase-heptulose 2-phosphate-oligosaccharide-AMP complex. J. Mol. Biol., 211, 645-61.

Klein, H. W., Im, M. J., & Palm, D. (1986). Mechanism of the phosphorylase reaction. Utilization of D-gluco-hept-1-enitol in the absence of primer. Eur. J. Biochem., 157, 107-14.

Klein, H. W., Im, M. J., Palm, D., & Helmreich, E. J. (1984). Does pyridoxal 5'-phosphate function in glycogen phosphorylase as an electrophilic or a general acid catalyst? Biochemistry, 23, 5853-61.

Klein, H. W., Palm, D., & Helmreich, E. J. (1982). General acid-base catalysis of alpha-glucan phosphorylases: stereospecific glucosyl transfer from D-glucal is a pyridoxal 5'-phosphate and orthophosphate (arsenate) dependent reaction. Biochemistry, 21, 6675-84.

McLaughlin, P. J., Stuart, D. I., Klein, H. W., Oikonomakos, N. G., & Johnson, L. N. (1984). Substrate-Cofactor Interactions for Glycogen Phosphorylase b: A Binding Study in the Crystal with Heptenitol and Heptulose-2-Phosphate. Biochemistry, 23, 5862-5873.

Palm, D., Klein, H. W., Schinzel, R., Buehner, M., & Helmreich, E. J. (1990). The role of pyridoxal 5'-phosphate in glycogen phosphorylase catalysis. Biochemistry, 29, 1099-107.

Phillips, D. C. (1966). The three-dimensional structure of an enzyme molecule. Sci.Am., 215(5), 75-80.

Schinzel, R., & Drueckes, P. (1991). The phosphate recognition site of Escherichia coli maltodextrin phosphorylase. Febs Lett., 286, 125-8.

Voet, J. G., & Abeles, R. H. (1970). The Mechanism of Action of Sucrose Phosphorylase. Isolation and properties of a beta-linked covalent glucose-enzyme complex. J. Biol. Chem., 245, 1020-1031.

Zundel, G., & Eckert, M. (1989). IR Continua of Hydrogen Bonds and Hydrogenbonded Systems. J. of Molecular Structure (Theochem), 200, 73-92.

Biochemistry of Vitamin B$_6$ and PQQ
G. Marino, G. Sannia and F. Bossa (eds.)
© 1994 Birkhäuser Verlag Basel/Switzerland

Binding mode of glucans to α–glucan phosphorylase isozymes and their chimeric enzymes

Toshio Fukui, Hiroyuki Mori and Katsuyuki Tanizawa

Institute of Scientific and Industrial Research, Osaka University, Ibaraki, Osaka 567, Japan

Summary

α-Glucan phosphorylases from various sources are characterized by the difference in glucan specificity, though they share similar primary structures. To investigate the molecular basis of the glucan specificity of phosphorylases, we have constructed two chimeric enzymes. A chimeric enzyme, in which a part of the sequence including the 78-residue long insertion and its flanking regions in the potato type-L isozyme was replaced by the corresponding part of the potato type-H isozyme lacking the insertion, showed affinity for glucans much higher than the type-L isozyme, comparable with that of the type-H isozyme. Another chimeric enzyme, in which the same part of the type-L isozyme was replaced by the corresponding part in the rabbit muscle enzyme including the glycogen-storage site, showed extraordinarily high affinity for all the glucans tested including glycogen, amylose, and maltodextrin. These results confirm the presence of a preferential binding site apart from the active site in the rabbit muscle enzyme, and suggest the presence of a similar binding site with high affinity in the potato type-H isozyme. In the potato type-L isozyme, the corresponding region is masked by the lengthy insertion so that glucans are bound directly to the active site that is located at the bottom of a deep cleft and contains the coenzyme pyridoxal phosphate. Therefore, this isozyme can use amylose and maltodextrin as well as amylopectin but not glycogen.

Introduction

α-Glucan phosphorylases that catalyze the reversible phosphorolysis of the α-1,4-glycosidic linkage in glucans exist as multiform in animal, plant, and microorganism. The enzymes from various sources are characterized by the difference in glucan specificity, though they all contain pyridoxal 5'-phosphate as coenzyme and share similar primary structures (Newgard et al., 1989). Rabbit muscle phosphorylase uses glycogen (branched glucan with longer chains) and amylopectin (branched glucan with shorter chains), as good substrate but poorly amylose (long linear glucan) and maltodextrin (short linear glucan). Glycogen is bound to the rabbit enzyme through two glucan-binding sites, the active site containing the coenzyme and the glycogen-storage site (Kasvinsky et al., 1978) with much higher affinity, as illustrated in Fig. 1.

168

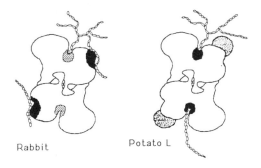

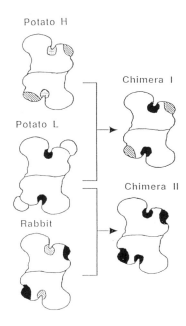

Figure 1. (upper) Hypothetical binding mode of linear and branched glucans to rabbit muscle phosphorylase dimer and potato type L phosphorylase isozyme dimer. See text for explanation.

Figure 2. (right) Schematic drawing for the preparation of the chimeric enzymes I and II from the parent phosphorylases (potato type L and H isozymes and rabbit muscle enzyme). Darker areas show higher affinity for glucans. See text for further explanation.

On the other hand, higher plant tissues contain two isozymes that are different from each other in the molecular size, the subcellular localization, and the substrate specificity (Fukui et al., 1987). The type L isozyme prefers maltodextrin, amylose, and amylopectin to glycogen as substrate, whereas the type H isozyme exhibits very high affinity for various glucans including glycogen and maltodextrin. The amino acid sequences of the two isozymes show considerably high similarity, except for a lengthy insertion consisting of 78 amino acid residues that occurs in the middle of the polypeptide chain of the type L isozyme (Mori et al., 1991). Thus, the low affinity for glycogen of the type L isozyme was explained by the presence of the 78-residue insertion, which is putatively located beside the mouth of the active-site cleft and exerts steric hindrance for large, highly branched glucans approaching the active site (Nakano and Fukui, 1986), as illustrated in Fig. 1. To prove this hypothesis and investigate the molecular basis for the glucan specificity of phosphorylases, we have constructed two chimeric enzymes (Fig. 2) and measured their kinetic parameters and dissociation constants to compare with those of the parent enzymes.

Chimeric Enzymes

For preparing the chimeric enzyme I, an about 570-base pair fragment encoding the 78-residue insertion (residue 414-491) and its flanking regions (residue 363-413 and 492-551) of the type L isozyme cDNA was replaced with an about 330-base pair fragment encoding the corresponding region (residue 363-474) of the type H isozyme (Mori et al., 1993a). Thus, the constructed plasmid encodes the chimeric enzyme consisting mainly of the type L isozyme with 112 residues from the type H isozyme in the middle of the polypeptide chain. On the other hand, an about 330-base pair fragment from the rabbit muscle enzyme cDNA encoding residues 363-474 of the animal enzyme involving the region for the glycogen-storage site was inserted into the type L isozyme cDNA at the same position as above (Mori et al., 1993b). The plasmid thus constructed encodes the chimeric enzyme II, consisting mainly of the type L isozyme with 112 residues from the rabbit enzyme that is located in the middle of the polypeptide chain. Both chimeric enzymes were expressed in *Escherichia coli* BL21(DE3) cells and purified by chromatographies on DEAE-cellulose and glycogen-Sepharose columns. The purified enzymes were homogeneous on sodium dodecyl sulfate-polyacrylamide gel electrophoresis, giving each single band of molecular weight 95,000. This value differed from the molecular weight of the type L isozyme (104,000) by about 9,000 due to the absence of the 78-residue insertion, as expected. The specific activities of the purified chimeric enzymes I and II were 5.7 and 26.5 units/mg, respectively, while that of the recombinant type-L isozyme was 28.7 units/mg (Mori et al., 1993a,b).

Kinetic Parameters

Steady-state kinetic parameters of the purified chimeric enzymes I and II were determined in the synthesis with maltopentaose as acceptor and the degradation of glycogen, amylopectin, and amylose as substrate. Table I summarizes the Michaelis constant (K_m) values of the two chimeric enzymes, in comparison with those of the parent enzymes. The chimeric enzyme I had the lowest K_m values for substrates including maltopentaose, while showing smaller V_{max} values than the parent isozymes (data not shown). The chimeric enzyme II had very high V_{max} values, comparable to that of the parent type L isozyme in glucan synthesis though less than half in the degradation (data not shown). All K_m values of chimeric enzyme I for maltopentaose, glucose-1-phosphate,

Table I. K_m values of α-glucan phosphorylases (Mori et al., 1993a,b)

Enzyme	K_m (mM)			K_m (μg/ml)		
	Glucose-1-*P*	P_i	Maltopentaose	Glycogen	Amylopectin	Amylose
Potato H	5.4	1.4	1.1	9.8	3.6	43
Chimera I	2.1	0.76	0.04	24	5.3	9.8
Potato L	3.0	1.4	0.13	10,000	82	37
Chimera II	3.0	0.78	0.14	6.2	4.3	19
Rabbit muscle	nd	nd	16	66	310	470

nd, not determined

and P$_i$ were all comparable with that of the type L isozyme. The chimeric enzyme I had K_m values for branched glucans much lower than the type L isozyme, and the values were comparable with those of the type H isozyme. In contrast, the K_m values of the chimeric enzyme I for linear glucans were much lower than those of the parent enzymes. The chimeric enzyme II showed an extraordinarily small K_m value for glycogen, which is even smaller than those of the rabbit muscle enzyme and potato type H isozymes. The V_{max} values of the chimeric enzymes I and II were mostly higher with linear glucans as substrate than with branched glucans (data not shown).

Dissociation Constants

Affinity of phosphorylase for various glucans are roughly estimated from electrophoretic mobilities of the enzyme in polyacrylamide gel containing glucans (Shimomura and Fukui, 1980). Because reciprocal plots of the measured mobilities of the two chimeric enzymes against concentrations of amylopectin or glycogen yielded straight lines (data not shown), apparent dissociation constant (K_d) values for those glucans were calculated from the slopes in these plots (Table II). Although the K_d values obtained did not perfectly coincide with the K_m values obtained, the two chimeric enzymes have much higher affinity for both glycogen and amylopectin than the parent enzymes. In particular, the K_d value for glycogen of the chimeric enzyme II was smallest even compared with the type H isozyme and the rabbit enzyme. The inhibition constant (K_i) values for a mobile ligand were also determined from the electrophoretic mobilities of the enzyme in the presence of a series of fixed concentrations of maltopentaose at various concentrations of immobilized glucan (Table II). The K_i values obtained also did not correspond with the K_m values for maltopentaose; the rabbit muscle enzyme as well as the type H isozyme had K_i values much smaller than their K_m values, indicating that the K_i for maltopentaose represents competition with glycogen binding at the storage site. Conversely, the type L isozyme and the two chimeric enzymes had K_i values considerably larger than the K_m values, which probably reflect the high affinity of the active site of the type L isozyme for maltopentaose.

Table II. Apparent K_d and K_i values (µg/ml) of α-glucan phosphorylases (Mori et al., 1993a,b)

Enzymes	Glycogen	Amylose	Maltopentaose
Potato H	5.6	1.3	27
Chimera I	79	7.5	45
Potato L	52,000	1,900	2,400
Chimera II	0.81	1.6	1,200
Rabbit muscle	75	15	780

Conclusion

The present results described above lead to the conclusion that the 78-residue insertion occurring apart from the active site of the type L isozyme causes steric hindrance for large, branched glucan molecules approaching the active site. The steric hindrance due to this bulky insertion over the active site also explains the marked discrepancy between K_m and K_d values determined for amylopectin of the type L isozyme. On the other hand, K_m values for maltopentaose of the chimeric enzyme I and the type L isozyme are much lower than that of the type H isozyme. This conclusion is consistent with the previous observation that the modification of the coenzyme site lowered the affinity for glucans of the potato type L isozyme but not of the rabbit muscle enzyme (Shimomura and Fukui, 1980), and suggests that the active site of the type L isozyme as well as that of the chimeric enzyme I consisting of residues of only the type L isozyme have high affinity for short sugar chains. The chimeric enzyme II showing extraordinarily high affinity for a variety of glucans is the first successful example in engineering of phosphorylase toward improvement of the substrate-binding properties. In this chimeric enzyme, the markedly increased affinity for large, branched substrates may be provided from the introduced glycogen-storage site of the rabbit enzyme and from the removal of the steric hindrance due to the 78-residue insertion of the parent type L isozyme, while the high affinity for linear glucans afforded by the active site of the type L isozyme is maintained.

References

Fukui, T., Nakano, K., Tagaya, M., and Nakayama, H. (1987) Phosphorylase isozymes of higher plants. In: Korpela, T., and Christen, P. (eds.): Biochemistry of Vitamin B$_6$, Birkhauser Verlag, Boston, pp. 267-276.

Kasvinsky, P.J., Madsen, N.B., Fletterick, R.J., and Sygusch, J. (1978) X-ray crystallographic and kinetic studies of oligosaccharide binding to phosphorylase. *J. Biol. Chem.* 253: 1290-1296.

Mori, H., Tanizawa, K., and Fukui, T. (1991) Potato tuber type H phosphorylase isozyme: Molecular cloning, nucleotide sequence, and expression of a full-length cDNA in *Escherichia coli*. *J. Biol. Chem.* 266: 18446-18453.

Mori, H., Tanizawa, K., and Fukui, T. (1993a) A chimeric α-glucan phosphorylase of plant type L and H isozymes. *J. Biol. Chem.* 268: 5574-5581.

Mori, H., Tanizawa, K., and Fukui, T. (1993b) Engineered plant phosphorylase showing extraordinarily high affinity for various α-glucan molecules. *Protein Sci.* 2: 1621-1629.

Nakano, K., and Fukui, T. (1986) The complete amino acid sequence of potato α-glucan phosphorylase. *J. Biol. Chem.* 261: 8230-8236.

Newgard, C.B., Hwang, P.K., and Fletterick, R.J. (1989) The family of glycogen phosphorylases: Structure and function. *Crit. Rev. Biochem. Mol. Biol.* 24: 69-99.

Shimomura, S., and Fukui, T. (1980) A comparative study on α-glucan phosphorylases from plant and animal: Interrelationship between the polysaccharide and pyridoxal phosphate binding sites by affinity electrophoresis. *Biochemistry* 19: 2287-2294.

Biochemistry of Vitamin B₆ and PQQ
G. Marino, G. Sannia and F. Bossa (eds.)
© 1994 Birkhäuser Verlag Basel/Switzerland

Slow conformational transitions of muscle glycogen phosphorylase *b*

B.I. Kurganov and E.I. Schors

A. N. Bach Institute of Biochemistry, Russian Academy of Sciences, Leninsky prospect 33, Moscow 117071, Russia

Summary

The effect of specific ligands (the substrate glucose 1-phosphate, AMP, and flavins) on the initial rate of tryptic digestion of muscle glycogen phosphorylase *b* has been studied (0.02 M HEPES, pH 6.8; 37°C). Differences were observed between the kinetic curves of the enzyme trypsinolysis initiated by the addition of a trypsin/ligand mixture and once trypsin was added to the enzyme preincubated with a ligand for 10 min. It was suggested that the specific ligands studied induce relatively slow conformational changes in the phosphorylase *b* molecule.

Introduction

Muscle glycogen phosphorylase (1,4-α-D-glucan: orthophosphate α-D-glucosyltransferase, EC 2.4.1.1) is the first enzyme for which the phenomenon of allosteric regulation was discovered. The allosteric regulation of the enzyme is realized via the binding of a metabolite-regulator at a definite site, spatially removed from the active site. Conformational changes induced by the binding of an allosteric effector cause changes in the enzyme catalytic efficiency. The glycogen phosphorylase molecule is a dimer consisting of two identical subunits with a molecular mass of 97 400 Da each. The enzyme's dephosphorylated form (form *b*) requires AMP to become catalytically active. The AMP-binding site (activatory allosteric site) is 3.2 nm distant from the active site. Apart from the active site and the activatory allosteric site, each subunit contains an inhibitory allosteric site capable of binding various heterocyclic compounds (adenosine, caffeine, flavins). Structural changes accompanying the allosteric transition of phosphorylase *b* from the inactive state into the active one were studied by Barford and Johnson (1989) by X-ray crystallography. The recent review by Johnson et al. (1989) summarizes the current knowledge on the structure and properties of phosphorylase *b*.

The goal of the present work is to study the conformational changes in muscle phosphorylase *b* induced by specific ligands (substrates and allosteric effectors) using the method of tryptic digestion of the enzyme.

Materials and Methods

Rabbit muscle phosphorylase *b* was prepared by the method of Fischer and Krebs (1962), using mercaptoethanol instead of cysteine, and recrystallized four times. A Sephadex G-25 column was used to separate AMP from the enzyme. HEPES was purchased from Serva (Germany), trypsin, AMP, and riboflavin from Reanal (Hungary), glucose 1-phosphate from Sigma (USA), FMN and FAD from Vitaminy (Moscow).

Phosphorylase *b* concentration was determined spectrophotometrically using an absorbance index of 13.0 for 1% protein solution. Flavin concentrations were detected spectro-photometrically using the following molar absorption coefficients: 1.23×10^4 $M^{-1}cm^{-1}$ for riboflavin (445 nm), 1.25×10^4 $M^{-1}cm^{-1}$ for FMN, and 1.13×10^4 $M^{-1}cm^{-1}$ for FAD.

Phosphorylase *b* was digested with trypsin at 37°C in 0.02 M HEPES, pH 6.8. Proteolytic digestion was followed by monitoring the decrease in the phosphorylase *b* fluorescence intensity at 335 nm (excitation at 290 nm) as described elsewhere (Kurganov, Lissovskaya and Livanova, 1972). Fluorescence was measured on a Hitachi fluorescence spectrophotometer MPF-4 (Japan) equipped with a thermostated cell holder. The values of fluorescence intensity of the phosphorylase *b*/trypsin mixture were corrected for the trypsin fluorescence intensity.

Results

The tryptic digestion of phosphorylase *b* is accompanied by a decrease in the protein fluorescence intensity (excitation at 290 nm) and a simultaneous bathochromic shift of the emission maximum. Such changes in the phosphorylase *b* fluorescence result from the exposure of the tryptophan residues of the enzyme molecule into the aqueous environment during proteolytic digestion. Therefore, we can monitor the digestion kinetics by the decrease in the enzyme fluorescence.

Figure 1,*a* illustrates the decrease in the relative fluorescence intensity of phosphorylase *b* (I/I_o) throughout the tryptic digestion process (curve *1*). It can be seen that the kinetic curve is linear at least within 400 s. The initial part of the kinetic curve remains linear when the enzyme is preincubated with 10 μM FAD for 10 min before the addition of trypsin (curve *2*). FAD appeared to protect phosphorylase *b* from proteolysis. Another pattern is observed when proteolysis is initiated by the addition of a trypsin/FAD mixture to phosphorylase *b* (curve *3*). In this case the kinetic curve was characterized by a continuously decreasing rate of trypsinolysis. As for the initial rate of trypsinolysis, it coincided with the corresponding value obtained in the absence of FAD. Riboflavin and FMN affect the rate of phosphorylase *b* digestion in a similar manner as FAD. However, the protective effect of FMN is more pronounced, compared to other flavins, so our further studies of the influence of flavins on tryptic digestion of phosphorylase *b* involved FMN. The results obtained indicate that flavin-induced conformational changes in the phosphorylase *b* molecule, leading to the enhancement of the enzyme resistance to the tryptic attack, progress slowly, with the time of half-conversion being of the order of tens of seconds.

Special experiments were performed to prove reversibility of the protective action of FMN (Fig. 2). The initial rate of trypsinolysis of phosphorylase *b* preincubated with 40 μM FMN for 10 min before the addition of trypsin (curve *3*) is 4.4 times lower than that in the absence of FMN (curve *1*). If phosphorylase *b* preincubated with 40 μM FMN for 10 min is 40-fold diluted and trypsin is added after 10-min incubation of the diluted solution (the final concentration of FMN is 1 μM), the initial trypsinolysis rate (curve *4*) is equal to that in the presence of 1 μM FMN (curve *2*; trypsinolysis is initiated by the trypsin addition to phosphorylase *b* preincubated with 1 μM FMN for 10 min). These results evidence the reversible character of the protective action of FMN. The rate of trypsinolysis initiated by the addition of phosphorylase *b* preincubated with 40 μM FMN for 10 min to trypsin solution (the final concentration of FMN is 1 μM) would be expected to rise due to the slow transition back into the initial conformational state, which is less resistant to the trypsin attack. The character of curve *5* confirms the prediction.

In order to characterize the velocity of the FMN-induced conformational changes in the phosphorylase *b* molecule, we studied the dependence of the initial rate of trypsinolysis

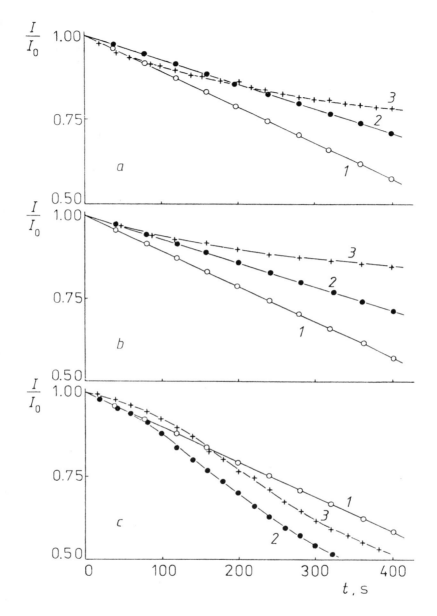

Fig. 1. Effect of FAD (10 μM, *a*), AMP (200 μM, *b*) and glucose 1-phosphate (20 mM, *c*) on the kinetics of tryptic digestion of phosphorylase *b*. Relative intensity of protein fluorescence (I/I_o) versus time *t* is plotted. 0.02 M HEPES, pH 6.8; 37°C. *1*, digestion in the absence of ligand; *2* and *3*, digestion in the presence of the ligand (trypsinolysis was initiated by the addition of trypsin or a trypsin/ligand mixture, respectively).

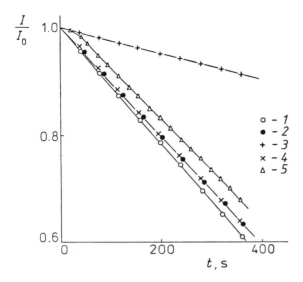

Fig. 2. Experiments demonstrating the reversibility of the protective action of FMN. *1*, trypsinolysis in the absence of FMN; *2*, trypsinolysis initiated by the addition of trypsin to phosphorylase *b* preincubated with 1 μM FMN for 10 min; *3*, trypsinolysis initiated by the addition of trypsin to phosphorylase *b* preincubated with 40 μM FMN for 10 min; *4*, phosphorylase *b* was preincubated with 40 μM FMN for 10 min, followed by a 40-fold dilution, whereupon trypsin was added; *5*, trypsinolysis initiated by the addition of phosphorylase *b* preincubated with 40 μM FMN for 10 min to a trypsin solution; the final concentration of FMN was 1 μM.

$w_0 = d(I/I_0)/dt$ $(t \rightarrow 0)$ on the duration of enzyme preincubation with FMN (Fig. 3). The decrease in the w_0 value is due to the transition of the enzyme into the state more resistant to trypsin attack. At 10 μM FMN, the time of half-conversion for conformational changes in phosphorylase *b* is about 2.4 min.

Our study of the effect of the allosteric activator (AMP) on the rate of phosphorylase *b* trypsinolysis revealed a difference between the kinetic curves of digestion: one curve characterizing the reaction started by the addition of trypsin to phosphorylase *b* preincubated with AMP (curve *2* in Fig. 1,*b*), and the other, by the addition of a trypsin/AMP mixture to phosphorylase *b* (Fig. 1,*b*, curve *3*). This indicates that AMP is able to induce relatively slow conformational changes in the phosphorylase *b* molecule.

Analysis of the influence of the substrate glucose 1-phosphate on the initial rate of trypsinolysis of phosphorylase *b* is complicated because of the gradual proteolysis acceleration. Nevertheless, the comparison of curves *2* and *3* in Fig. 1,*c* that feature the proteolytic processes

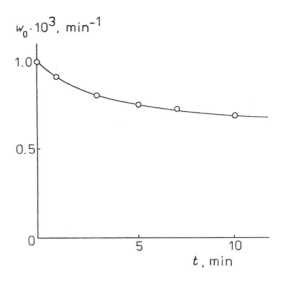

Fig.3. The initial rate of tryptic digestion (w_0) as a function of the time of phosphorylase b incubation with FMN (10 μM).

initiated by the addition of trypsin to phosphorylase b preincubated in the presence or in the absence of glucose 1-phosphate, respectively, shows that the substrate binding induces slow conformational changes in the enzyme molecule.

Discussion

The study of the effects of specific ligands on the rate of proteolysis of an enzyme may help to characterize the ligand-induced conformational changes in the enzyme molecule. The approach was used, for example, by Marshall and Fahien (1988) for rat carbamoyl-phosphate synthetase I and by Smith and Wilson (1991) for rat brain hexokinase. The present paper demonstrates other possibilities of this approach once the proteolytic process is traced continuously. Measurements of the initial rate of tryptic digestion of muscle glycogen phosphorylase b allowed us to observe relatively slow conformational changes in the enzyme molecule induced by the binding of the substrate glucose 1-phosphate and the allosteric effectors (flavins and AMP), with the time of half-conversion being of the order of a few minutes.

It should be noted that there are many sites for tryptic attack in the phosphorylase b molecule. This means that the initial rate of trypsinolysis and the character of action of specific ligands on digestion depend on the method used for recording the digestion kinetics. If the kinetics of digestion is followed by a decrease in phosphorylase b fluorescence, the relative initial rate of proteolysis w_0 is equal to 1.0×10^{-3} min^{-1} (pH 6.8; 37°C). Meanwhile, under the same conditions the enzymatic activity of phosphorylase b declines markedly faster: the relative initial rate of the enzymatic activity decrease is equal to 0.2 min^{-1} (Kurganov et al., 1993).

There are numerous experimental data demonstrating that the kinetics of conformational changes induced by specific ligands may be characterized by the time of half-conversion being of the order of several minutes (Kurganov, 1982). Slow conformational transitions of the enzyme molecule are manifested as a lag-period or a burst on the curves of the time-dependent accumulation of the enzymatic reaction product. The physiological significance of slow changes in the conformation of the enzyme molecule (and, consequently, of slow changes in the catalytic properties of the enzyme) is that such "hysteretic" properties smooth over the alterations of enzyme activities when concentrations of metabolites change drastically (Frieden, 1970, 1979; Neet and Ainslie, 1980).

According to the findings the present study, muscle glycogen phosphorylase b may be classified as a "hysteretic" enzyme. Further studies are needed to elucidate the role of slow conformational transitions in the enzymatic process catalyzed by phosphorylase b.

This work was supported by Grant 93-04-7784 from the Russian Foundation for Basic Research.

References

Barford, D., and Johnson, L.N. (1989) The allosteric transition of glycogen phosphorylase. *Nature* 340: 609-616.

Johnson, L.N., Hajdu, J., Acharya, K.R., Stuart, D.I., McLaughlin, P.I., Oikonomakos, N.G., and Barford, D. (1989) Glycogen phosphorylase b. In: Herve, G. (ed.): *Allosteric Enzymes*, CRC Press, Boca Raton, pp. 81-127.

Fisher, E.H., and Krebs, E.G. (1962) Muscle phosphorylase b. In: Kaplan, N.O. (ed.): *Methods in Enzymology*, vol.5, Academic Press, New York, pp. 369-373.

Kurganov, B.I., Lissovskaya, N.P., and Livanova, N.B. (1972) On the spatial distinction of ligand-binding sites in phosphorylase b. *Biokhimiya* 37: 289-298 (In Russian).

Marshall, M., and Fahien, L.A. (1988) Proteolysis as a probe of ligand-associated conformational changes in rat carbamyl phosphate synthetase I. *Arch. Biochem. Biophys.* 262: 455-470.

Smith, A.D., and Wilson, J.E. (1991) Effect of ligand binding on the tryptic digestion pattern of rat brain hexokinase: relationship of ligand-induced conformational changes to catalytic and regulatory functions. *Arch. Biochem. Biophys.* 291: 59-68.

Kurganov, B.I., Schors, E.I., Livanova, N.B., Chebotareva, N.A., Eronina, T.B., Andreeva, I.E., Makeeva, V.Ph., and Pekel', N.D. (1993) Effect of flavins on the rate of proteolytic digestion of muscle glycogen phosphorylase *b*. *Biochimie* 75: 481-485.

Kurganov, B.I. (1982) *Allosteric Enzymes. Kinetic Behaviour*. John Wiley & Sons, Chichester, 344 pp.

Frieden, C. (1970) Kinetic aspects of regulation of metabolic processes. The hysteretic enzyme concept. *J. Biol. Chem.* 245: 5788-5799.

Frieden, C. (1979) Slow transitions and hysteretic behavior in enzymes. *Annu. Rev. Biochem.* 48: 471-489.

Neet, K.E., and Ainslie, G.R. (1980) Hysteretic enzymes. In: Purich, D.L. (ed.): *Methods in Enzymology*, vol.64, *Enzyme Kinetics and Mechanisms*, Part B, Academic Press, New York, pp.192-226.

OTHER PYRIDOXAL-DEPENDENT ENZYMES

Biochemistry of Vitamin B$_6$ and PQQ
G. Marino, G. Sannia and F. Bossa (eds.)
© 1994 Birkhäuser Verlag Basel/Switzerland

X-ray study of tryptophanase at 2.1 Å resolution

M. Isupov[1], I. Dementieva[2], L. Zakomirdina[2], K.S. Wilson[3], Z. Dauter[3], A.A. Antson[4], G.G. Dodson[4] and E.G. Harutyunyan[1]

[1] *Shubnikov Institute of Crystallography, Moscow, Russia;* [2] *Engelhardt Institute of Molecular Biology, Moscow, Russia;* [3] *EMBL, Hamburg, Germany;* [4] *University of York, Dept.of Chemistry, York, England*

Summary

Holotryptophanase from *Proteus vulgaris* was crystallized in the presence of K$^+$. The structure was solved at 2.1 Å resolution by molecular replacement technique and refined to descrepancy factor R=15.6%. Each subunit of the tetramer consists of a large and a small domain. The folding of the PLP-binding domain is similar to that of some PLP-dependent enzymes. PLP-binding site is formed by two subunits. Potassium ions (one per subunit) are localized in the interior between two subunits of "catalytical" dimer.

Tryptophanase (Tnase, tryptophan indole-lyase; EC 4.1.99.1) is a bacterial pyridoxal-P (PLP)-dependent enzyme which catalyzes α,β-elimination and β-replacement reactions on interaction with L-tryptophan and many other β-substituted L-amino acids (Snell, 1975). The active molecule consists of four identical subunits with one molecule of PLP per subunit bound through a Schiff base linkage to ε-amino group of lysine residue. The monovalent cations (NH$_4^+$, K$^+$ or Rb$^+$) are essential for Tnase activity, Na$^+$ ions inactivate the enzyme.

Crystals of holoTnase from *P.vulgaris* with P2$_1$2$_1$2$_1$ space group, a=113.6 Å, b=114.6 Å, c=151.4 Å were obtained by hanging-drop technique using polyethylene glycol 4000 as precipitant in the presence of potassium ions. Asymmetric unit contains one molecule of the enzyme. The 2.1 Å data set (117863 unique reflections) was collected on EMBL wiggler beam line BW7, at DESY, Hamburg.

Atomic model of tyrosine phenol-lyase (TPL) (Antson et al., 1993) having 50% similarity in amino acid sequence with Tnase (Kamath et al., 1993) was used for structure solution of Tnase by molecular replacement method (Navaza, 1992). All residues 2-466, except the N- and C-terminal ones, in each of the four subunits were localized and refined. Final model includes 14712 protein atoms, 4 coenzyme molecules, 1750 water molecules and 4 potassium ions. Discrepancy factor R=15.6%. Accuracy of atomic co-ordinates is better than 0.2 Å.

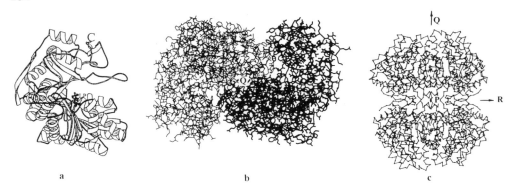

Figure 1. Ribbon representation of the Tnase subunit. PLP-molecule is shown (a). Scheleton model of "catalytical" dimer viewed along Q molecular double axis (b). C_α-tracing of polypeptide chain in the Tnase tetramer viewed along P molecular double axes (c). "Catalytical" dimers are connected by horizontal R molecular double axis.

Each α/β type subunit comprises PLP-binding large domain (residues 51-320), small domain (residues 20-50 and 321-467), and the N-terminal segment (Fig.1,a). The structure of the large PLP-binding domain is conserved in most of the studied PLP-dependent enzymes (transaminases, TPL, dialkylglycine decarboxylase). It consists of seven-stranded β-sheet of mixed type, surrounded by α-helices. The small domain core is formed by a four-stranded antiparallel β-sheet. The overall number of α-helices in the subunit equals 14. The two subunits form the so-called "catalytical" dimer. Active sites of these subunits are located between the small and the large domains of the subunit and the large domain of the neighbor one (Fig.1,b). The N-terminal segments of each subunit of the "catalytical" dimer and fragments 57-59 form an intersubunit four-stranded β-sheet with analogous fragments of the neighbor dimer. The tertiary structure of Tnase molecule is rather similar to that of TPL. Four subunits occupy the vertices of tetrahedron with 222 point symmetry (Fig.1,c). They form a common hydrophobic cluster in the center of the molecule.

Spatial arrangement of the amino acid residues at the PLP-binding site (Fig.2) is also similar to those in the other PLP-dependent enzymes. Phosphate group of coenzyme makes hydrogen bonds with the main chain nitrogens of Gly 100 and Arg 101, side chains of Arg 101, Gln 99, Ser 263 and via ordered water molecules with Ser 52, Lys 265, Tyr 72 and Tyr 301. The last two residues belong to neighboring subunits. The C5'-O5'-phosphate bond of PLP is nearly perpendicular to the plane of the pyridine ring as in aspartate aminotransferase and tryptophan synthase. Internal Schiff base is formed by Lys 266. As in some other PLP enzymes the aromatic residue (Phe 132) forms a stacking pair with the pyridine ring

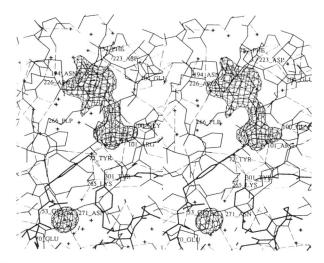

Figure 2. Stereo pairs of the difference electron density map at the binding sites of PLP-molecule and K^+. The map is contoured at the 5 σ level.

of PLP molecule. The pyridine nitrogen atom interacts with the β-carboxyl group of Asp 223; O3' oxygen of PLP ring is close to side chains of Asn 194 and Arg 226. The Arg 414 of Tnase lies closest to the substrate α-carboxyl binding residue Arg 386 of aspartate aminotransferase when these structures are superimposed by β-sheets of large domains. The potassium ions are located between the two subunits of the "catalytical" dimer. Each K^+ is linked by carbonyl and carboxyl oxygen atoms of GLu 70 of one subunit and carbonyl oxygen atoms of Gly 53 and Asn 271 of the other one and binds three water molecules. Interactions K^+ — W $\cdots$ N_ε Lys 265 $\cdots$ W $\cdots$ PO_4 (PLP) are found in the active site region.

Structural bases of Tnase catalytical mechanism are under study. X-ray investigation of crystalline complexes with α-methyl-DL-tryptophan (Michaelis complex) and oxindolyl-L-alanine (quinonoid intermediate) is in progress.

This work was supported partly by the Russian Foundation for Fundamental Research grant (93-04-7923) and the NATO Collaboration Research grant (920962).

References

Antson, A.A., Demidkina, T.V., Gollnick, P., Dauter, Z., Von Tersch, R.L., Long, J., Berezhnoy, S.N., Phillips, R.S., Harutyunyan, E.H. & Wilson, K.S. (1993). Three-dimensional structure of tyrosine phenollyase. *Biochemistry* 32:4195-4206.

Kamath, A.V. & Yanofsky, C. (1992). Characterization of the tryptophanase operon of *Proteus vulgaris*. Cloning, nucleotide sequence, aminoacid homology and *in vitro* synthesis of the leader peptide and regulatory analysis. *J.Biol.Chem.* 267: 19978-19985.

Navaza, J. (1992). AMoRe: A new package for molecular replacement. In: *Proc.of the CCP4 Study Weekend*. SERC Daresbury Laboratory. U.K., pp.87-90.

Snell, E.E. (1975). Tryptophanase: structure, catalytic activities, and mechanism of action. *Advan.Enzymol.* 42:287-333.

Biochemistry of Vitamin B$_6$ and PQQ
G. Marino, G. Sannia and F. Bossa (eds.)
© 1994 Birkhäuser Verlag Basel/Switzerland

Crystallographic studies of tyrosine phenol-lyase

A.A. Antson, G.G. Dodson, K.S. Wilson[1], S.V. Pletnev[2], E.G. Harutyunyan[2]
and T.V. Demidkina[3]

York University, York, UK
[1]*European Molecular Biology Laboratory, Hamburg Outstation, Germany*
[2]*Shubnikov Institute of Crystallography, Moscow, Russia*
[3]*Engelhardt Institute of Molecular Biology, Moscow, Russia*

Summary

Monovalent cation binding site of the enzyme was determined using X-ray data obtained from apoenzyme crystals soaked in K$^+$ and Cs$^+$ containing solutions. Glu 69 is involved in formation of that site and is conserved in all other tyrosine phenol-lyases and tryptophan indol-lyases with known sequence. Three dimensional structures of holoenzyme and its complex with 3-(4-hydroxyphenyl)propionic acid were solved and refined at 2.7Å and 2.5 Å respectively. The structures explicitly reveal the cofactor and substrate binding pockets.

Introduction

Tyrosine phenol-lyase (TPL) (EC.4.1.99.2) from *Citrobacter intermedius* is pyridoxal-P (PLP) dependent enzyme catalyzing series of β-elimination, β-replacement and racemization reactions (Yamada and Kumagai, 1975) and side transamination reaction (Demidkina et al., 1987). The enzyme consists of four identical subunits (Kazakov et al., 1987). Monovalent cations are obligatory for the functioning of TPL (Toryata et al., 1976; Demidkina et al., 1989). Three-dimensional structure of apoenzyme has been recently solved and refined at 2.3Å resolution and Lys 257 has been shown to be PLP binding residue (Antson et al., 1993). The tetrameric molecule of TPL can be subdivided into two equivalent dimers each having domain architecture similar to that found in molecule of aspartate aminotransferase (Ford et al., 1980). Each subunit of TPL could be subdivided into a small and a large domain. Lys 257 is located at the interface between large and small domains of one subunit and large domain of adjacent subunit of the dimer. The three dimensional structure of apo-TPL resembles a matrix which is now being used for structural studies of other tyrosine phenol-lyases and a number of tryptophan indol-lyases (Tnases) (EC 4.1.99.1) (Dementieva et al., 1994). Here we described crystallographic studies of TPL from *Citrobacter intermedius* to find out monovalent cation, PLP and substrate binding residues. These studies were performed by soaking the apoenzyme crystals and also via co-crystallization of TPL with PLP and substrate analogue, 3-(4-hydroxyphenyl)propionic acid.

Results and discussion

Location of the monovalent cation binding site

Crystals of holoenzyme, containing K^+ or Cs^+ cations were obtained by soaking the apoenzyme crystals with PLP in the presence of KCl or CsCl. Diffraction data from crystals which belong to the space group $P2_12_12$, were collected using synchrotron radiation. Cation binding sites were determined from a difference Fourier synthesis calculated with coefficients $(|F_{Cs}|-|F_K|) \exp(i\alpha_K)$, where $|F_{Cs}|$ and $|F_K|$ are amplitudes of the structure factors for the complexes with PLP in KCl and CsCl containing solutions respectively; α_K are phases calculated from refined model of the complex in KCl. Highest peaks on that synthesis which were ascribed to the cation sites, with maximum at a level of about 10 r.m.s., are at least 2.5 times higher than any other peaks. Crystal structure of the complex with cofactor and K^+ has been refined to a crystallographic R-factor of 17.2% at 2.5Å. Cations are bound between the two subunits in the dimer (two cations per each dimer). Each is co-ordinated by two main chain oxygens of Gly 52 and Asn 262 from one subunit and by main chain and one of the side chain oxygens of Glu 69 from crystallographically related subunit. Monovalent cation binding site is in about 10Å from the phosphate of PLP. Glu 69, the only residue which contributes its side chain to the cation binding site is conserved in àll other TPLs and Tnases with known primary structure. Conformation of the cation binding site is conserved in recently solved *Proteus vulgaris* Tnase crystal structure (Isupov, 1994). Absence of monovalent cations would course weakening contacts between the two subunits in the diner. Substitution of K^+ by Na^+ might course conformational changes in the active site, like it was observed in the crystal structure of dialkylglycine decarboxylase (Toney et al., 1993).

Structure of holoenzyme

Crystals of the holoenzyme obtained with 5000 monomethyl ether polyethylene glycol as a precipitant, diffract up to 2.0Å resolution. However, they were of small size and so far the X-ray data have been collected to 2.7Å resolution using synchrotron radiation. Three-dimensional structure of holoenzyme has been refined to crystallographic R-factor of 19.9%.

Cofactor forms Schiff base with ε-amino group of Lys 257. Phosphate group of PLP is H-bonded by main chain nitrogens of Gly 99 and Arg 100 and also by side chain of Ser 254. C5'-O5'-phosphate bond of PLP is nearly orthogonal to the plane of pyridine ring. Like in pig cytosolic aspartate aminotransferase (Arnone et al., 1985) and Tnase from *Proteus vulgaris* (Isupov, 1994) the "phosphate handle" is placed behind pyridine ring. Nitrogen of pyridine ring is H-bonded to Asp 214 and O3' oxygen of PLP is H-bonded to Arg 217. Pyridine ring of cofactor makes a stacking interaction with phenol ring of Phe 123 which is nearly parallel to the plane of the pyridine ring.

Substrate binding site

Crystals of holoenzyme complex with 3-(4-hydroxyphenyl)propionic acid were obtained under conditions similar to those of holoenzyme. Three-dimensional structure of this complex has been refined to crystallographic R-factor of 18.9% at 2.5Å resolution. We believe that this complex mimics Michaelis complex as the ligand has all features of the natural substrate, L-tyrosine, except α-amino group. Figure 1 shows part of the active site where 3-(4-hydroxyphenyl)propionic acid is bound. Earlier the three-dimensional structures of aspartate aminotransferase and apo-TPL were compared. We postulated that Arg 404 should be responsible for the α-carboxylate binding (Antson et al., 1993). In fact carboxyl group of that tyrosine analogue is H-bonded by guanidinium group of Arg 404 and also by hydroxy group of Thr 49. Arg 404 is conserved in primary structures of TPL from *Citrobacter intermedius* and *Erwinia herbicola*, and also in primary structures of Tnase from *E. coli*, *Proteus vulgaris* and *Symbiobacterium thermophilum* (Isupov, 1994). The hydroxy group of the analogue is within hydrogen-bonding distance from guanidinium group of Arg 381, the only charged group which is close to the hydroxy group of 3-(4-hydroxyphenyl)propionic acid. It was postulated (Faleev et al., 1988) that substrate specificity of TPL is controlled on the stage of the elimination of the phenol moiety by two factors: one is the steric restrictions for a volume of the aromatic moieties of the substrates another is a basic group which abstracts the proton of phenol p-hydroxy group and should be strictly located at the active site of the enzyme. This base was shown to exhibit a pK of 8.0-8.2 (Kiick and Phillips, 1988a). On first glance it looks curious that Arg 381 may be this basic group as the pK value for an arginine side chain is normally 12.5. But we believe that a net of interactions in the vicinity of guanidinium group of Arg 381 which involves H-bounds between Glu -380, Ser 385 and Arg 381 is decreasing the pK of the Arg 381 to enable it to abstracts p-hydroxy proton of substrate. Further evidence that the Arg 381 may control the substrate specificity of TPL comes from the fact that it is conserved in *Citrobacter intermedius* and *Erwinia herbicola* enzymes, but not conserved in all Tnases mentioned above (Isupov, 1994). In *E. coli* Tnase a group with pK of 6.0 abstracts

190

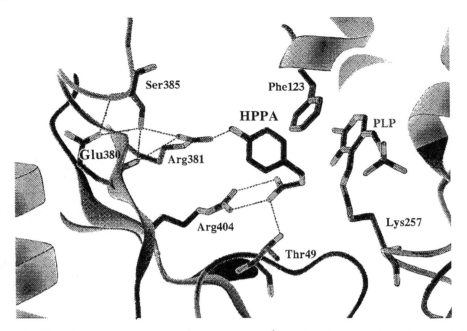

Figure 1. Ribbon diagram of TPL in the region of substrate binding cleft with some of the residues highlighted. Hydrogen bonds are shown by dashed lines. 3-(4-hydroxyphenyl)propionic acid is designated as HPPA.

the ring nitrogen proton of tryptophan (Kiick and Phillips, 1988b). In general, TPL and Tnase are characterized by broad substrate specificity towards a number of non physiological aromatic substrates. But they are strictly specific for their own natural substrates. Thus we believe that the substrate specificity in TPL is controlled by Arg 381 and in Tnase it is controlled by some other basic group.

This work was supported by NATO Collaborative Research Grants Programme (grant CRG920962) to T.V.D. and E.G.H., by the Russian Foundation for Fundamental Investigations (grant 93-04-7922) to T.V.D., and by the SERC (UK).

References

Antson, A.A, Demidkina, T.V., Gollnick, P., Dauter, Z., Von Tersch, R.L., Long, Y., Bereznoy, S.N., Phillips, R.S., Harutyunyan, E.H., and Wilson, K.S. (1993) Three-dimensional structure of tyrosine phenol-lyase. *Biochemistry* 32:4195-4206.

Arnone, A., Rogers, P.H., Hyde, C.C., Briley, P.D., Metzler, C.M. & Metzler, D.E. (1985). Pig cytosolic aspartate aminotransferase: the structures of the internal aldimine, external aldimine and ketimine and of the β-subform. In: P. Christen & D.E. Metzler (eds.): *Transaminases*, John Wiley & Sons, New York, pp. 138-155.

Dementieva, I.S., Zakomirdina, L.N., Sinitzina, N.I., Antson, A.A., Wilson, K.S., Isupov, M.N., Lebedev, A.A. and Harutyunyan, E.H. (1994) Crystallization and preliminary X-ray investigation of holotryptophanases from *Escherichia coli* and *Proteus vulgaris*. *J.Mol.Biol.* 235: 783-786.

Demidkina, T.V., Myagkikh, I.V. and Azhayev, A.V. (1987) Transamination catalyzed by tyrosine phenol-lyase from *Citrobacter intermedius*. *Eur.J.Biochem.* 170: 311-316.

Demidkina, T.V. and Myagkikh, I.V. (1989) The activity and reaction specificity of tyrosine phenol-lyase regulated by monovalent cations. *Biochimie* 71: 565-571.

Faleev, N.G., Ruvinov, S.B., Demidkina, T.V., Myagkikh, I.V., Gololobov, M.Yu., Bakhmutov, V.I. and Belikov, V.M. (1988) Tyrosine phenol-lyase from *Citrobacter intermedius*. Factors controlling substrate specificity. *Eur.J.Biochem.* 177: 395-401.

Ford, J.C., Eichele, G., Jansonius, J.N. (1980) Three-dimensional structure of a pyridoxal-phosphate dependent enzyme, mitochondrial aspartate aminotransferase. *Proc. Natl. Acad. Sci. US,.* 77: 2559-2563.

Isupov, M.N. (1994) Ph.D. thesis, Shubnikov Institute of Crystallography, Moscow.

Kazakov, V.K., Myagkikh, I.V., Tomina, I.I. and Demidkina, T.V., (1987) Identity of the subunits of *Citrobacter intermedius* tyrosine phenol-lyase. *Biokhimia* (Russian) 52: 1319-1323.

Kiick, D.M., Phillips, R.S. (1988a) Mechanistic deductions from kinetic isotope effect and pH studies of pyridoxal phosphate dependent carbon-carbon lyases: *Erwinia herbicola* and *Citrobacter freundii* tyrosine phenol-lyase. *Biochemistry* 27: 7333-7338.

Kiick, D.M., Phillips, R.S. (1988b) Mechanistic deductions from multiple kinetic and solvent deuterium isotope effects and pH studies of pyridoxal phosphate dependent carbon-carbon lyases: *Escherichia coli* tryptophan indole-lyase. *Biochemistry* 27: 7339-7344.

Toney, M.D., Hohenester, E., Cowan, S.W., Jansonius, J.N. (1993) Dialkylglycine decarboxylase structure: bifunctional active site and alkali metal sites. *Science* 261: 756-759.

Toraya, T., Nihira, T., and Fukui, S. (1976) Essential role of monovalent cations in the firm binding of pyridoxal-5'- phosphate to tryptophanase and β-tyrosinase. *Eur.J.Biochem.* 69: 411-419.

Yamada, H., and Kumagai, H. (1975) Synthesis of L-tyrosine related amino acids by β-tyrosinase. *Adv.Appl.Microbiol.* 19: 249-288.

Biochemistry of Vitamin B_6 and PQQ
G. Marino, G. Sannia and F. Bossa (eds.)
© 1994 Birkhäuser Verlag Basel/Switzerland

Studies of the Mechanism of Tyrosine Phenol-lyase: Kinetics and Site-Directed Mutagenesis

Robert S. Phillips, Haoyuan Chen and Paul Gollnick[1]

Departments of Chemistry and Biochemistry, and Center for Metalloenzyme Studies, University of Georgia, Athens, Georgia 30602, USA
[1]*Department of Biological Sciences, State University of New York at Buffalo, Buffalo, New York 14260, USA*

Summary

The binding of phenol and analogues to complexes of *Citrobacter freundii* tyrosine phenol-lyase (TPL) with L-alanine and D-alanine affects the equilibria between external aldimine and quinonoid complexes. The results demonstrate that there are two distinct quinonoid intermediates formed from either D- or L-alanine, and suggest that the interconversion of quinonoid intermediates is rate-limiting in the racemization of alanine. Histidine-343 is in the active site of TPL, and it was mutated to alanine to evaluate the role in catalysis. H343A TPL is active, indicating that this group is not one of the essential bases. However, the pH dependence of k_{cat} is changed, and the isotope effects with α-[^{2}H]-3-fluoro-L-tyrosine are greater for H343A TPL. Thus, His-343 appears to assist in promoting the conformational changes when substrates bind. Tyrosine-71 was also mutated to phenylalanine; however, the resultant mutant TPL has no detectable activity ($<10^{-4}$ %) with L-tyrosine. The Y71F mutant enzyme binds amino acids strongly and forms quinonoid intermediates very slowly, with intense absorbance at 500 nm. Thus, Tyr-71 appears to play an essential role in the mechanism of TPL.

Introduction

Tyrosine phenol-lyase (TPL) is a PLP-dependent enzyme which catalyses the reversible hydrolytic cleavage of L-tyrosine to produce phenol and ammonium pyruvate (Kumagai et al., 1970). TPL has been isolated from a number of microorganisms, including *Citrobacter intermedius (Escherichia intermedia)* (Kumagai et al., 1970; Demidkina et al., 1984), *Citrobacter freundii* (Carman and Levine, 1977), and *Erwinia herbicola* (Enei et al., 1973), and has recently been cloned from *C. freundii* and overexpressed in *E. coli* (Antson et al., 1993). This enzyme has been of considerable interest, not only because the mechanism involves a β-elimination with concomitant carbon-carbon bond cleavage, but also because the enzyme can be used for the *de novo* synthesis of L-tyrosine, L-dopa, and analogues by reversal of the reaction (Yamada et al., 1972). In addition to the physiological reaction, TPL also efficiently catalyses the β-elimination of a number of β-substituted amino acids with good leaving groups, such as S-methyl-L-cysteine, β-chloroalanine (Kumagai et al., 1970), and S-(*o*-nitrophenyl)-L-cysteine (SOPC) (Phillips, 1987). Moreover, TPL has been shown to catalyse the racemization of alanine, but at a much slower rate than the β-elimination reactions (Kumagai et al., 1970).

Experimental

Tyrosine phenol-lyase and mutants were purified from cells of *E. coli* SVS370 containing plasmid pTZTPL as described elsewhere (Chen and Phillips, submitted). The mutants were prepared using either the method of Eckstein (Taylor et al., 1985), using the kit purchased from Amersham, or the method of Kunkel (1985), using the kit purchased from Bio-Rad. Mutations were confirmed by DNA sequencing of the mutated region. Enzyme activity was measured either using SOPC at 370 nm (Phillips, 1987), or by following pyruvate ion formation at 340 nm using lactate dehydrogenase and NADH. Steady-state kinetic measurements were performed on either a Gilford Response or a Cary 1E, equipped with thermoelectric cell blocks. Rapid-scanning and single-wavelength stopped-flow kinetic measurements were performed using an instrument described previously (Phillips, 1991).

Results and Discussion

We have examined the racemization of alanine catalysed by *C. freundii* TPL using both steady-state and stopped-flow kinetic methods. The steady-state kinetic parameters for alanine racemization are: k_{cat}^D=.008 s^{-1}, K_m^D=32 mM, k_{cat}^L=.03 s^{-1}, K_m^L=11 mM, at pH 8 and 25 ° C (Chen and Phillips, 1993). Addition of either D- or L-alanine to solutions of TPL results in a prominent absorption band at 500 nm, assigned to a quinonoid intermediate. However, addition of K$^+$ *increases* the intensity of the quinonoid peak formed from L-alanine, but *decreases* it with D-alanine. Addition of phenols and analogues to these solutions also affects the intensity of the quinonoid band, indicating that phenols bind to the TPL-alanine complexes. Phenol decreases the quinonoid absorbance peak at 500 nm formed with either D- or L-alanine, while pyridine N-oxide and 4-hydroxypyridine increase the 500 nm absorbance. Rapid-scanning and single-wavelength stopped-flow spectrophotometry was then used to probe the mechanism of these effects. Phenol binds to all of the intermediates, but most strongly to the external aldimine, while pyridine N-oxide binds only to the quinonoid intermediate. The reaction of 4-hydroxypyridine is complex, with an absorbance *decrease* occurring in the fast phase, and a large absorbance *increase* occurring in a much slower second phase. Addition of 4-hydroxypyridine to TPL complexes of either L-alanine or D-alanine results in large increases in ellipticity of the 500 nm bands, and the CD spectra of these ternary complexes are identical. These data are consistent with the existence of two distinct quinonoid intermediates formed from D- or L-alanine. Since the rate constants for formation of the second quinonoid intermediate measured by stopped-flow methods are in good agreement with the steady-state k_{cat} values for the racemization reaction, we propose that the formation of this central quinonoid intermediate is the rate-determining step in the racemization of alanine (Chen and Phillips, 1993).

Recently, the three dimensional structure of apoTPL from *C. intermedius* was solved by x-ray crystallography (Antson et al., 1993), and this structure showed that His343 is near the PLP-binding residue, Lys257. This histidine residue is conserved in the sequences of TPL from other species, and in the sequences of tryptophan indole-lyase, a closely related enzyme. Previously, we demonstrated that TPL has two catalytically essential basic groups, with average pK_a values of 7.8, in the pH profile of k_{cat}/K_m for L-tyrosine. It seemed possible that His343 was one of these catalytic groups. Furthermore, since it had been proposed that TPL contains an essential histidine, as it is inactivated by modification with diethylpyrocarbonate (Kumagai et al., 1975), we mutated His343 to alanine using site-directed mutagenesis. The resultant H343A TPL exhibits about 10% of the activity of the wild-type enzyme with L-tyrosine (Table I), and also shows two pK_a's with average values of 7.8 in the pH profile of k_{cat}/K_m. Thus, His343 is not one of the catalytically essential bases. However, k_{cat} is pH independent for wild-type TPL, but is pH dependent for H343A TPL. The H343A mutant TPL also exhibits a significantly greater primary kinetic isotope effect ($^{H}k_{cat}/^{D}k_{cat}$=5.8) in the reaction of α-[^{2}H]-3-fluoro-L-tyrosine than does wild-type TPL ($^{H}k_{cat}/^{D}k_{cat}$=4.0). Compared with wild-type TPL, the H343 mutant TPL forms very weak absorbance at 500 nm when complexed with amino acids, indicating that the formation of quinonoid intermediates is unfavorable. In addition, the H343A TPL is inactivated by diethylpyrocarbonate in a pseudo-first order process, faster than the wild type TPL, which is inactivated in a pseudo-second order process. Thus, we conclude that His343 plays an important role in catalysing the conformational changes required for efficient formation of the quinonoid intermediates during catalysis (Chen and Phillips, submitted).

Table I. Steady-state Kinetic Constants for Wild-type and Mutant Forms of Tyrosine Phenol-lyase

Substrate	Wild-type TPL		H343A TPL		Y71F TPL	
	k_{cat}, (s^{-1})	k_{cat}/K_m (M^{-1} s^{-1})	k_{cat}, (s^{-1})	k_{cat}/K_m (M^{-1} s^{-1})	k_{cat}, (s^{-1})	k_{cat}/K_m (M^{-1} s^{-1})
L-Tyrosine	3.5	1.75×10^4	0.42	1.9×10^2	$<1.3 \times 10^{-5}$	
3-Fluoro-L-tyrosine	1.4	1.40×10^4	0.18	1.45×10^2		
SOPC	5.1	4.6×10^4	1.55	3.2×10^3	1.1×10^{-2}	1.6×10^2
S-Methyl-L-cysteine	0.9	2.8×10^2	0.15	12	3.8×10^{-4}	0.72
S-Ethyl-L-cysteine	3.9	4.9×10^2	1.4	1.2×10^3	2.2×10^{-4}	0.72
S-Benzyl-L-cysteine	0.5	2.7×10^3	0.02	17	1.2×10^{-4}	2.4
L-Serine	0.17	9.5	0.07	6		
L-Alanine	0.03	2.7				
D-Alanine	0.01	0.3	0.004	0.04		

Tyrosine 71 is also located in the active site region of TPL (Antson et al., 1993), in a location similar to that of Tyr-70, which hydrogen bonds to the phosphate of PLP in aspartate aminotransferase. Mutation of Tyr-71 to phenylalanine in TPL results in an enzyme which has no detectable activity with tyrosine as substrate (Table I), and very low but measurable activity with S-alkyl-L-cysteines and SOPC (Chen and Phillips, unpublished). This result is in sharp contrast to *E. coli* aspartate aminotransferase, the Y70F mutant of which has 8% activity (Toney and Kirsch, 1991; Inoue et al., 1991). In contrast to wild-type TPL and the H343A mutant, Y71F TPL forms very stable quinonoid complexes with L-tyrosine and other amino acids. Thus, this mutant may be useful for NMR and X-ray studies of the structures of amino acid complexes of TPL. These results suggest that Tyr-71 plays an essential role in the mechanism of TPL.

Acknowledgments

This work was partially supported by a grant from the National Institutes of Health (GM42588) to RSP.

References

Antson, A. A., Demidkina, T. V., Gollnick, P., Dauter, Z., Von Tersch, R. L., Long, J., Berezhnoy, S. N., Phillips, R. S., Harutyunyan, E. H. and Wilson, K., "Three-dimensional Structure of Tyrosine Phenol-lyase," (1993) *Biochemistry*, **32**, 4195-4206.

Carman, G. M. and Levine, R. E., "Partial Purification and some Properties of Tyrosine Phenol-lyase from *Aeromonas phenologenes* ATCC 29063," (1977) *Appl. Envir. Microbiol.*, **33**, 192-198.

Chen, H. and Phillips, R. S., "Binding of Phenol and Analogues to Alanine Complexes of Tyrosine Phenol-lyase from *Citrobacter Freundii*: Implications for the Mechanism of β-Elimination and Alanine Racemization", (1993), *Biochemistry*, **32**, 11591-11599.

Demidkina, T. V., Myagkikh, I. V., Faleev, N. G. and Belikov, V. M., "Isolation and Certain Properties of Tyrosine Phenol-lyase from *Citrobacter intermedius*," (1984) *Biokhim.*, **49**, 27-31 (Eng. Trans.).

Enei, H., Yamashita, K., Okumura, S. and Yamada, H., "Distribution of Tyrosine Phenol-lyase in Microorganisms," (1973) *Agric. Biol. Chem.*, **36**, 1861-1868.

Inoue, T., Kuramitsu, S., Okamoto, A., Hirotsu, K., Higuchi, T. and Kagamiyama, H., "Site-directed Mutagenesis of *Escherichia coli* Aspartate Aminotransferase: Role of Tyr70 in the Catalytic Process," (1991) *Biochemistry*, **30**, 7796-7801.

Kiick, D. M. and Phillips, R. S., "Mechanistic Deductions from Kinetic Isotope Effects and pH Studies of Pyridoxal Phosphate-dependent Carbon-carbon Lyases: *Erwinia herbicola* and *Citrobacter freundii* Tyrosine Phenol-lyase," (1988), *Biochemistry*, **27**, 7333-7338.

Kumagai, , H., Matsui, H., Ohkishi, H., Ogata, K., Yamada, H., Ueno, T. and Fukami, H., "Synthesis of 3,4-Dihydroxyphenyl-L-alanine from L-Tyrosine and Pyrocatechol by crystalline β-Tyrosinase," (1970) *Biochem. Biophys. Res. Comm.* **39**, 796-801.

Kumagai, H., Utagawa, T. and Yamada, H., "Studies on Tyrosine Phenol-lyase: Modification of Essential Histidyl Residues by Diethylpyrocarbonate," (1975), *J. Biol. Chem.*, **250**, 1661-1667.

Kumagai, H., Yamada, H., Matsui, H., Ohkishi, H. and Ogata, K., "Tyrosine Phenol-lyase: I. Purification, Crystallization, and Properites," (1970), *J. Biol. Chem.*, **245**, 1767-1772.

Kunkel, T. A. "Rapid and Efficient Site-specific Mutagenesis Without Phenotypic Selection," (1985) *Proc. Natl. Acad. Sci. (USA)*, **82**, 488-492.

Phillips, R. S., "The Reaction of Indole and Benzimidazole with Amino Acid Complexes of *E. coli* Tryptophan Indole-lyase: Detection of a New Reaction Intermediate," (1991) *Biochemistry*, **30**, 5927-5934.

Phillips, R. S., "Reactions of O-Acyl-L-serines with Tryptophanase, Tyrosine Phenol-lyase and Tryptophan Synthase", (1987), *Arch. Biochem. Biophys.*, **256**, 302-310.

Taylor, J. W., Ott, J. and Eckstein, F., "The Rapid Generation of Oligonucleotide-directed Mutations at High Frequency Using Phosphorothioate-modified DNA." (1985) *Nucl. Acids Res.* **13**, 8765-8785.

Toney, M. and Kirsch, J. F., "Tyrosine 70 Fine-tunes the Catalytic Efficiency of Aspartate Aminotransferase." (1991) *Biochemistry*, **30**, 7456-7461.

Yamada, H., Kumagai, H., Kashima, N., Torii, H., Enei, H. and Okumura, S., "Synthesis of L-Tyrosine from Pyruvate, Ammonia and Phenol by Crystalline Tyrosine Phenol-lyase," (1972), *Biochem. Biophys. Res. Comm.*, **46**, 370-374.

Biochemistry of Vitamin B$_6$ and PQQ
G. Marino, G. Sannia and F. Bossa (eds.)
© 1994 Birkhäuser Verlag Basel/Switzerland

The role of pyridoxal phosphate in the refolding of serine hydroxymethyltransferase

Kang Cai and Verne Schirch

Department of Biochemistry, Virginia Commonwealth University, Richmond, Virginia 23298-0614, USA

Summary

Escherichia coli serine hydroxymethyltransferase is reversibly unfolded in 1 to 8 M urea solutions in Tris buffer, pH 7.3. Three methods were used to study the refolding process; fluorescence of tryptophan residues, circular dichroism of both secondary structure and pyridoxal phosphate binding, and size separation by high performance liquid chromatography. During unfolding the earliest event is the dissociation of pyridoxal phosphate which occurs in solutions between 1 and 2 M urea. Separation of the dimer subunits occurs between 2.5 and 6 M urea. Complete loss of secondary and tertiary structure occurs above 6.5 M urea. Refolding studies were done at 0.8 M urea in both the presence and absence of pyridoxal phosphate. Greater than 95% of the catalytic activity could be recovered from fully unfolded enzyme in 10 minutes at 30 °C. There was a lag period of 30 seconds before the appearance of active enzyme. The addition of pyridoxal phosphate did not cause a significant change in the refolding kinetics. When refolding was done at 4 °C no active enzyme was formed in a period of several hours, but both secondary and tertiary structure appeared to be like native enzyme. Analysis on high performance liquid chromatography size exclusion gels showed that after a few minutes of refolding at 4 °C the enzyme was a mixture of monomer and dimer species. After one hour the enzyme was all dimer. Analysis by circular dichroism and Trp fluorescence during this period showed that pyridoxal phosphate did not bind to either the monomer or dimer formed at 4 °C. We conclude that pyridoxal phosphate binds only to the native apoenzyme and does not play a role in the refolding process of this enzyme.

Introduction

Studies have established that the primary sequence of a protein determines its biologically active three-dimensional structure. However, attempts to predict three-dimensional folding from the primary sequence have failed for even small single domain proteins (Dill and Shortle, 1992). Formulation of models to predict three-dimensional structures from primary sequences is a current major area of research. Pyridoxal phosphate (PLP) enzymes offer another problem in that the coenzyme must be added at some step during the folding process to yield the native holoenzyme. How and when PLP is added to these enzymes during biosynthesis is not known. It is unlikely that PLP is added as the free aldehyde since this reactive form of the coenzyme would form imines nonspecifically with amino groups on other proteins. Rather, there is most likely a targeting mechanisms to add PLP only to those enzymes which use it as a cofactor during catalysis.

In *E. coli,* PLP is synthesized from common small precursor molecules (Dempsey, 1971). The metabolic pathway is not yet completely known. However, it has been estimated that there are only 60,000 to 80,000 molecules of PLP in an *E. coli* cell. Apparently the cell makes PLP only as it is needed and does not keep a pool of free PLP available for adding to newly synthesized B_6 requiring enzymes. Little work has been done on the mechanism of the addition of PLP to apoenzymes *in vitro*. But with serine hydroxymethyltransferase (SHMT) the formation of holoenzyme takes as long as 30 min if the PLP and apoenzyme concentrations are both in the low μM range. It is unlikely that *in vivo* the cell takes this amount of time to convert newly synthesized apoenyme to holoenzyme.

To investigate the mechanism of formation of holoSHMT in *E. coli* cells we have studied the mechanism of addition of free PLP to apoenzyme *in vitro*. We have asked the following questions. Does SHMT reversibly refold from a random coil *in vitro*? What are the intermediates on the refolding pathway? Which intermediates are capable of binding PLP? Does PLP increase or decrease the rate of refolding? After establishing the mechanism of refolding *in vitro* and determining how free PLP adds during the refolding process, we will be in a position to investigate the mechanism of refolding and addition of PLP in *E. coli* extracts. We want to pursue the possibility that there is a donor molecule which adds PLP in the cell by a more specific and rapid process than occurs in the purified *in vitro* system described in this study.

Materials and Methods

All chemicals were of the highest purity that could be obtained. Ultra pure urea was obtained from Boehringer Mannheim and solutions were made in 50 mM Tris buffer, pH 7.3, immediately before being used in the refolding studies. ApoSHMT was prepared my incubating holoenzyme (in 20 mM potassium phosphate, pH 7.3) with 100 mM L-cysteine for 10 min and then adding ammonium sulfate to 75% of saturation (Schirch, *et al.*, 1973). After another 10 min incubation the solution was centrifuged for 15 min at 13,000*g*. The pellet was dissolved in 100 mM L-cysteine containing 500 mM potassium phosphate, pH 7.3, and again precipitated with ammonium sulfate. This procedure was repeated 3 times. Ammonium sulfate was removed by dialysis overnight in 2 liters of 20 mM potassium phosphate, pH 7.3, containing 5 mM 2-mercaptoethanol. The protein concentration of these stock apoenzyme solutions was usually about 10 mg per ml.

Unfolding was performed by diluting stock holo- or apoenzyme solutions in 8 M urea containing 20 mM Tris•HCl, pH 7.3 with 5 mM 2-mercaptoethanol. The final concentration of enzyme was in the range of 0.05 to 2 mg per ml depending on the experiment to be performed. The enzyme was kept in the 8 M urea for varying lengths of time at either room temperature or 4 °C. Refolding was initiated by diluting the enzyme 10-fold into the appropriate buffer and temperature.

Fluorescence spectra were obtained with a Shimadzu RF5000U spectrofluorophotometer. Excitation wavelength was 280 nm and emission spectra were recorded from 300 nm to 400 nm. Temperature was controlled at 30 °C. Protein concentration was usually 0.05 mg per ml in a 3 ml cell with a 1 cm pathlength. Circular dichroism spectra were recorded with a JASCO J-500 spectropolorimeter. For far uv spectral studies, cells with a pathlength of 1.0 mm and protein concentrations of 0.3 mg per ml were used. For visible spectra in the 350 to 500 nm wavelength range a cell with a 1 cm pathlength and protein concentrations of 0.6 mg per ml were used. Temperature was controlled at either 4 °C or 30 °C.

Formation of native holoenzyme was determined by either enzymatic assay with L-serine and tetrahydrofolate as substrates or my monitoring the formation of an abortive complex at 502 nm of enzyme, glycine, and 5-formyltetrahydrofolate. This abortive complex exhibits a unique absorption peak at 502 nm which has a molar absorbtivity coefficient of 40,000 $M^{-1}cm^{-1}$. Use of this complex permitted a continuous trace of the return of active holoenzyme during refolding.

Results and Discussion

Unfolding-The rate and extent of unfolding were monitored by both Trp fluorescence and far uv circular dichroism. At room temperature, the complete loss of optical activity at 220 nm was obtained in the few minutes that it required to take a spectrum. There was essentially no observable differences between holo- and apoenzyme using this technique. With solutions of apoenzme, we observed that fluorescence emission decreased about 50% during unfolding and the maximum emission wavelength shifted from 335 nm to 352 nm. This shows that the Trp residues (3 in SHMT) are being transferred from a hydrophobic environment to a hydrophilic environment during unfolding. The rate of change in fluorescence after adding either the apo- or holoenzyme to 8 M urea was very rapid. Even at 4 °C the total change in Trp fluorescence occurred in 120 sec.

Holoenzyme exhibits only about 60 % of the Trp fluorescence observed with the apoenzyme.

We were able to confirm that this is the result of the bound PLP quenching the Trp fluorescence. This quenching of fluorescence proves to be a valuable method for observing the binding of PLP to apoenzyme.

Refolding-When unfolded apoenzyme in 8 M urea is diluted 10-fold there is a rapid recovery of the far uv circular dichroism spectrum to the value of the native apoenzyme. This is complete within 20 sec, even at 4 °C. This suggests that essentially all secondary structure has been recovered rapidly. When refolding is monitored by Trp fluorescence there is a rapid burst in the increase in fluorescence followed by a slower rate of increase. After about 2 min the fluorescence signal is about the same as observed with apoenzyme. This suggests that the return of tertiary structure, as determined by the burying of the 3 Trp residues into their hydrophobic environment, occurs in several stages and the overall process is slower than the return of secondary structure.

When unfolded enzyme is diluted 10-fold into a solution containing excess PLP the return of secondary structure and Trp fluorescence follows the same pattern as observed in the absence of PLP for the first several minutes. However, after Trp fluorescence approaches the values observed for apoenzyme there is a decrease in the signal to values characteristic of the fluorescence of the holoenzyme. These results suggest that PLP adds to the apoenzyme only after it is formed from the random coil state.

When the unfolded enzyme is diluted 10-fold into a buffer with excess PLP at 4 °C the secondary structure and Trp fluorescence returned within a few minutes. However, no active holoenzyme returns, even after an incubation of 1 hour. Some intermediate containing secondary structure and some tertiary structure has accumulated at this low temperature. To determine the quaternary structure of this intermediate at various time points after renaturation at the low temperature we passed the enzyme through a BIOSEP SEC-S3000 high performance liquid chromatography column (300 x 7.5 mm) at 4 °C. The first sample taken after only 30 sec of renaturation showed that the enzyme was about 50% monomer and 50% dimer. Succeeding experiments showed that the monomer was converted to dimer and after 1 hour of incubation at 4 °C the protein was completely converted to the dimer.

Unfolded SHMT that was renatured at 4 °C for one hour showed the Trp fluorescence properties and dimeric structure of native apoSHMT. When the temperature of these 4 °C incubated solutions was quickly raised to 30 °C in the presence of PLP, the enzyme formed active holoenzyme at essentially the same rate when starting with random coil SHMT. This suggests that the dimer formed at 4 °C is on the folding pathway between random coil and native enzyme.

Addition of PLP to Folding Intermediates- The accumulation of the monomeric and dimeric folding intermediates at 4 °C allows a determination of when PLP adds to SHMT during the refolding process. The unfolded enzyme in 8 M urea was diluted 10-fold into buffer at 4 °C containing PLP in a 10-fold excess over enzyme concentration. PLP binding was monitored both by Trp fluorescence and optical activity at 420 nm, which is characteristic of bound PLP. The circular dichroism spectra in the 350 to 500 nm range did not show any increase in optical activity even after 1 hour of incubation at 4 °C. This suggests that PLP was not forming the internal aldimine at the active site of the enzyme. However, when the temperature of the solution was raised to 30 °C the optical activity at 420 nm increased in a few minutes to the value characteristic of holoenzyme.

Dilution of the unfolded enzyme into the PLP containing buffer at 4 °C showed a rapid return of the Trp fluorescence to a level characteristic of the apoenzyme. Again no additional change in fluorescence was observed during the next 60 min. After increasing the temperature to 30 °C the Trp fluorescence signal decreased to a level characteristic of holoenzyme. These results further support the circular dichorism results that PLP does not bind to either the monomer or dimer species that accumulate at 4 °C, and that PLP binds only to the native apoenzyme that is formed on raising the temperature to 30 °C.

Conclusions- Our ultimate goal is to determine the mechanism of PLP binding to *E. coli* SHMT during biosynthesis *in vivo*. Our first goal was to demonstrate that the folding of the enzyme could be studied *in vitro* and that intermediates on the folding pathways could be detected. We have demonstrated that the unfolding and refolding of *E. coli* SHMT is a reversible process. Furthermore, we have shown that at 4 °C both a monomeric and dimeric species accumulate. Neither of these can bind PLP, but they have the secondary structure, Trp fluorescence properties, and quaternary structure of native apoenzyme. These studies suggest that free PLP binds only to native apoenzyme and not to any folding intermediate. This now defines the system to explore when PLP binds to enzyme *in vivo* during the folding process.

Acknowledgments

This work was supported by Grant GM 28143 from the National Institutes of Health.

References

Dempsey, W. (1971) *J. Bacteriol.* **108**, 1001-1007

Dill, K. A., and Shortle, D. (1992) *Annu. Rev. Biochem.* **60**, 795-825

Biochemistry of Vitamin B$_6$ and PQQ
G. Marino, G. Sannia and F. Bossa (eds.)
© 1994 Birkhäuser Verlag Basel/Switzerland

The Mechanism of O-Acetylserine Sulfhydrylase from *Salmonella typhimurium*

K.D. Schnackerz and P. F. Cook*

*Theodor-Boveri-Institut für Biowissenschaften, Physiologische Chemie I, Am Hubland, D-97074 Würzburg, Germany and *Dept. of Biochemistry and Molecular Biology, University of North Texas Health Science Center, Fort Worth, Texas 76107-2690, U.S.A.*

Summary

The pyridoxal 5'-phosphate dependent enzyme O-acetylserine sulfhydrylase catalyzes the final step in the biosynthesis of L-cysteine in enteric bacteria, from O-acetyl-L-serine (OAS) and inorganic sulfide. The enzyme has been studied in the absence and presence of reactants and reactant analogues using absorbance, fluorescence, circular dichroism, and ^{31}P NMR spectroscopy. Addition of L-cysteine gives the external Schiff base, while addition of L-serine gives a mixture of the *gem*-diamine and the external Schiff base, and OAS gives the a-aminoacrylate intermediate. Formation of the external Schiff base with either cysteine or serine results in an increase in the energy transfer from an active site tryptophan to the protonated Schiff base as a result of an induced conformational change. Induced circular dichroism spectra of the bound cofactor indicate that a significant change in the orientation of the bound cofactor is realized when the a-aminoacrylate Schiff base is formed. The above data are corroborated by the ^{31}P NMR spectra which suggest a further tightening of the binding of the cofactor in the cysteine external Schiff base, and an equilibrium between two species with serine present.

Introduction

The biosynthetic pathway for L-cysteine in *Escherichia coli* and *Salmonella typhimurium* consists of two enzyme-catalyzed reactions as illustrated below:

$$L\text{-serine} + acetylCoA \;\rightarrow\; O\text{-acetyl-L-serine} + CoA \qquad (1)$$
$$O\text{-acetylserine} + sulfide \;\rightarrow\; L\text{-cysteine} + acetate \qquad (2)$$

The first reaction is catalyzed by serine transacetylase, while the second is carried out by O-acetylserine sulfhydrylase (OASS; EC 4.2.99.8). The latter protein consists of two identical subunits each containing 1 mol pyridoxal-P covalently bound as a Schiff base (Kredich and Tomkins, 1966). The native dimeric enzyme has a molecular mass of 68.9 kDa (Becker et al., 1969).

The kinetic mechanism for OASS-A has been determined using several alternative substrates to be ping pong with competitive inhibition by both substrates indicative of E:sulfide and E:O-acetylserine (OAS) dead end complexes (Cook and Wedding, 1976; Tai et al., 1993). The ultraviolet-visible spectrum of OASS-A exhibits an absorption maximum at 412 nm due to the formation of a protonated Schiff base between an active site lysine (K-42; Rege et al., 1994) and pyridoxal-P (Cook and Wedding, 1976; Cook et al., 1992). Addition of OAS to native OASS results in the disappearance of the absorbance at 412 nm concomitant with the appearance of new absorption maxima at 320 and 470 nm indicating the formation of a protonated Schiff base between pyridoxal-P and α-aminoacrylate upon the β-elimination of acetate (Cook and Wedding, 1976; Nalabolu et al., 1992). Michael addition of sulfide to the β-carbon of the α-aminoacrylate Schiff base generates L-cysteine.

In the present study amino acid substrates and analogues are used in an attempt to stop the OASS reaction at specific points along the reaction pathway. The spectral properties of intermediates are characterized using ultraviolet-visible, fluorescence, circular dichroic, and ^{31}P NMR spectroscopy.

Materials and Methods

Enzyme.   OASS-A from Salmonella typhimurium LT-2 was purified by a procedure described by Hara et al. (1990) and modified according to Tai et al. (1993).

Enzyme assay.   Two assays were used to monitor the OASS reaction. Either the disappearance of sulfide observed using a computer-assisted sulfide ion selective electrode (Hara et al., 1990) or the disappearance of TNB was followed spectrophotometrically at 412 nm (Cook et al., 1991).

Spectral Studies. All absorbance spectra were collected at 25°C in either 100 mM Hepes, pH 7 (enzyme alone or plus OAS), or 100 mM Ches, pH 9 (enzyme plus 4 mM cysteine or 40 mM L-serine) in cuvettes of 1 cm pathlength and 1 mL volume. Spectra were obtained using a Hewlett Packard diode array spectrophotometer and an enzyme subunit concentration of about 8 μM. Fluorescence spectra were collected using a Shimadzu RF-5000 spectrofluorometer exciting at 298 nm and scanning the emission monochromator from 300 to 600 nm. A bandwidth of 5 nm was used for both monochromators. Spectra were taken using a 3 mL cuvette with a 1 cm pathlength in the buffers given above with an enzyme subunit concentration of 2.5 μM. Circular dichroism spectra were recorded on an AVIV 62 HDS spectropolarimeter using 0.5 mL cuvettes with a 0.2 cm pathlength. Spectra were collected with a 1.5 nm bandwidth with a 3 sec dwell time for signal averaging every 1 nm. Triplicate runs were averaged to give the final spectra. Far UV-CD spectra were obtained in 10 mM phosphate buffer with a protein concentration of ≤80 μg/mL, while visible spectra were obtained using 500 μg/mL in the buffers used for absorbance spectra. ^{31}P NMR spectra were collected at 121.4 MHz on a Bruker AM300 SWB superconducting spectrometer using a 10-mm multinuclear probehead. The enzyme sample (2 mL) and D_2O (0.2 mL) was kept at 20 ± 0.1°C using a thermostatted continuous air flow. A spectral width of 2000 Hz was acquired in 8K data points with a pulse angle of 60°. Positive chemical shifts in parts/million are downfield changes with respect to 85% H_3PO_4.

Results and Discussion

Absorbance Spectra. Addition of L-cysteine to OASS-A gives no increase in the formation of the α-aminoacrylate intermediate, despite the fact that it is a product of the reaction. Instead, a shift in the λ_{max} from 412 to 424 nm is observed indicative of formation of the external Schiff base with the active site PLP (Morozov et al. 1982). The extinction coefficient for the external Schiff base has been estimated as 7,800 $M^{-1}cm^{-1}$. A plot of the fractional change in absorbance at 440 nm against the concentration of L-cysteine gives a dissociation constant about 1.5 mM at pH 7. The external Schiff base is also formed with L-alanine and glycine.

The presence of L-serine gives a more complex spectrum than that obtained with L-cysteine. There is again no formation of the α-aminoacrylate intermediate detected, rather a decrease in the absorbance at 412 nm by about 50% and a shift in the λ_{max} of the remaining absorbance to 424 nm. In addition, there is the appearance of a new species absorbing in the range 320-330 nm, suggested to represent the *gem*-diamine intermediate. Thus, replacement of the thiol group of L-cysteine with the hydroxyl group of L-serine results in an equilibrium distribution of *gem*-diamine and external Schiff base. The inability of serine to be completely converted to the external Schiff base is likely a result of a hydrogen-bonding interaction with the hydroxyl of serine that is not possible with the thiol of cysteine. The equilibrium constant between the *gem*-diamine and external Schiff base must be very close to unity, assuming that the extinction coefficients for the internal and external Schiff bases are not much different, a reasonable assumption given the above data for L-cysteine. Titration of the change at 330 nm allows estimation of a dissociation constant of 15 mM for the *gem*-diamine at pH 7.

Fluorescence Spectra. The fluorescence emission spectrum of OASS-A exciting at 298 nm exhibits λ_{max} values at 337 and 500 nm (McClure and Cook, 1994). The 337 nm band reflects intrinsic tryptophan fluorescence, while the longer wavelength band is attributed to energy transfer between an active site tryptophan and the PLP protonated Schiff base. Addition of either cysteine or acetate causes an enhancement of the long wavelength band as a result of a conformational change that reorients the tryptophan and PLP with respect to one another, and/or the distance between the two species (Federiuk and Shafer, 1983). The conformational change is thought to result from occupancy of the amino acid α-carboxyl subsite upon formation of the external Schiff base with L-cysteine or via dead-end complex formation with acetate (McClure and Cook, 1994).

Addition of L-serine to OASS-A also results in an enhancement of the long wavelength fluorescence. However, the enhancement obtained with serine is only half that observed with cysteine. These data are consistent with the above absorbance spectra that indicate only 50% of the enzyme is present as the external Schiff base in the presence of added serine.

Circular Dichroism Spectra. Enzyme exhibits a broad minimum in the circular dichroism spectrum between 210 and 220 nm with a negative Cotton effect. No change in the far-UV CD is observed upon addition of OAS, L-cysteine, or L-serine.

The protein induces circular dichroism of the bound PLP, which is observed in the visible region centered on the visible absorption band of the cofactor. Formation of the external Schiff base by the addition of L-cysteine results in a shift in the λ_{max} of the visible CD band to 424 nm with little to no change in the molar ellipticity. Also consistent with the above absorption data, L-serine gives a shift in the λ_{max} of the visible band to 424 nm, but with only half the intensity observed for L-cysteine. The greatest change in the visible CD spectrum is observed upon addition of OAS. A new band appears centered on the visible absorption band at 470 nm as expected, but the Cotton effect is of opposite sign. Similar results are reported for tryptophan synthase despite the fact that the α-aminoacrylate intermediate absorbs in the near UV at 330 nm (Kayastha et al., 1991).

The above CD data indicate that there is no significant change in the manner in which the protein binds the cofactor in the internal and external Schiff bases. This is despite the fact that there is a conformational change detected by enhancement of the Schiff base fluorescence upon formation of the external Schiff base by addition of amino acid to the internal Schiff base. However, there is a significant change in the way the cofactor is bound to protein upon formation of the α-aminoacrylate intermediate. Data suggest that there are either different faces of the cofactor bound in internal and external Schiff bases, or at least a rotation of the cofactor as the intermediate is formed.

31P NMR Spectra. Native OASS-A shows a pH independent ^{31}P NMR signal of the cofactor phosphate group at 5.1 ppm with a line width of 20.5 Hz (Cook et al., 1992). Data were interpreted to suggest that the cofactor is rigidly bound to the enzyme via one or more salt bridges. In the presence of 10 mM L-cysteine, the signal is further downfield at 5.3 ppm suggesting an even tighter binding of the cofactor phosphate. These data are consistent with the conformational change proposed based on the enhancement of the fluorescence energy transfer between an active site tryptophan and the protonated Schiff base (see above).

Addition of L-serine produces a significant upfield shift in the resonance of the cofactor phosphate to 4.4 ppm and an increase in the line width to about 50 Hz. As discussed above, the presence of serine gives an equilibrium mixture of *gem*-diamine and external Schiff base. The broad resonance at 4.4 ppm thus likely reflects a relatively rapid equilibration of the two species giving an average value of the chemical shifts for the two species. If the chemical shift of the external Schiff base is taken to be 5.3 ppm, the chemical shift of the gem-diamine is expected to be 3.5 ppm. A study of the temperature dependence of the ^{31}P NMR spectrum in the presence of serine should provide a test of the hypothesis.

Conclusions

The above spectral studies present a self consistent picture of the changes that occur along the OASS reaction pathway. Apparently none of the steps along the reaction pathway are accompanied by significant changes in the gross structure of the protein as seen in the far UV-CD. The formation of the *gem*-diamine is accompanied by a change in the tightness of the bound cofactor as suggested by ^{31}P NMR data, and a further change in the cofactor is observed upon formation of the external Schiff base as suggested by an increase in the amount of fluorescence energy transfer and a downfield shift in the ^{31}P NMR resonance. The most significant change in the orientation of the bound cofactor occurs upon formation of the α-aminoacrylate intermediate as supported by a change in the sign of the Cotton effect of the induced cofactor CD.

References

Becker, M.A. Kredich, N.M., and Tomkins, G.M. (1969) The Purification and Characterization of O-Acetylserine Sulfhydrylase-A from *Salmonella typhimurium. J. Biol. Chem.* 244. 2418-2427.

Cook. P.F., and Wedding, R.T. (1976) A Reaction Mechanism for O-Acetylserine Sulfhydrylase from *Salmonella typhimurium* LT-2. *J. Biol. Chem.* 251: 2023-2027.

Cook, P.F., Hara, S., Nalabolu, S. R., and Schnackerz, K.D. (1992) pH Dependence of the Absorbance and ^{31}P-NMR Spectra of O-Acetylserine Sulfhydrylase in the Absence and Presence of O-Acetylserine. *Biochemistry* 31: 2298-2303.

Cook, P.F., Nalabolu, S.R., and Tai, C.H. (1991) In Enzymes Dependent on Pyridoxal Phosphate and Other Carbonyl Compounds as Cofactors (Fukui,T., Kagamiyama, H., Soda, K., and Wada, H., Eds) pp 321, Pergamon Press, Tokyo.

Federiuk, C.S., and Shafer, J.A. (1983) .A Reaction Pathway for Transimination of the Pyridoxal 5'-Phosphate in D-Serine Dehydratase by Amino Acids. *J. Biol. Chem.* 258: 5372-5378.

Hara, S., Payne, M.A., Schnackerz, K.D., and Cook, P.F. (1990) A Rapid Purification and Computer-Assisted Sulfide Ion Selective Electrode Assay for O-Acetylserine Sulfhydrylase from Salmonella typhimurium. *Protein Expression Purif.* 1: 70-76.

Kayastha, A.M., Sawa, Y., Nagata, S., Kanzaki, H., and Miles, E. W. (1991) Circular dichroism studies of the coenzyme environment in the active sites of mutant forms of the β–subunit in the tryptophan synthase $\alpha_2\beta_2$ complex. *Ind. J. Biochem. & Biophys.* 28: 352-357

Kredich, N.M., and Tomkins, G.M. (1966) The Enzymic Synthesis of L-Cysteine in *Escherichia coli* and *Salmonella typhimurium*. *J. Biol. Chem.* 241: 4955-4965.

McClure, G.D., Jr., and Cook, P.F. (1994) Product Binding to the α-Carboxyl Subsite Results in a Conformational Change at the Active Site of O-Acetylserine Sulfhydrylase A: Evidence from Fluorescence Spectroscopy. *Biochemistry* 33: 1674-1683.

Nalabolu, S.R., Tai, C.H., Schnackerz, K.D., and Cook, P.F. (1992) Mechanism of O-Acetylserine Sulfhydrylase from *Salmonella typhimurium* LT-2. *Amino Acids* 2: 119-125.

Rege, V., Schnackerz, K.D., Kredich, N.M., Karsten, W.E., and Cook, P.F. (1994) unpublished.

Tai., C.H. Nalabolu, S.R., Jacobson, T.M., Minter, D.E., and Cook, P.F. (1993) Kinetic Mechanisms of the A and B Isozymes of O-Acetylserine Sulfhydrylase from *Salmonella typhimurium* LT-2 Using the Natural and Alternative Reactants. *Biochemistry* 32: 6433-6442.

Involvement of PLP in biological formation iron–sulfur clusters

Limin Zheng and Dennis R. Dean

Department of Biochemistry and Anaerobic Microbiology, Virginia Polytechnic Institute and State University, Blacksburg, Virginia 24061, USA

Summary

The *nifS* gene product is a pyridoxal phosphate binding enzyme which catalyzes the desulfuration of L-cysteine to yield L-alanine and sulfur. This activity is required for the full activation of the two nitrogenase component proteins called Fe protein and MoFe protein. Because both Fe protein and MoFe protein have metalloclusters comprised of metals and inorganic sulfide, we have suggested that NIFS might supply the inorganic sulfide for Fe–S core formation. The mechanism for the desulfurization of L–cysteine catalyzed by NIFS was determined in several ways. The substrate analogs, L–allylglycine and L–vinylglycine, were shown to irreversibly inactivate NIFS by formation of a γ–methylcystathionyl or cystathionyl residue, respectively, through nucleophilic attack by an active site cysteinyl residue on the corresponding pyridoxal phosphate–analog adduct. The reactive cysteinyl residue, which is required for cysteine desulfurization activity, was identified as Cys[325] by the specific alkylation of that residue and by site–directed mutagenesis experiments. Also, the formation of an enzyme–bound cysteinyl persulfide was identified as an intermediate in the NIFS–catalyzed reaction. Finally, evidence was obtained for an enamine intermediate in the formation of L–alanine. These results support a mechanism for NIFS–catalyzed desulfurization of L–cysteine which involves formation of a substrate cysteine–pyridoxal phosphate ketimine adduct and subsequent nucleophilic attack by the thiolate anion of Cys[325] on the sulfur of the substrate cysteine. This leads to formation of a protein–bound persulfide, which is the proposed sulfur donor in Fe–S core formation, and a pyridoxal phosphate–bound enamine which is ultimately released as L–alanine. Using L–cysteine, ferrous ion, DTT, and MgATP, NIFS is able to catalyze the reactivation of the apo-Fe protein *in vitro*. The Fe$_4$S$_4$ cluster of the Fe protein reconstituted by NIFS is identical to the native one, as indicated by EPR analysis in the presence or absence of MgATP.

Introduction

Pyridoxal phosphate (PLP)–containing enzymes commonly use amino acids as substrates. During catalysis the PLP cofactor binds to the substrate amino acid by forming a Schiff's base. The electron–withdrawing property of the PLP subsequently allows the extraction of the α–proton of the bound substrate, permitting replacement or elimination reactions to occur at the α, β, or γ position of the PLP amino acid adduct. Some well–known functions of PLP–containing enzymes include transamination, decarboxylation, and racemization. In this brief review we discuss the identification, characterization, and proposed physiological function of a new member of the PLP family of enzymes. The product of the *nifS* gene, hereafter called NIFS, catalyzes the desulfurization of L–cysteine which results in an enzyme–bound activated sulfur species that is proposed to provide the inorganic sulfide required for formation of the nitrogenase associated metalloclusters. Nitrogenase catalyzes the MgATP–dependent reduction of atmospheric nitrogen and it is a complex metalloenzyme comprised of two component proteins usually referred to as Fe protein and MoFe protein. The Fe protein is a homodimer that contains a single Fe_4S_4 cluster, whereas the MoFe protein is a hetrotetramer that contains two pairs of novel metalloclusters, called P clusters and FeMo–cofactors (See Kim and Rees, 1994 for a review). During catalysis, electrons are delivered one at a time from the Fe protein to the MoFe protein in a process which requires association–dissociation of the component proteins and hydrolysis of two MgATP per electron transfer. The MgATP binding and hydrolysis sites are located on the Fe protein whereas the substrate binding and reduction sites are contained within the MoFe protein. Binding of MgATP causes Fe protein to undergo a conformational change resulting in exposure of its Fe_4S_4 cluster (reviewed by Dean *et al.*, 1993), which is proposed to assist in the intermolecular electron transfer event. The primary products of the structural genes which encode the nitrogenase component proteins are not active, but rather require the activities of several *nif*–specific gene products involved in various aspects of the formation and insertion of their associated metalloclusters (Dean and Jacobson, 1992). NIFS is one such gene product. In *Azotobacter vinelandii,* deletion of the *nifS* gene results in reduction of both Fe protein and MoFe protein activities (Jacobson *et al.*, 1989). Thus, we suggested that NIFS is involved in a step common to maturation of both the Fe protein and the MoFe protein, i.e., it might be involved in the mobilization of the Fe or S required for metallocluster formation.

NIFS is a PLP–dependent cysteine desulfurase

Because NIFS is accumulated at only very low levels in *A. vinelandii*, it was hyperproduced by heterologous expression in *Escherichia coli* and was purified by ammonium sulfate fractionation and Q Sepharose and Phenol Sepharose column chromatographies. Purified NIFS was shown to have a yellow cofactor which was isolated and identified as PLP by UV–visible spectroscopy, ^{1}HNMR and GC/MS analysis (Zheng *et al.*, 1993). Different amino acids were incubated with NIFS to test whether or not formation of a specific PLP–amino acid adduct results in an alteration in the visible spectrum. In this way, L–Cysteine was identified as the specific NIFS substrate and the products were found to be L–alanine and sulfur, or under reducing conditions, sulfide. Thus, the reaction catalyzed by NIFS is as shown in Fig. 1.

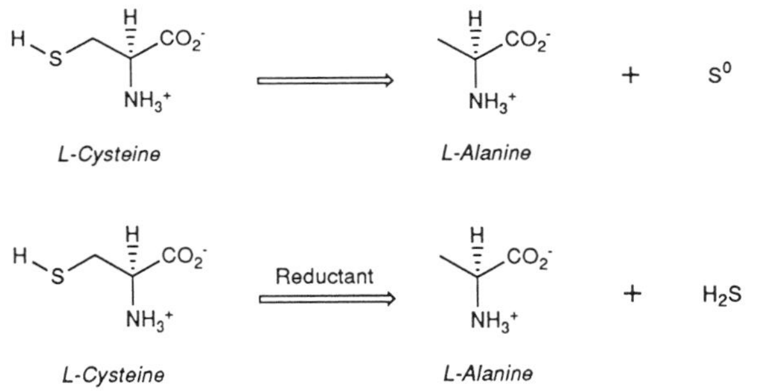

Figure 1. Cysteine desulfurization reaction catalyzed by NIFS.

Catalytic mechanism of NIFS

1. Cys[325] is the reactive cysteinyl residue in NIFS.

The desulfurase activity of NIFS can be dramatically inhibited by preincubation of the enzyme with equimolar amounts of alkylating reagents such as p–chloromercuribenzoic acid, iodoacetamide, or N–(iodoacetyl)–N'–(5–sulfo–1–naphthyl)ethylenediamine (1,5–I–AEDANS). This observation indicated that NIFS has an active site cysteinyl residue that is required for cysteine desulfurization activity. Using the fluorescent property of 1,5–I–AEDANS, we determined that NIFS binds to the thiol–specific reagent at only a 1 to 1 ratio, even though there are four cysteinyl residues in each NIFS monomer. To identify this reactive cysteine, the derivatized NIFS was digested with trypsin and the resulting oligopeptides separated by reverse–phase HPLC chromatography. A single fluorescent oligopeptide was subsequently isolated and the sequence of the peptide determined by automated amino acid sequencing. By comparison of the amino acid sequence of the isolated oligopeptide to the primary sequence of NIFS deduced from gene sequence data it was shown that Cys[325] is the hyper–reactive cysteinyl residue (Zheng *et al.*, 1994). The fact that Cys[325] is the reactive cysteine was further confirmed by site–directed mutagenesis experiments where Cys[325] was substituted by Ala[325]. NIFS–Ala[325] has no cysteine desulfurase activity and can no longer be labeled by the fluorescent alkylating reagent 1,5–I–AEDANS (Zheng *et al.*, 1994).

2. A γ–methylcystathioninyl or cystathioninyl residue is formed at the Cys[325] position when L–allylglycine or L–vinylglycine, respectively, is used as NIFS substrate.

Unsaturated amino acids are often used to probe the mechanism of PLP–binding enzymes. Incubation of NIFS with L–allylglycine or L–vinylglycine resulted in a time–dependent loss of NIFS–catalyzed cysteine desulfurase activity (Zheng *et al.*, 1994). The cause of such inactivation was identified as formation of a γ–methylcystathioninyl or a cystathioninyl residue at the Cys[325] position as shown by GC/MS analysis of the acid hydrolysis products of L–allylglycine or L–vinylglycine treated NIFS samples, respectively. Thus, it appears that during the reaction, a nucleophilic attack by the reactive Cys[325] thiolate occurs at the γ–position of the PLP amino acid analog adduct. This results in formation of either a γ–methylcystathioninyl or cystathioninyl residue when either L–allylglycine or L–vinylglycine are respectively used as substrate (Fig. 2). When cysteine is used as substrate, nucleophilic attack results in formation of an enzyme–bound persulfide (see below) and an enamine that is ultimately released as L–Alanine (Fig. 2).

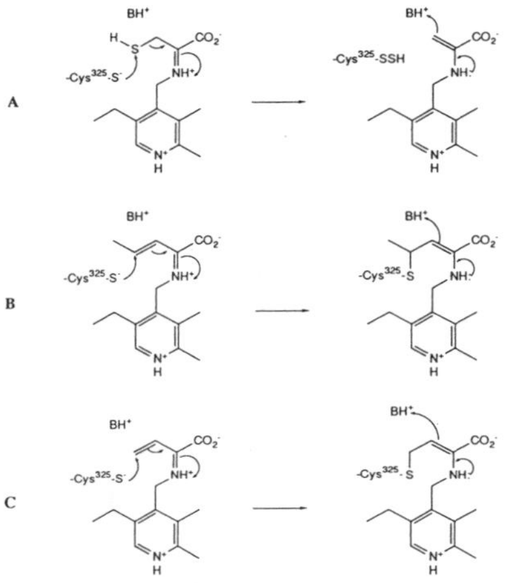

Figure 2. Proposed NIFS mechanism. Nucleophilic attack by the Cys[325] thiolate occurs at the γ–position of the PLP–cysteine adduct resulting in formation of an enzyme–bound persulfide and an enamine (A). The same mechanism can be used to explain γ–methylcystathionyl (B) or cystathionyl (C) formation when L–allylglycine or L–vinylglycine are respectively used as substrates.

3. An enzyme–bound persulfide is formed during the catalysis.

The fluorescence property of 1,5–I–AEDANS was also used to establish that an enzyme–bound persulfide is an intermediate in the cysteine desulfurization reaction. The rationale of the experiment was that if a persulfide is formed during catalysis, it should react with 1,5–I–AEDANS to form a disulfide bond that can subsequently be cleaved using a reductant. However, if there is no persulfide formed as an intermediate, reaction with 1,5–I–AEDANS should form a thio–ether that cannot be cleaved by a reductant. Using ultrafiltration, it was possible to separate more than 80% of the fluorescence from the enzyme that had been sequentially treated with cysteine, 1,5–I–AEDANS, and DTT. Under the same conditions, less than 2% of the fluorescence could be separated from the enzyme if the cysteine treatment step was omitted (Zheng et al., 1994). Thus, an enzyme–bound persulfide is an intermediate in the cysteine desulfurization reaction catalyzed by NIFS (Fig. 2).

NIFS can be used to catalyze a biologically active FeS cluster

Can the NIFS–bound persulfide formed during the cysteine desulfurization reaction be used as the source of inorganic sulfide required for FeS cluster formation? To test this possibility, apo–Fe protein was prepared by removal of its Fe_4S_4 cluster by chelation in the presence of MgATP. The purified apo–Fe protein prepared in this way had virtually no activity but could be reconstituted to near full activity by incubation with NIFS, cysteine, DTT and Fe^{2+} (Fig. 3). The reactivated Fe protein also has an Fe_4S_4 cluster identical to that of the native enzyme, as indicated by EPR spectroscopic analysis and enzymatic activity comparison. This result shows that NIFS can provide the acid labile sulfide in Fe_4S_4 cluster formation.

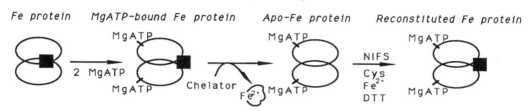

Figure 3. Scheme for preparation of the apo–Fe protein and reconstitution of the Fe protein using NIFS enzyme.

NIFS was also successfully used to reconstitute metal–chelated *A. vinelandii* NIFU, which is a protein having a Fe_2S_2 cluster, and apo–ferredoxin I from *A.vinelandii* (our unpublished results). Considering that *nifS*–like genes and NIFS activity has now been found in several organisms, it seems reasonable to propose that NIFS activity could represent a universal mechanism involving PLP chemistry in providing the inorganic sulfide in metallocluster formation.

References

Dean, D. R., and Jacobson, M. R. (1992) Biochemical genetics of nitrogenase. p.763–834 in G. Stacey, R. H. Burris and D. J. Evans (ed.) Biological nitrogen fixation. Chapman & Hall, New York.

Dean, D. R., Bolin, J. T., and Zheng, L. (1993) Nitrogenase metalloclusters: structures, organization, and synthesis. *J. Bacteriol.* 175: 6737–6744.

Jacobson, M. R., Brigle, K. E., Bennett, L. Y., Setterquist, R. A., Wilson, M. S., Cash, V. L., Beynon, J., Newton, W. E., and Dean, D. R. (1989) Physical and genetic map of the major gene cluster from Azotobacter vinelandii. *J. Bacteriol.* 171:1017–1027.

Kim, J. and Rees, D. C. (1994) Nitrogenase and biological nitrogen fixation. *Biochemistry*, 33:389–397.

Zheng, L., White, R.H., Cash, V.L., and Dean, D. R. (1994) Mechanism for the desulfurization of L–cysteine catalyzed by the *nifS* gene product. *Biochemistry*, in press.

Zheng, L., White, R.H., Cash, V.L., Jack, R. F., and Dean, D. R. (1993) Cysteine desulfurase activity indicates a role for NIFS in metallocluster biosynthesis. *Proc. Natl. Acad. Sci. USA* 90:2754–2758.

Iron-sulfur clusters as alternatives to pyridoxal-5'-phosphate in bacterial L-serine dehydratases: Cloning of the gene encoding the β-subunit of the enzyme from *Peptostreptococcus asaccharolyticus*

A.E.M. Hofmeister, R. Grabowski[1] and W. Buckel

Laboratorium für Mikrobiologie, Fachbereich Biologie, Philipps-Universität, D-35032 Marburg, Germany
[1]*Max-Planck-Institut für Biophysikalische Chemie, Abteilung Molekulare Genetik, Am Fassberg, D-37077 Göttingen, Germany*

Summary

L-Serine dehydratases from the strictly anaerobic bacteria Peptostreptococcus asaccharolyticus *and* Clostridium propionicum *were shown to contain [4Fe-4S]clusters but no pyridoxal-5'-phosphate. Both enzymes are inactivated by oxygen and reactivated by ferrous ion under anaerobic conditions. In combination with EPR-studies, the data indicate an aconitase-like mechanism of the dehydration of L-serine. Both enzymes are composed of two different subunits (α, 30 kDa and β, 25 kDa). The gene coding for the β-subunit from* P. asaccharolyticus *was cloned and sequenced. The N-terminus of the deduced amino acid sequence shows significant identities to that of the β-subunit of* C. propionicum *as well as to the N-termini of both L-serine dehydratases from* Escherichia coli.

Introduction

L-Serine dehydratase (EC 4.2.1.13) from the strictly anaerobic Gram-positive bacterium *Peptostreptococcus asaccharolyticus* is novel in the class of deaminating hydro-lyases in that it is an iron-sulfur protein and lacks pyridoxal-5'-phosphate. The enzyme is highly specific for L-serine, K_m = 0.8 mM, k_{cat} = 330 s^{-1}, whereas k_{cat}/K_m for threonine is 500-times lower. L-Serine dehydratase contains 3.8 ± 0.2 mol non-heme iron and 5.6 ± 0.3 mol inorganic sulfur/heterodimer (α, 30 kDa; β, 25 kDa). The molecular mass of the native enzyme was estimated at approx. 200 kDa. The dehydratase is inactivated by exposure to air ($T_{1/2}$ = 4 h) and can be specifically recativated by incubation with ferrous ion under anaerobic conditions (Grabowski & Buckel, 1991).

Anaerobic preparations of purified L-serine dehydratase from *P. asaccharolyticus* yielded EPR spectra characteristic of a [3Fe-4S]$^+$ cluster constituting 1% of the total cluster concentration. Upon incubation of the enzyme under air the increase in intensity of the [3Fe-4S]$^+$ signal correlated with the loss of enzymatic activity. Addition of L-serine prevented the increase in intensity of the [3Fe-4S]$^+$ signal and the concomitant loss of activity. Hence, active L-serine dehydratase probably contains a diamagnetic [4Fe-4S]$^{2+}$ cluster which is converted to the paramagnetic [3Fe-4S]$^+$ cluster of the inactive enzyme upon oxidation by loss of an iron atom (A.E.M. Hofmeister, S. Albracht & W. Buckel, in preparation). In analogy to the mechanism elucidated for aconitase (Beinert & Kennedy, 1989) it is proposed that L-serine is coordinated *via* its hydroxyl and carboxyl group to a specific iron atom of the [4Fe-4S] cluster (Fig. 1). This iron atom would thus act as a Lewis acid and facilitate the β-elimination of the hydroxyl group, an otherwise poor leaving group. The resulting enamine would escape from the cluster and should be protonated randomly from both sides yielding a ketimine which hydrolyses to pyruvate and ammonia (Grabowski et al. 1993).

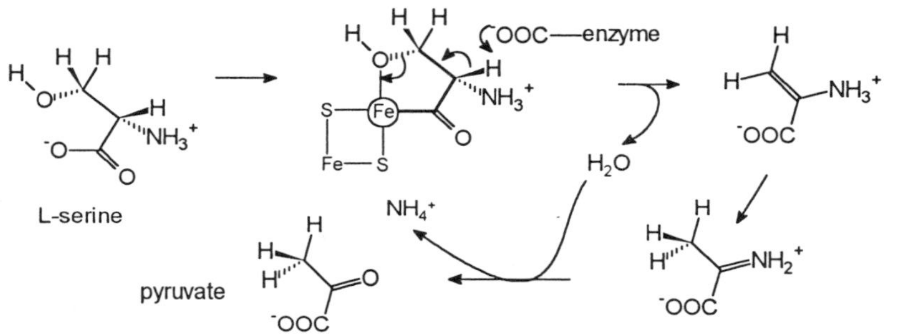

Fig. 1. Proposed mechanism of action of iron-sulfur cluster-containing L-serine dehydratases

In order to get more insight into the mechanism of the deamination, the stereochemistry of this protonation at C-3 was investigated using L-threonine as substrate. For this purpose the enzymatic reaction was carried out with unlabelled L-threonine in ^2H_2O and with L-[3-^{3}H]threonine in ^1H_2O. Isotopically labelled 2-oxobutyrates thus formed were enzymatically reduced to their corresponding 2-hydroxybutyrates which were then subjected to conformational analyses of their labelled methylene groups. The deuterated compound was analyzed by ^{1}H-NMR while the ^{3}H-labelled compound was oxidatively decarboxylated by permanganate to propionate which was subsequently analysed by propionate CoA-transferase and transcarboxylase in the presence of acetyl-CoA. The results obtained by both methods consistently indicated that the overall deamination of L-threonine proceeds with 67% inversion and 33% retention. In a control experiment with the PLP-dependent L-threonine dehydratase from *Clostridium propionicum* 96% retention was observed. The considerable racemisation (67%) observed with the iron-sulfur-dependent enzyme suggests that the primary dehydration product 2-aminocrotonate is liberated from the enzyme but protonation still occurs in the vicinity of the enzyme (Hofmeister et al. 1992). In the

PLP-dependent enzyme, however, protonation occurs at a stage at which the enamine is still bound to the prosthetic group (Vederas et al. 1978).

   C. propionicum, another strictly anaerobic Gram-positive bacterium, was shown to contain both an iron-sulfur-dependent L-serine dehydratase and a PLP-dependent L-threonine dehydratase (Hofmeister et al. 1993). This finding demonstrated the existence of the two independent mechanisms for the deamination of 3-hydroxy amino acids in one organism. Although L-threonine dehydratase also deaminated L-serine, k_{cat}/K_m was 118-fold higher for L-threonine. L-Serine dehydratase, however, was absolutely specific for its substrate. Inactivation of this enzyme upon exposure to air, its ability to be specifically reactivated by ferrous ion and the results obtained by EPR-spectroscopy indicated that L-serine dehydratase contains an iron-sulfur cluster important for catalysis. Hence, the question arises why L-threonine is dehydrated by PLP, whereas L-serine requires an iron-sulfur cluster. A possible answer may be that the leaving of the hydroxyl group of threonine is favoured by the methyl group which stabilizes the resulting secondary carbocation at C-3. Therefore it may be more efficient for the enzyme to facilitate the removal of the proton at C-2 by PLP rather than to activate the hydroxyl group. In serine, however, the hydroxyl group is more firmly attached, since the corresponding primary carbocation is less stable, and may require activation by an iron-sulfur cluster.

   Like L-serine dehydratase from *P. asaccharolyticus*, the corresponding enzyme from *C. propionicum* is composed of two different subunits (α, 30 kDa; β, 26 kDa). The *N*-terminal amino acid sequences of the small subunits of both enzymes as determined by Edman degradation (30 residues) were found to be 47% identical. In addition, between 35% and 48% identities with the *N*-termini of the two L-serine dehydratases, SdaA and SdaB, present in *Escherichia coli* (Shao & Newman, 1993) were detected. Together with the biochemical similarities this finding supports the notion that iron-sulfur-dependent L-serine dehydratases are widespread among *bacteria* but have escaped intensive characterization due to their oxygen lability (Hofmeister et al., 1993).

Materials and Methods

   Amplification of a DNA-segment from genomic DNA of *P. asaccharolyticus* (ATCC 14963) was achieved by polymerase chain reaction (PCR). A 25-μl amplification reaction contained 10 mM Tris-HCl, 1.5 mM $MgCl_2$, 50 mM KCl, gelatine (0.1 mg/ml) pH 8.3, 0.8 μg genomic DNA, 50 pmol of each heterologous oligonucleotide primer (derived from the N-terminal amino acid sequences of the α- and β-subunits of L-serine dehydratase from *P. asaccharolyticus*), 160 μM of each dNTP and 16.7 nkat *Taq* DNA polymerase. Following the initial denaturation of double stranded DNA at 94°C for 5 min, 30 cycles of PCR were performed using the following tempera-

220

ture profile: denaturation at 94°C for 1 min, primer annealing at 55°C for 1 min and primer extension at 72°C for 2 min. Cycling concluded with a final extension at 72°C for 5 min. Reactions were stopped by chilling to 4°C. The PCR products were cloned in *Escherichia coli* according to the procedure supplied with the TA Cloning® kit. Nucleotide sequencing was carried out according to the dideoxy-mediated chain termination method using the Sequenase kit (USB). Both strands of three independently amplified and cloned PCR-products were sequenced.

Results and Discussion

In order to amplify the gene coding for one subunit of L-serine dehydratase, polymerase chain reaction (PCR) was applied using genomic DNA from *P. asaccharolyticus* as template and oligonucleotides derived from the *N*-terminal amino acid sequences of both subunits in the forward and reverse directions as primers. Only the experiment with the forward β- and the reverse α-primer

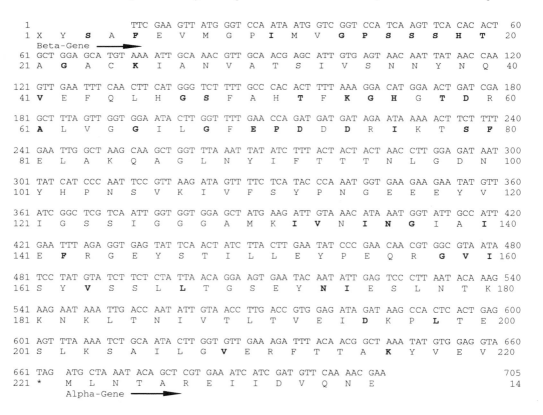

Fig.2. Deduced amino acid sequence of the β-subunit of the L-serine dehydratase from *P. asaccharolyticus*

yielded significant amounts of DNA, 705 bp in length. This result indicates that the genes coding for the subunits of L-serine dehydratase lie close together in the order *sdaBA*. Similar results were obtained with the genes coding for L-serine dehydratase from *C. propionicum*. The DNA-fragment derived from *P. asaccharolyticus* was inserted into the TA Cloning® vector pCR™II, cloned in *E. coli* and sequenced (Fig. 2). Of the deduced amino acid sequence, only the first 80 residues of SdaB from *P. asaccharolyticus* show a significant number of identities (bold letters) and similarities to those of SdaB from *C. propionicum* as well as to those of the L-serine dehydratases SdaA and SdaB from *E. coli*, each of which is composed of one kind of subunits (49 kDa; Shao and Newman, 1993). Curiously, the *C*-terminus of SdaB from *P. asaccharolyticus* contains a significant number of identities to the *C*-terminus of 3-phosphoglycerate dehydrogenase from *Bacillus subtilis* (EC 1.1.1.97; Sorokin et al. 1993). Since the sequence of SdaB from *P. asaccharolyticus* contains only one cysteine, the iron-sulfur cluster which requires three cysteines may be located either at the α-subunit or between both subunits. The occurrence of similar L-serine dehydratases in Gram-negative as well as in Gram-positive *bacteria* suggests that this type of iron-sulfur cluster-containing enzymes might be widespread among this domain.

Acknowledgements

The EPR-spectra were obtained in collaboration with Dr. Simon Albracht, Amsterdam (unpublished results). This work was supported by grants from the Deutsche Forschungsgemeinschaft and the Fonds der Chemischen Industrie.

References

Beinert, H. and Kennedy, M.C. (1989) Engineering of protein bound iron-sulfur clusters. *Eur. J. Biochem.* 186: 5-15.

Grabowski, R. and Buckel, W. (1991) Purification and properties of an iron-sulfur-containing and pyridoxal-phosphate-independent L-serine dehydratase from *Peptostreptococcus asaccharolyticus*. *Eur. J. Biochem.* 199: 89-94.

Grabowski, R., Hofmeister, A.E.M. and Buckel, W. (1993) Bacterial L-serine dehydratases: a new family of enzymes containing iron-sulfur clusters. *Trends Biochem. Sci.* 18: 297-300.

Hofmeister, A.E.M., Berger, S. and Buckel, W. (1992) The iron-sulfur-cluster-containing L-serine dehydratase from *Peptostreptococcus asaccharolyticus*. Stereochemistry of the deamination of L-threonine. *Eur. J. Biochem.* 205: 743-749.

Hofmeister, A.E.M., Grabowski, R., Linder, D. and Buckel, W. (1993) L-Serine and L-threonine dehydratase from *Clostridium propionicum*. Two enzymes with different prosthetic groups. *Eur. J. Biochem.* 215: 341-349.

Shao, Z. and Newman, E.B. (1993) Sequencing and characterisation of the *sdaB* gene from *Escherichia coli* K-12. *Eur. J. Biochem.* 212: 777-784.

Sorokin, A., Zumstein, E., Azevedo, V., Ehrlich, S.D. and Serror, P. (1993) The organisation of the *Bacillus subtilis* 168 chromosome region between the *spoVA* and *serA* genetic loci, based on sequence data. *Molecular Microbiol.* 10: 385-395.

Vederas, J.C., Schleicher, E., Tsai, M.-D. and Floss, H.G. (1978) Stereochemistry and mechanism of reactions catalysed by tryptophanase from *Escherichia coli*. *J. Biol. Chem.* 253: 5350-5354.

Biochemistry of Vitamin B$_6$ and PQQ
G. Marino, G. Sannia and F. Bossa (eds.)
© 1994 Birkhäuser Verlag Basel/Switzerland

Phosphorescence of Pyridoxal Kinase at Room Temperature: The Effects of Ligands Bound to the Nucleotide Site

Manuel Blazquez, Teresa Pineda, Francis Kwok and Jorge Churchich
University of Tennessee, Department of Biochemistry, Knoxville, TN 37996

Summary. Ligands bound to the nucelotide site of pyridoxal kinase influence the phosphorescence properties of tryptophanyl residues. Binding to the substrate ATP perturbs the triplet state of the protein leading to a significant decrease in phosphorescence lifetime from 0.9 to 0.3ms. The effect is attributed to changes in the flexibility of the embedding macromolecular matrix elicited by binding of the substrate. The probe DANS-GABA inhibits the enzyme by displacing ATP from the nucleotide binding site and quenches protein phosphorescence by a mechanism of triplet-singlet energy transfer. Ligand bonds to specific sites on proteins are suitable to study specific quenching mechanisms leading to deactivation of the triplet state at room temperature.

Introduction. The reaction catalyzed by pyridoxal kinase involves the transfer of a phosphoryl group from ATP to pyridoxal, thus forming the products ADP and pyridoxal-5-P. The monomer of the kinase (40kDA) is folded into two structural domains which can be cleaved by limited chymotryptic digestion (Dominici). One of the fragments, characterized by a molecular mass of 24kDA, binds ATP analogues with affinity constants comparable to those of the undigested monomer (Dominici [1989], Pineda [1993]).

The large distance separating the substrates bound to the enzyme as measured by resonance energy transfer (Kwok [1991]) and NMR spectroscopy (Wolkers [1991]), has led to the hypothesis that a hinge bending movement of the substrate domains facilitate the catalytic cycle. However, the nature of the structural fluctuations induced by binding of ATP to the nucleotide site remains to be elucidated. The phosphorescence emitted by tryptophanyl residues in protein can provide unique information on the dynamics of the macromolecule, since the quantum yield and phosphorescence lifetime are sensitive to the chromophore environment and to quenching interactions with distal centers in the macromolecule. Phosphorescence is readily detected for most proteins at room temperature in the absence of O$_2$, a powerful quencher of the triplet state (Konev [1967], Saviotti [1974]).

In the present work, we have examined the effects of ligands bound to the nucleotide site of pyridoxal kinase on the phosphorescence properties of the tryptophanyl residues.

Results and Discussion

Phosphorescence of Pyridoxal Kinase. Pyridoxal kinase exhibits a structureless phosphorescence band when excited at either 280 or 290nm. The phosphorescence emitted at 430nm decays in a monoexponential manner with a lifetime of 0.9ms (Table I). Phosphorescence emission is only detected when O_2 molecules are displaced from the solvent by bubbling N_2 gas. When the phosphorescence properties of pyridoxal kinase (10 μM) were examined in the presence of ATP (20μM) in 20mM potassium phosphate (pH 7), and O_2 excluded from the solution, it was found that a reduction in the phosphorescence yield of the tryptophanyl residues is paralleled by a significant decrease in phosphorescence lifetime (Figure 1, Table I). The results included in Table I are the average of three independent experiments performed on deoxygenated samples of pyridoxal kinase at room temperature.

Triplet Singlet Energy Transfer. The dansyl chromophore, N-dansyl-4-aminobutyrate, DANS-GABA, behaves as a competitive inhibitor with respect to ATP (K_I=4μM) at saturating concentrations of pyridoxal. The binding of DANS-GABA to the enzyme is easily detected by a dramatic increase in the fluorescence emitted at 480 nm (excitation 340nm or 290nm) (Fig. 2). As shown in Figure 2, the presence of bound DANS-GABA induces quenching of the protein fluorescence which can be attributed to a mechanism of radiationless energy transfer taking place between molecules in their singlet excited state. In view of the preceding results, it was though of interest to investigate whether the phosphorescence properties of the tryptophanyl residues are also influenced by the binding of DANS-GABA. When the phosphorescence of pyridoxal kinase (10μM) was examined in the presence of DANS-GABA (10μM) in 20mM phosphate (pH 7) under deoxygenated conditions, it was found that quenching of protein phosphorescence results in the appearance of sensitized luminescence which coincides with the fluorescence band displayed by the inhibitor (Fig. 1).

That a specific mechanism of quenching (i.e., triplet-singlet) is operative in the binary complex DANS-GABA-kinase is shown from the observations that (a) the phosphorescence yield of the tryptophanyl residues of the protein is reduced; (b) the phosphorescence lifetime of the protein is decreased from 0.9 to 0.4ms; and (c) the long-lived luminescence of bound DANS-

Table I.

Luminescence of pyridoxal kinase at room temperature. The effects of ligands bound to the nucelotide site

Sample	λ_a (nm)	λ_f (nm)	λ_p (nm)	τ_p
PK	280	340	430	0.9
PK-ATP	280	340	410	0.3
PK-DAN	280	340/510	410/510	0.4
	340	510	510	1.6
DAN	340	560	560	

All parameters were determined at room temperature. λ_a is the excitation wavelength; λ_f is the maximum wavelength of fluorescence emission; λ_p is the maximum wavelength of phosphorescence; and τ_p is phosphorescence lifetime.

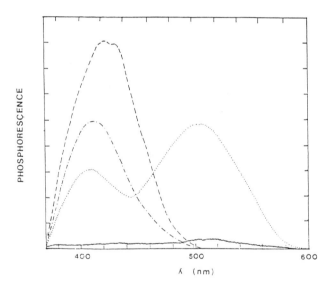

Fig. 1. Luminescence of pyridoxal kinase. Phosphorescence emission spectra of pyridoxal kinase (-----), pyridoxal kinase-ATP (-·-·-), pyridoxal kinase-N-dansyl-4-aminobutyrate (· · · ·) and free N-dansyl-4-aminobutyrate (–). The concentration of protein and N-dansyl-4-aminobutyrate are 10 and $10\mu M$, respectively, whereas the concentration of ATP is $10\mu M$. Experiments conducted in 20mm K. phosphate buffer (pH 7) at 25°. Excitation 290 nm.

226

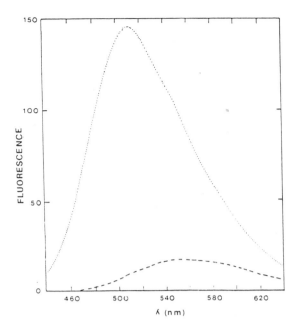

Fig. 2. Binding of N-dansyl-4-aminobutyrate to pyridoxal kinase. Emission spectra of N-dansyl-4-aminobutyrate (10μM) in the absence (-----) and presence ($\cdot\,\cdot\,\cdot\,\cdot$) of enzyme ($10\mu$M). Excitation was at 340 nm.

GABA (τ=1.6ms) is characterized as delayed fluorescence.

In this type of luminescence quenching, the efficiency of energy transfer depends on the sixth power of the distance (R) separating the donor/acceptor pair triplet tryptophan/singlet DANS-GABA- and on the critical distance of transfer (Ro) as indicated in Equation 1:

$$E = \frac{Q_D - Q_{DA}}{Q_D} = \frac{1}{1 + \left(\dfrac{R}{Ro}\right)^6} \qquad (1)$$

According to Forster's theory of Radiationless Energy Transfer (Forster [1965], Ermolaev [1963]), the critical distance of transfer (Ro) can be determined with the aid of Equation 2:

$$Ro = 9.7 * 10 \left[x^2 * Q_D * n^{-4} * J(v) \right]^{\frac{1}{6}} \qquad (2)$$

when the overlap integral $J(v) = 1.3 \times 10^{-15} cm^{-6} mmol^{-1}$, the quantum yield of the donor $Q_D = 4.2 \times 10^{-4}$, the orientation factor $x^2 = 0.67$ and the refractive index $n = 1.33$, the critical distance of transfer approaches a value $R_0 = 10\text{Å}$. For an efficiency of energy transfer of $E = 0.2$, the actual distance of transfer for the donor/acceptor pair tryptophan/DANS-GABA is $R = 13\text{Å}$.

Discussion. In analyzing the effect of ATP and DANS-GABA on the phosphorescence of the tryptophanyl residues of pyridoxal kinase, it is important to consider "environmental" effects (Knr) and "specific" quenching mechanisms (Kpq) leading to deactivation of the triplet state.

The observed phosphorescence lifetime (τp) depends upon the rate constants Knr, Kp and Kpq corresponding to non-radiative, radiative and specific quenching mechanisms, respectively.

$$\frac{1}{\tau p} = K_{nr} + K_p + K_{pq} [Q] \qquad (3)$$

The triplet lifetime and phosphorescence yield of proteins display a strong dependence on the microviscosity of the embedding macromolecular matrix (9), therefore any change in the microviscosity of the tryptophanyl residues due to conformational changes of the protein would affect Knr and the observed phosphorescence lifetime. The quenching effect exerted by binding of ATP to the kinase is assumed to proceed through a change in the non-radiative rate constant Knr. In the case of binding of DANS-GABA to the protein, a specific quenching mechanism (Kpq) influences the phosphorescence yield and decay time of the tryptophanyl residues.

That a specific mechanism of quenching (i.e., triplet-singlet transfer) is operative in the binary complex DANS-GABA-kinase is shown from the observation that (a) the phosphorescence yield of the tryptophanyl residues of the protein is reduced; (b) the phosphorescence lifetime of the protein is decreased from 0.9 to 0.4ms; and (c) the long-lived luminescence of bound DANS-GABA has been characterized as delayed fluorescence.

The method of energy transfer was applied to deduce proximity relationship between the DANS-GABA bound to the nucleotide site and the tryptophanyl residues participating in phosphorescence emission.

228

References

Dominici P, Kwok F and Churchich JE (1989) Proteolytic Cleavage of Pyridoxal Kinase into Two Structural Domains *Biochimie* **71**:585-590.

Ermolaev VL (1963) Energy Transfer in Organic Systems Involving the Triplet State *Russian Physics* **80**:333-358.

Forster T (1965) in *Modern Quantum Chemistry*, Part III, Sinanoglu O, ed., Academic Press, New York.

Konev SV (1967) *Fluorescence and Phosphorescence of Proteins and Nucleic Acids*, Plenum Press, New York.

Kwok F and Churchich JE (1991) The Interaction of Paramagnetic Ions Chelated to ATP with Pyridoxal Analogues *Eur J Biochem* **199**:157-162.

Pineda T and Churchich JE (1993) Reversible Unfolding of Pyridoxal Kinase *J Biol Chem* **268**:20218-20222.

Saviotti ML and Galley WC (1974) Room Temperature Phosphorescence and the Dynamic Aspects of Protein Structure *Proc Natl Acad Sci USA* **71**:4154-4158.

Strambini GB and Gonnelli M (1985) The Indole Nucleus Triplet State Lifetime and its Dependence on Solvent Microviscosity *Chem Phys Lett* **115**:196-200.

Wolkers WF, Gregory JD, Churchich JE and Serpersu EH (1991) Arrangement of the Substrates at the Active Site of Brain Pyridoxal Kinase *J Biol Chem* **267**:20761-20766.

The Schiff base of pyridoxal-5'-phospate with ethylenediamine and ethylamine: Species in solution

J.M. Sevilla, C. Hidalgo, T. Pineda, F. Garcia-Blanco and M. Blazquez

Departamento de Química Física y Termodinámica Aplicada, Universidad de Córdoba, 14004 Córdoba, Spain

Introduction

Elucidation of intermediates in the transamination reactions has been widely studied on the basis of model reactions between pyridoxal (PL) and pyridoxal 5'-phosphate (PLP) with amines and diamines. H-NMR and UV-visible data [1-4] suggested the presence of carbinolamine and/or geminaldiamine together with Schiff base. The present work deals with a contribution to the study of the reaction mixtures of PLP and ethylenediamine (Etd) and PLP and ethylamine (Et) by electrochemical techniques and UV-visible and fluorescence spectroscopies.

Experimental

Material and experimental procedures were essentially the same as described previously [4,5].

Results and discussion

The electrochemical results in aqueous buffered solutions at neutral pH show that the formation of the Schiff base PLP-Etd is favoured as compared to PLP-Et Schiff base. This fact is mainly concerning with the existence of an enolimine tautomer and a geminaldiamine in basic solution, the last one being electroactive after a fast conversion to imine at the electrode interface. Changes of the electrochemical order with respect to the proton on the electroreduction kinetic of the Schiff base [6] are consistent with the presence of a high concentration of enolimine with a cyclic structure [4].

In Table 1 are summarized UV-visible and fluorescence properties of the reaction mixture of PLP with Etd. Absorption spectra revealed three main species, enolimine (335 nm), ketoenamine (414-418 nm) and in basic media, geminaldiamine (315 nm). Fluorescence results show emission bands centered at 430 and 500 nm for enol and keto tautomers, respectively, together with a 373-380 nm emission band for geminaldiamine, this species having the highest quantum yield. Additionally, one observes an emission centered at 471 nm (by excitation at 371 nm) that strongly suggest the formation of a multipolar form in the singlet excited state (Scheme 1). Fast interconversion in the excited state can be explained by the concurrence of a high enolimine concentration on the reaction mixture with a high basicity of the ring nitrogen of the Schiff base in the excited state.

Table 1

UV-visible and fluorescence properties of the mixture of PLP with ethylenediamine in buffered aqueous solutions at 25°C

pH	Specie[*]	λ_{abs}/nm	ε/$M^{-1}cm^{-1}$	λ_{exc}/nm	λ_{em}/nm	$\phi \cdot 10^3$
4.0	SH_3^{2+}	418	4200	425	500	4.4
		336	2350	335	430	8.5
					471	9.0
				371	471	13.7
7.0	SH_2	418	1800	425	485	4.9
		335	2860	335	471	5.3
				371	471	16.8
10.0	SH	414	2900	425	489	2.0
				371	471	10.5
	GH	313	2500	315	380	7.9
13.3	S^-	345(s)	1600	355	471	4.5
				371	471	9.2
	G^-	312	4400	315	373	76.9

(*) S: Schiff base, G: Geminaldiamine

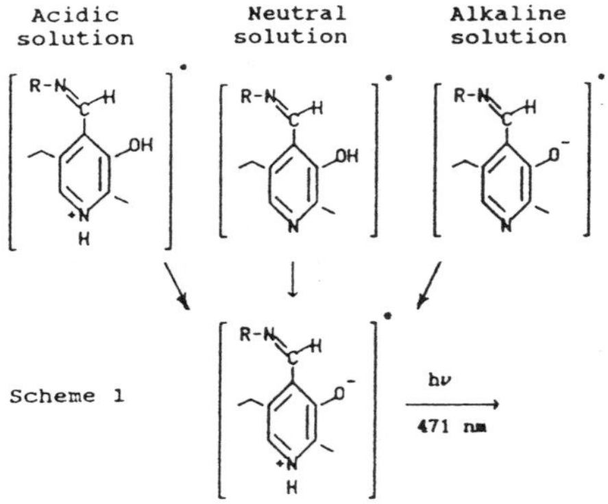

Scheme 1

Understanding the conditions in which these reactions are favoured in the excited state may help to interpret PLP environment in protein binding site.

Acknowledgements

Financial support from Spanish DGICYT (Project PB91-0833) and the Junta de Andalucia is gratefully acknowledged.

References

1. Abbot, E.H. and Martell, A.H. (1971) J.Am.Chem.Soc., 93, 5852.
2. Tobias, P.S. and Kallen, R.G. (1975) J.Am.Chem.Soc., 97, 6530.
3. Metzler, C.M., Cahill, A. and Metzler, D.E. (1980) J.Am.Chem.Soc., 102, 6075.
4. Robitaille, P.M., Scott, R.O., Wang, J. and Metzler, D.E.(1989) J.Am.Chem.Soc., 111, 3034
5. Sevilla, J.M., Blazquez, M., Dominguez, M. and García-Blanco, F. (1992) J.Chem.Soc. Perkin Trans.2, 921
6. Hidalgo, C., Pineda, T., Sevilla, J.M. and Blazquez, M. (1994) J.Electroanal.Chem. 364, 199-207

AMINE OXIDASES

Biochemistry of Vitamin B$_6$ and PQQ
G. Marino, G. Sannia and F. Bossa (eds.)
© 1994 Birkhäuser Verlag Basel/Switzerland

Biological role and reactivity of TPQ containing amine oxidases

Bruno Mondovì

University of Rome "La Sapienza", Dept. of Biochemical Sciences "A. Rossi Fanelli" and CNR Center of Molecular Biology, Rome, Italy

Some properties of the trihydroxyphenylalanine quinone (TPQ) containing amine oxidases (TAOs) will be outlined in order to better focus on the main current problems concerning this class of enzymes.

Biological role

TAOs are deaminating oxidases which act on primary amines, whereas the FAD dependent monoamine and polyamine oxidases can also act on secondary amines. The catalytic products of TAOs are: aldehyde, hydrogen peroxide and ammonia. The physiological function is essentially related to the functions proper of their substrates and reaction products: high polyamine levels are typical of actively proliferating cell populations, while oxidized polyamines have in some way opposite metabolic effects, i.e. impairment of cell growth and proliferation both *in vitro and in vivo* (Bachrach et al, 1967). In this respect, TAOs should be considered as regulatory enzymes of the balance between biosynthetic and catabolic reactions. Polyamines are involved in transcription and translation by interacting with DNA and RNAs(Mc Intire, 1993).

Pig kidney diamine oxidase (PKDAO) immobilized on Concanavalin A-Sepharose was able to inhibit tumor growth when injected intraperitoneally into mice with Ehrlich ascites tumors. Since these cells contain elevated levels of polyamines, injected PKDAO presumably produced cytotoxic aldehydes and H_2O_2 (Mondovì et al, 1982). In agreement with this hypothesis it was demonstrated that bovine serum amine oxidase (BSAO), obtained as homogeneous protein, caused cytotoxicity in cultured CHO cells in the presence of exogenous spermine (Averill-Bates et al, 1993). Both aldehydes and H_2O_2 appear to participate in generating the observed toxic effect, but at different levels and times: the presence of catalase abolished cytotoxicity completely during the first 20 min. and partially up to 60 min., whereas aldehyde dehydrogenase (ADH) exerted no protective effect up to 30 min. and very low protection up to 60 min. With both catalase and ADH present, cytotoxicity was completely abolished throughout 60 min. incubation. These results indicate that H_2O_2 is the only species contributing to cytotoxicity at early stages of the reaction, while aldehydes may contribute to the cytotoxic effect at longer incubation times (Averill-Bates et al, 1994).

When the major sources of polyamines were systematically blocked by inhibiting ornithine decarboxylase (biosynthetic route) and polyamine oxidase (interconversion route), an almost complete inhibition of tumor growth was observed (Claverie et al, 1987). On the other hand, inhibition of TAOs activity seems to promote tumor growth: administration of the DAO inhibitor aminoguanidine to rats increased the tumor promotion by azoxymethane from zero to 66% (Kusche et al, 1989), after one year of observation. In this context, we can hypothesize that the carcinogenic activity of metronidazole (a well known synthetic antibacterial and antiprotozoal imidazole derivative) observed in rodents could be imputable to its inhibitory effect on DAO (Befani, Turini, Gerosa and Mondovì to be published).

Elevation of DAO activity, indicating an activation of polyamine metabolism, was observed in the liver showing early and persistent preneoplastic nodules of hepatomas (Sessa et al, 1990).

TAOs are also involved in membrane functions; it was recently demonstrated (Rigobello et al, 1993) that polyamines decrease the inner mitochondrial membrane permeability and, by preventing mitochondrial glutathione loss, also act as protective agents against oxidative stress. In physiological conditions the concentration of phosphate ion regulates the polyamine concentration by binding to them, giving an apparent competitive inhibition of BSAO activity (Corazza et al, 1992). The amine oxidase activity is strongly ionic strenght-dependent: an increase of Km values at high ionic strenght was observed (Stevanato et al, 1994).

An other important role of TAOs is the protection against pseudoallergic and allergic reactions. A protective role of PKDAO in anaphylactic shock was demonstrated in guinea pig (Mondovì et al, 1975). When DAO (histaminase) activity is blocked, plasma histamine levels are much higher and severe clinical symptoms appear (hypotension, flush, vomiting) (Moneret-Vautrin, 1991). It should be emphasized that many commonly used drugs are DAO inhibitors (Sattler et al, 1988).

A post translational modification of proteins imputable to TAOs has to be taken in account. The role of lysyloxidase in elastin formation is discussed in another session of this Symposium (Narashiman and Kagan, 1994). Oxidation of ε-amino groups of lysyl residues by BSAO was observed (Oda et al, 1981). We recently demonstrated (Mateescu, Wang and Mondovì, to be published) a H_2O_2 production from polylysine in the presence of BSAO. By extention of this model, the aldehyde groups formed by oxidation of exposed NH_2 groups of protein amino acids become reactive and could give cross-link reactions. Other important functions of TAOs are related to H_2O_2 formed during polyamine oxidation. An insulin-like effect was observed in several model systems: stimulation of glucose and amino acids transport and glycogen synthesis and inhibition of intracellular protein degradation (Mc Intire, 1993). TAO inhibitors prevent the stimulation of lipogenesis, which is mediated by H_2O_2 (Livingston et al, 1977). Moreover, H_2O_2 is able to enhance human platelet aggregation induced by either soluble or particulate stimulating agents at less than micromolar concentration (Del Principe et al, 1985). Recently Novotny et al (1994) identified the human kidney DAO with the amiloride-binding protein, which is involved in the active transport of Na^+ from the luminal side to the blood.

Reactivity of TAOs

While a general consensus was recently reached on the presence of TPQ in these enzymes (Klinman et al, 1991), some controversy still exists on the stoichiometry and reactivity. Two or only one TPQ mol/dimer were titrated with phenylhydrazine in BSAO by Janes et al (1991) and Morpurgo et al (1992) respectively. Only one TPQ mol/dimer was titrated in pig serum amine oxidase (PSAO) with substrate or phenylhydrazine (Lindstrom et al, 1978). Two TPQ mol/dimer were titrated in the enzyme from lentil seedlings (Padiglia et al, 1992) with a number of different inhibitors. However both in PSAO (Collison et al, 1989) and BSAO (Morpurgo et al, 1992) two TPQ mol/dimer were evidenced with other inhibitors. In these cases the second molecule reacted at a much slower rate than the first one. Half-site reactivity was suggested (Morpurgo et al, 1992) admitting intrinsic difference between the sites. This hipothesis was supported by the following results (Morpurgo et al, 1994). Doubly derivatized BSAO adducts were examined and the identity of the sites was established by proteolytic degradation, chromatographic purification of derivatized fragments, and amino-acid analysis. The optical spectra of intact and proteolyzed BSAO adducts were significantly different. The protein environment appears to considerably influence the structure of the TPQ derivatives.

The catalysis appears to occur by an aminotransferase mechanism, in stepwise reactions involving proton abstraction and concomitant enzyme reduction, hydrolysis of an imine intermediate and, finally, reoxidation of reduced cofactor by dioxygen to produce hydroperoxide (Janes and Klinmann, 1991). Mammalian and plant enzymes seem to differ in the catalytic mechanism. Reduction of copper and appearance of a free radical, which detected in anaerobiosis by both ESR and optical spectroscopy, was clearly observed only in the plant enzymes (Dooley et al, 1991 Bellelli et al, 1991), imputable to the formation of amino-6-hydroxydopa semiquinone. The radical was detected only in very small amount in the mammalian TAOs (Dooley et al, 1991) and no evidence was found of its presence in BSAO by anaerobic rapid scanning stopped-flow spectroscopy (Hartmann et al, 1993, Bellelli et al, unpublished results).

Several TAOs are reported to exist as isoenzymes; this may in part explain the heterogeneity seen for undenaturated forms (Mc Intire, 1993). BSAO appears to have two types of microheterogeneity: a first one is imputable to differences in the carbohydrate moiety and a second one observable in each isoform imputable to a possible conformational equilibrium stabilizing the protein or a different exposure of charged aminoacids due to the masking effects of the carbohydrate moiety in each form (Shiozaki et al, 1994). The role of carbohydrates maintaining a correct conformation in BSAO and PKDAO is also supported by the results obtained by treating these enzymes with lectins. When BSAO and SKDAO are immobilized on concanavalin A-sepharose, their susceptibility to proteolysis is enhanced probably because of conformational changes of the protein imputable to the binding of carbohydrate to the solid phase support (Mondovì et al, 1992).

The 3D structure of TAOs is not known, but crystallization and preliminary crystallographic characterization of the pea seedlings enzyme was recently published (Vignevich et al, 1993). The results of this paper are in agreement with the literature; the protein consists of two identical subunits of about 66 kDa each. Some TAO genes have been cloned and the sequence of yeast amine oxidase from Hansenula Polymorpha (Bruinberg et al, 1989), lentil seedlings (Rossi et al, 1992), bacterial methylamine oxidase (Zhang et al, 1993), bovine serum, human and pig kidney (Mu et al, 1994) have been determined. It is confirmed that TPQ derives from a tyrosine residue, which is in position 470 and corresponds to the post-translationally modified TPQ. Three conserved histidine residues are likely to be ligands to copper, in agreement with previous results (Mondovì et al, 1967, 1987).

Acknowledgements
This work was partially supported by funds from Consiglio Nazionale delle Ricerche. Progetto speciale ACRO n° 93.02203.39 and Ministero Università e Ricerca Scientifica e Tecnologica. We thank Mr. Amleto Ballini for skilfull technical assistence.

References

Averill-Bates, D.A., Agostinelli, E., Przybytkowski, E., Mateescu, M.A., and Mondovì, B. (1993) Arch. *Biochem. Biophys.* 300: 75-79.

Averill-Bates, D.A., Agostinelli, E., Przybytkowski, E., and Mondovì, B. (1994) The role of aldehydedehydrogenase in protection against cytotoxicity induced by bovine serum amine oxidase and spermine in chinese hamster ovary cells, Biochem. Cell. Biol. in press.

Bachrach, U., Abzug, S., and Bekierkunst, A. (1967) Cytotoxic effect of oxidized spermine on Ehrilich ascites cells. *Biochim. Biophys. Acta* 134: 174-181.

Bellelli, A., Finazzi-Agrò, A., Floris, G., and Brunori, M. (1991) On the mechanism and rate of substrate oxidation by amine oxidase from lentil seedlings. *J. Biol. Chem.* 266: 20654-20657.

Bruinenberg, P.G., Evers, M., Waterham, H.R., Kuipers, J., Arnberg, A.C., and Geert, A.B. (1989) Cloning and sequencing of the peroxisomal amine oxidase gene from Hansenula polymorpha. *Biochim. Biophys. Acta* 1008: 157-167.

Claverie, N., Wagner, J., Knoedgen, B., and Seiler, N. (1987) Inhibition of polyamine oxidase improves the antitumoral effect of ornithine decarboxylase inhibitors. *Cancer Lett* 7: 765-772.

Collison, D., Knowles, P. F., Mabbs, F. E., Rius, F. X., Singh, I., Dooley, D. M., Cote, C. G. and McGuirl, M. (1989) Studies on the active site of pig plasma amine oxidase. *Biochem. J.* 264: 663-669.

Corazza, A., Stevanato, R., Di Paolo, M.L., Scarpa, M., Mondovì, B., and Rigo,A. (1992) Effect of phosphate ion on the activity of bovine plasma amine oxidase. *Biochem. Biophys. Res. Comm.* 189: 722-727.

Del Principe, D., Menichelli, A., De Maeis, M.L., Di Corpo, L., Di Giulio, S., and Finazzi-Agrò, A. (1985) Hydrogeperoxide has a role in the aggregation of human platelets. *FEBS Lett.* 185: 142-146.

Dooley, D.M., Mc Guirl, M.A., Brown, D.E., Turowski, P.N., Mc Intire, W.S., and Knowles, P.F. (1991) A Cu(I)-semiquinone state in substrate-reduced amine oxidases. *Nature* 349: 262-264.

Hartman, C., Brzovic, P., and Klinman, J.P. (1993) Spectroscopic detection of chemical intermediates in the reaction of para-substituted benzylamines with bovine serum amine oxidase. *Biochemistry* 32: 2234-2241.

Janes, S.M., and Klinman, J.P. (1991) An investigation of bovine serum amine oxidase active site stoichiometry: evidence for an aminotransferase mechanism involving two carbonyl cofactor per enzyme dimer. *Biochemistry* 30: 4599-4605.

Klinman, J., Dooley, D.M., Duine, J.A., Knowles, P.F., Mondovi, B., and Villafranca, J.J. (1991) Status of the cofactor identity in copper oxidative enzymes. *FEBS Lett* 282: 1-4.

Kusche, J., Mennigen, R., Günther, M., and Leisten, L. (1989) Large bowel tumor promotion by inhibition of mucosal diamine oxidase in rats. 6: I Morphological Aspects 15-26.

Lindstrom, A., and Petterson, G. (1978) Active site titration of pig-plasma benzylamine oxidase. *Eur. J. Biochem.* 83: 131-135.

Livingston, J.N., Gurny, P.A., and Lockwood, D.H. (1977) Insulin like effect of polyamines in fat cells. *J. Biol. Chem.* 252: 560-562.

Mc Intire, W.S. (1993) Copper containing amine oxidases in: Principles and applications of quinoproteins. Davidson, V.L. ed. Dekker, M. publ. New York, Basel, Hong Kong 97-171.

Mondovì, B., Rotilio, G., Costa, M.T., Finazzi-Agrò, A., Chiancone, E., Hansen, R., and Beinert, H. (1967) Diamine oxidase from pig kidney: improved purification and properties. *J. Biol. Chem.* 242: 1160-1167.

Mondovì, B., Scioscia-Santoro, A., Rotilio, G., Costa, M.T., and Finazzi-Agrò, A. (1975) In vivo anti-histaminic activity of histaminase. *Agents and Action* 5: 460.

Mondovì, B., Gerosa, P., and Cavaliere, R. (1982) Studies on the effect of polyamines and their products on Ehrlich ascites tumours. *Agents Actions* 12: 450-451.

Mondovì, B., Morpurgo, L., Agostinelli, E., Befani, O., Mc Cracken, J., and Peisach, J. (1987) A comparison of the local enviroment of Cu(II) in native and half-Cu-depleted bovine serum amine oxidase. *Europ. J. Biochem.* 168: 503-507.

Mondovì, B., Befani, O., and Mateescu, M.A. (1992) Enhanced susceptibility to proteolysis of copper amineoxidases immobilized on Con A sepharose. *Life Chem. Rep.* 10: 151-155.

Moneret-Vautrin, D.A. (1991) In: Somogyi, J.C., Mülller, H.R. and Ockhuizen Th (eds.): Food allergy and food intolerance Nutritional Aspects and development *Bibl. Nutr. Dieta Publ.*, Basel, Kager 48: 61-71.

Morpurgo, L., Agostinelli, E., Mondovì, B., Avigliano, L., Silvestri, R., Stefancich, G., and Artico, M. (1992) Bovine serum amine oxidase: half-site reactivity with phenylhydrazine, semicarbazide and aromatic hydrazides. *Biochemistry* 31: 2615-2621.

Morpurgo, L., De Biase, D., Agostinelli, E. and Mondovì, B. (1994) Half-site reactivity of bovine serum amine oxidase. *This Symposium.*

Mu, D., Medzihradszky, K.F., Adams, G.W., Mayer, P., Hines, W.M., Burlingame, A.L., Smith, A.J., Cai, D., and Klinman, J.P. (1994) *J. Biol. Chem.* 269: 9926-9932.

Narasimhan, and Kagan, H.M. (1994) Modulation of lysyl oxidase activity toward lysine in synthetic oligopeptides by vicinal anionic residues. Implications for collagen crosslinking. *This Symposium.*

Novotny, W.F., Chassande, O., Baker, M., Lazdunski, M. and Barby, P. (1994) Diamine oxidase is the amiloride-binding protein and is inhibited by amiloride analogues. *J. Biol. Chem.* 269: 9921-9925.

Oda, O., Manube, T., and Okuyama, T. (1981) Oxidation of ε-amino group of lysyl peptides by bovine serum amine oxidase. *J. Biochem.* 86: 1317-1323.

Padiglia, A., Medda, R. and Floris, G. (1992) Lentil seedling amine oxidase: interaction with carbonyl reagents. *Biochem. Intern.* 28: 1097-1107.

Rigobello, M.P., Toninello, A., Siliprandi, D., and Bindoli, A. (1993) Effect of spermine on mitochondrial glutathione release. *Biochem. Biophys. Res. Comm.* 194: 1276-1281.

Rossi, A., Petruzzelli, R., and Finazzi-Agrò, A. (1992) cDNA-derived aminoacid sequence of lentil seedlings amine oxidase. *FEBS Lett-* 301: 253-257.

Sattler, J., Hafner, D., Klotter, H.J., Lorenz, W., and Wagner, P.K. (1988) Food-induced histaminosis as an epidemiological problem: plasma histamine elevatyion and hemodynamic alterations after oral histamine administration and blockade of diamino oxidase (DAO). *Agent Actions* 23: 361-365.

Sessa, A., Desiderio, M.A., and Perin, A. (1990) Diamine oxidase activity in a model of multistep hepatocarcinogenesis. *Cancer Lett.* 51: 75-78.

Shiozaki, T. S., Befani, O., Loreti, P., Mondovì, B. and Graziani, M. T. (1994) Microheterogeneity in isoforms of bovine serum amine oxidase. Symposium on Polyamines: Biological and Clinical aspects. Alberé di Tenna, Trento.

Stevanato, R., Mondovì, B., Befani, O., Scarpa, M., and Rigo, A. (1994) Electrostatic control of oxidative deamination catalyzed by bovine serum amine oxidase. *Biochem. J.* 299: 317-320.

Vignevich, V., Dooly, M.D., Guss, J.M., Harvey, I., Mc Guirl, M.A., and Freeman, H. (1993) Crystallization and preliminary crystallographic characterization of the copper containing amine oxidase from pea seedlings. *J. Mol. Biol.* 229: 243-245.

Zhang, X., Fuller, J.H., and Mc Intire, W.S. (1993) Cloning, sequencing, expression, and regulation of the structural gene for the copper/topa quinone-containing methylamine oxidase from Arthrobacter strain P1, a gram-positive facultative methyllotroph. *J. Bacteriol.* 175: 5617-5627.

Biochemistry of Vitamin B$_6$ and PQQ
G. Marino, G. Sannia and F. Bossa (eds.)
© 1994 Birkhäuser Verlag Basel/Switzerland

Two distinct quinoprotein amine oxidases are functioning in *Aspergillus niger*

I. Frebort, H. Toyama, K. Matsushita, H. Kumagai[1], P. Pec[2], L. Luhova[2] and O. Adachi

Yamaguchi University, Department of Biological Chemistry, 1677-1 Yoshida, Yamaguchi 753, Japan
[1]*Kyoto University, Department of Food Science and Technology, Sakyo-ku, Kyoto 606-01, Japan*
[2]*Palacky University, Department of Analytical and Organic Chemistry, Tr.Svobody 8, 771 46 Olomouc, Czech Republic*

Summary

Two distinct copper-quinoprotein amine oxidases (EC 1.4.3.6), AO-I and AO-II, were isolated from the soluble fraction of homogenized *Aspergillus niger* mycelia grown on butylamine medium. AO-I is a dimmer consisting of two 75 kDa subunits, while AO-II is a monomer of 80 kDa. Purified AO-I and AO-II show pink (490 nm) and yellow (420 nm) colors, respectively. The enzymes show comparable substrate specificity and sensitivity to inhibitors. Hexylamine, butylamine, benzylamine, tyramine and histamine are preferred substrates. Both enzymes are inhibited by substrate analogs, copper chelating agents, some alkaloids and carbonyl reagents. Enzymes labeled with *p*-nitrophenylhydrazine showed different absorption maxima at 465 and 440 nm for AO-I and AO-II, respectively, in neutral pH. These maxima were shifted to 585 nm under alkali conditions. Absorption and fluorescence spectra of synthesized model compound - topaquinone hydantoin *p*-nitrophenylhydrazone and labeled enzymes were in very good agreement, while PQQ *p*-nitrophenylhydrazone showed significant difference. After digestion by thermolysin, labeled cofactor containing peptides were purified using reverse phase HPLC and sequenced by Edman degradation, resulting typical topaquinone containing sequence, Asn-topa-Glu-Tyr, for AO-II and a noncofactor peptide, Val-Val-Ile-Glu-Pro, which contained topaquinone linked to γ-carboxyl of Glu, for AO-I. Cofactor structures were confirmed by mass spectrometry. N-Terminal amino acid sequences of AO-I and II were found to be different and peptide mapping showed some distinct patterns for both enzymes. A gene encoding AO-I has been cloned already and the second gene for AO-II is now under processing.

Introduction

Amine oxidase of *Aspergillus niger* is a copper-carbonyl enzyme, which was found in the middle of 1960s, crystallized and characterized (Yamada et al., 1965; Adachi and Yamada, 1969). Recently, the importance of the fungal amine oxidase has risen again, because the enzyme can be applied to monitor histamine contents in fishery products. The discovery of topaquinone as the cofactor of eukaryotic copper-containing amine oxidases (Janes et al., 1990) and also amine oxidases from yeast (Mu et al., 1992) and bacteria (Cooper et al., 1992) has inspired us to search for the structure of the cofactor of *Aspergillus niger* amine oxidase. Recently, we have found two distinct quinoprotein amine oxidases (EC 1.4.3.6), AO-I and AO-II, in *Aspergillus niger* mycelia grown on *n*-butylamine medium. AO-I is the enzyme previously reported, consisting of two 75 kDa subunits, while AO-II is a novel one of 80 kDa similar to amine oxidases from yeast and bacteria. We would like to present our latest results on the isolation and characterization of these two amine oxidases from *Aspergillus niger*.

Materials and Methods

Purification of amine oxidases from *Aspergillus niger*

Cultivation of *Aspergillus niger* AKU 3302 mycelia in nitrate medium and induction of amine oxidase by *n*-butylamine was performed using routine method (Yamada et al., 1965).

Mycelia were collected, washed with water and crushed in a mill. Enzymes were extracted twice by 10 mM potassium phosphate buffer (KPB), pH 7, then the extracts were combined and fractionated with ammonium sulfate (55 % sat.). Precipitate was suspended in the same buffer, treated with charcoal powder to remove lipids and insoluble material and centrifuged. Supernatant was fractionated again with ammonium sulfate and centrifuged. Precipitate was suspended in 10 mM KPB, pH 7, and dialyzed against the same buffer for 12 hours. Dialyzed sample was applied onto a DEAE-cellulose column (4 cmID x 17 cm) equilibrated with 10 mM KPB, pH 7, and washed with the same buffer. Then enzyme was eluted by 0.1 M KPB, pH 7. Activity fractions were combined, fractionated with ammonium sulfate and centrifuged. Precipitate was suspended in 1 mM KPB, pH 7, and dialyzed against the same buffer for 12 hours. Dialyzed sample was applied onto a hydroxylapatite column (3 cmID x 6.5 cm) equilibrated with 1 mM KPB, pH 7. Enzyme was eluted in two fractions, by 1 mM and 100 mM KPBs, pH 7. Both fractions were combined and fractionated with ammonium sulfate and centrifuged. Precipitate was suspended in the least volume of 10 mM KPB, pH 7.0, and filtrated through a Sephadex G-100 column (3.8 cmID x 80 cm) with the same buffer as a mobile phase. Fractions of separated AO-I and II were pooled. Usual yield of complete purification was 70-80 % of total enzyme activity.

Results and Discussion

Fundamental properties of both amine oxidases are shown in Table I. For purified amine oxidases, two distinct protein bands very close each other, corresponding to 75 kDa (subunits of separated AO-I) and 80 kDa (AO-II), were found by SDS PAGE. On native enzyme PAGE, two distinct activity bands identical to two protein bands were observed. Resolution of the bands highly exceeded SDS PAGE. In agreement with higher molecular mass of dimmer, AO-I showed lower mobility than AO-II, quite opposite to SDS PAGE, where AO-I had been separated into subunits. These two activity bands were detected in a crude extract and throughout all purification steps. By isoelectric focusing, isoelectric points at pI 6.0 were found for both enzymes. In absorption spectra, besides absorption maximum at 280 nm, AO-I shows "pink" maximum at 490 nm, while AO-II is of yellow color with maximum absorption at 420 nm. In fluorescence emission spectra with excitation at 365 nm, both show maxima at 420 and 440-450 nm. Copper content of AO-I indicates one copper ion per dimmer of 150 kDa. Low copper content in AO-II is similar to that observed with purified amine oxidase from *Klebsiella aerogenes* (Yamashita et al., 1993). No significant activations (5-10 %) were observed with 0.5 μM Cu^{2+} for both amine oxidases. Micromolar concentration of Cu^{2+} then had an inhibitory effect.

Table I. Comparison of properties of *Aspergillus niger* amine oxidases

	AO-I	AO-II
molecular mass	150 kDa	80 kDa
molecular structure	dimmer (2 x 75 kDa)	monomer
color	pink	yellow
maximum absorption	280, 490 nm	280, 420 nm
pI	6.0	6.0
Cu atoms per mole	1.01	0.09
carbohydrates	< 0.5 %	< 0.5 %
specific activity (hexylamine)	128 nkat/mg	29 nkat/mg
specific activity (benzylamine)	46 nkat/mg	12 nkat/mg
pH optimum (hexylamine)	7.5	7.5
K_m (hexylamine)	0.15 mM	0.15 mM

Different N-terminal sequences of *Aspergillus niger* amine oxidases result also some small differences in peptide maps obtained by SDS PAGE with specific proteases as shown in Fig.1.

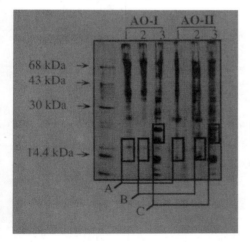

N-terminal amino acid sequences:

AO-I (35):
Met-Leu-Pro-Xaa-Pro-Leu-Ala-Ile-Leu-Ser-Glu-Glu -Glu-Thr-Asn-Ile-Ala-Arg-Asn-Val-Ile-Leu-Ala-Gln -His-Pro-Asn-Thr-Val-Ile-Asp-Phe-Arg-Glu-Ile-

Xaa - an unknown residue, previously determined as His

AO-II (11):
Asn-Asp-Ser-Pro-Ala-Leu-Asn-Asp-Leu-Ser-Leu-

Figure 1. Peptide mapping performed by double SDS PAGE. Protein bands of purified enzymes after staining with Coomassie brilliant blue from the first gel (not shown) were cut off and inserted into the second gel, in which denatured enzymes were digested by specific proteases - arginylendopeptidase (1), asparaginylendopeptidase (2) and protease V8 from *Staphylococcus aureus* (3) (Takara Biomedicals, Japan). Peptide bands on the second gel were stained by silver staining (Wako Ltd., Japan). Peptide maps show differences in regions marked A, B, C.

Kinetic properties of both amine oxidases were compared. Generally, both amine oxidases oxidize more likely alkyl- and aralkylmonoamines as hexylamine or benzylamine, than diamines

244

and polyamines, do not showing any remarkable differences in substrate specificity. AO-I and AO-II, are inhibited by substrate analogs as 1,5-diamino-3-pentanone and ethylenediamine, typical copper chelating agents as o-phenanthroline, 2,2'-bipyridyl, diethylenetriamine and triethylenetetramine, carbonyl reagents as phenylhydrazine, and some alkaloids.

Cofactor of both amine oxidases reacts with p-nitrophenylhydrazine, forming an orange hydrazone of irreversibly inactivated enzyme with the absorption maximum at 465 nm and 440 nm, for AO-I and AO-II, respectively, as shown in Fig.2. The shift of this maximum to 585 nm under alkali conditions suggests the presence of topaquinone as a cofactor (Janes et al., 1992).

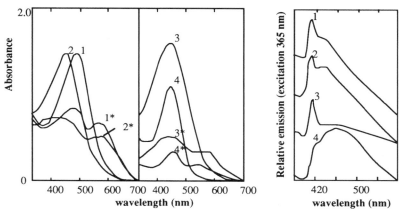

Figure 2. Absorption and fluorescence emission spectra of p-nitrophenylhydrazones of *Aspergillus niger* amine oxidases and model compounds in 10 mM KPB, pH 7 and pH 12 (adjusted by sodium hydroxide).
Left panel: Absorption maxima - pH 7: AO-I - 465 nm (1), AO-II - 440 nm (2), topaquinone hydantoin - 440 nm (3), PQQ - 440 nm (4); - pH 12: AO-I - 450 and 585 nm (1*), AO-II - 420 and 485 nm (2*), topaquinone hydantoin - 440 and 585 nm (3*), PQQ - 460 and 540 nm (4*). Right panel: Emission maxima: AO-I - 420 and 440 nm (1), AO-II - 420 and 440 nm (2), topaquinone hydantoin - 420 nm (3) and PQQ - 430 and 470 nm (4).

Synthesized model compound, topaquinone hydantoin p-nitrophenylhydrazone, shows the same spectral characteristics as the amine oxidases, rising a new absorption maximum at 585 nm in pH 12, while PQQ p-nitrophenylhydrazone shows only a maximum at 540 nm. Also both amine oxidases and topaquinone hydantoin p-nitrophenylhydrazones show fairly similar fluorescence emission spectra (excitation at 365 nm) with a sharp emission maximum at 420 nm and a flat one at 440 nm, while PQQ p-nitrophenylhydrazone spectrum is quite different.

Labeled enzymes were digested by thermolysin; labeled peptides were isolated by HPLC as shown in Fig.3, sequenced by Edman degradation. The structures were investigated by tandem mass spectrometry and topaquinone was found as a cofactor of both enzymes. The AO-I peptide, Val-Val-Ile-Glu-Pro, shows a ester linkage to the cofactor, N-terminal of which was blocked and could not be sequenced. AO-II does not contain such a linkage. Its sequence, Asn-topa-Glu-Tyr, is identical to topaquinone containing yeast *Hansenula polymorpha* (Mu et al., 1992), *Escherichia coli* (Cooper at al., 1992) and *Klebsiella aerogenes* (Yamashita et al., 1993) amine oxidases, all monomers of 80 kDa.

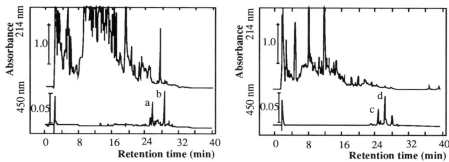

Figure 3. HPLC analyses of *p*-nitrophenylhydrazine labeled thermolytic peptides on a Shimadzu LC 6AD liquid chromatograph equipped with Capcell Pak C18 column (4.6 mmID x 25 cm, equilibrated with 0.3 % triethylamine acetate buffer, pH 7) and SPD M6A photodiode array detector, monitored at 214 and 450 nm. Purified enzymes, placed in 10 mM KPB, pH 7, were labeled with 1.1 fold of *p*-nitrophenylhydrazine (1 mM solution in ethanol) and dialyzed against the same buffer overnight. Then solid urea was added to 2 M concentration and enzymes were digested by thermolysin (3 %) for 48 hours at 37°C with shaking. Labeled peptides were purified by linear gradient to 20 % of the same buffer containing 60 % of acetonitrile in 10 min, followed by an increase to 45 % in 35 min, at flow rate of 1.4 ml/min, and sequenced by Edman degradation. Left panel: AO-I a) Val-Ile-Glu-Pro (25.7 min), b) Val-Val-Ile-Glu-Pro (28.4 min). Right panel: AO-II c) Asn-unk-Glu (25.3 min), d) Asn-unk-Glu-Tyr (26.8 min).

It is interesting that there are two genes for methylamine oxidase and only one gene is expressed in *Arthrobacter* strain P1 (Zhang et al., 1993). Different from that case, it is promising, that two genes are expressed to command two different quinoprotein amine oxidases in *Aspergillus niger*. A gene encoding AO-I has already been cloned and the second gene for AO-II is now under processing.

References

Adachi, O. and Yamada, H. (1969) Amine oxidase of microorganisms. VII. An improved purification procedure and further properties of amine oxidase of *Aspergillus niger*. *Agric. Biol. Chem.* 33: 1707-1716.

Cooper, R.A., Knowles, P.F., Brown, D.E., McGuirl, M.A. and Dooley, D.M. (1992) Evidence for copper and 3,4,6-trihydroxyphenylalanine quinone cofactors in an amine oxidase from the Gram-negative bacterium *Escherichia coli* K12. *Biochem. J.* 288: 337-340.

Janes, S. M., Palcic, M. M., Scaman, C. H., Smith, A. J., Brown, D. E., Dooley, D. M., Mure and M., Klinman, J. P. (1992) Identification of topaquinone and its consensus sequence in copper amine oxidases. *Biochemistry* 31: 12147-11254.

Janes, S.M., Mu, D., Wemmer, D., Smith, A.J., Kaur, S., Maltby, D., Burlingame, A.L. and Klinman, J.P. (1990) A new redox cofactor in eukaryotic enzymes: 6-hydroxydopa at the active site of bovine serum amine oxidase. *Science* 248: 981-987.

Mu, D., Janes, S.M., Smith, A.J., Brown, D.E., Dooley, D.M. and Klinman, J.P. (1992) Tyrosine codon corresponds to topa quinone at the active site of copper amine oxidases. *J. Biol. Chem.* 267: 7979-7982.

Yamada, H., Adachi, O. and Ogata, K. (1965) Amine oxidase of microorganisms. II. Purification and crystallization of amine oxidase of *Aspergillus niger*. *Agric. Biol. Chem.* 29: 649-654.

Yamashita, M., Sakaue, M., Iwata, N., Sugino, H. and Murooka, Y. (1993) Purification and characterization of monoamine oxidase from *Klebsiella aerogenes*. *J. Ferment. and Bioeng.* 76: 289-295.

Zhang, X., Fuller, J.H. and McIntire, W.S. (1993) Cloning, sequencing, expression, and regulation of the structure gene for the copper/topa quinone-containing methylamine oxidase from *Arthrobacter* strain P1, a Gram-positive facultative methylotroph. *J. Bacteriol.* 175: 5617-5627.

Biochemistry of Vitamin B$_6$ and PQQ
G. Marino, G. Sannia and F. Bossa (eds.)
© 1994 Birkhäuser Verlag Basel/Switzerland

The catalytic competence of cobalt-amine oxidase

Enzo Agostinelli, Laura Morpurgo, Changqing Wang, Bruno Mondovi and Anna Giartosio

Department of Biochemical Sciences, University of Rome "La Sapienza" and C.N.R. Center of Molecular Biology, Rome, Italy

Summary

Bovine serum amine oxidase is a dimer containing two equivalents of TPQ and two copper atoms, both of which are essential for full enzymatic activity and can be reversibly removed. Half copper depleted and fully copper depleted amine oxidase samples reconstituted with either copper or cobalt were studied by visible spectrophotometry, by enzyme activity analysis and by high sensitivity scanning calorimetry, The visible spectrum of the oxidized TPQ, which is bleached by Cu removal, is restored to approximately the same level by the addition of either copper or cobalt. The shape of the calorimetric profiles of cobalt substituted derivatives is extremely similar to that of the copper reconstituted species. Activity measurements show that in cobalt substituted amine oxidase the organic cofactor is reactive and the enzyme is catalytically competent, although kinetically less efficient.

Introduction

Bovine serum amine oxidase is an enzyme belonging to the wide class of deaminating oxidases (amine: oxygen oxidoreductases EC 1.4.3.6). It is only active on primary amines, which are oxidized by dioxygen to the corresponding aldehyde with production of hydrogen peroxide and ammonia. The enzyme is a dimer and contains two copper atoms and two molecules of the redox cofactor trihydroxyphenylalanine quinone or TPQ (Janes et al., 1990). The enzyme shows half-site reactivity: only one molecule of phenylhydrazine is bound per dimer (Morpurgo et al., 1992) and one molecule of benzaldehyde is produced in the reaction with benzylhydrazine, acting as a pseudo-substrate (Morpurgo et al., 1989).

Also the two Cu ions exhibit a different reactivity since only one or both are removed depending on conditions. The enzyme activity, 80% decreased in the half copper depleted from

(Morpurgo et al., 1987) and practically abolished in the fully copper depleted protein, can be partially recovered by copper or cobalt reincorporation (Suzuki et al., 1981; Morpurgo et al., 1990). The role of the metal cofactor in the catalytic mechanism of amine oxidases is not clear, since another metal can substitute for copper (Suzuki et al., 1983).

The relationship between copper and TPQ and the electron transfer in the enzyme are so far not well established. In order to obtain further information on this point some catalytic, chemical and physico-chemical properties of the enzyme with different contents of copper or cobalt were examined.

Materials and Methods

All chemicals were commercial reagents of analytical grade and were used without further purification, with the exception of N,N-diethyldithiocarbamate (DDC) and phenylhydrazine which were recrystallized from ethanol.

Purification of bovine serum amine oxidase, assay of the enzymatic activity, titration of reactive carbonyl groups and protein concentration determination were performed as described by Morpurgo et al. (1992).

Copper and cobalt were determined by atomic absorption spectrometry, with a Perkin-Elmer 3030 apparatus equipped with an HGA-400 graphite furnace.

Half copper depleted amine oxidase was prepared by the procedure of Morpurgo et al. (1987). The fully copper depleted protein was prepared according to Suzuki et al. (1983). Reconstitution of half and fully copper depleted species was achieved by dialysis against 2.0 mM $CuCl_2$ or 2.0 mM $CoCl_2$ in 0.1 M TRIS-HCl buffer, pH 7.2, for 48 hours at 4°C followed by dialysis against 1 mM EDTA to remove excess metal.

Microcalorimetric measurements were carried out at a heating rate of 60°C/h with a MicroCal MC-2D instrument (MicroCal Inc., Northampton, MA) , as described by Giartosio et al. (1988). Thermodynamic parameters were obtained by standard procedures (Privalov & Potekhin, 1986) using the Origin software package.

Results and Discussion

The fully copper depleted protein reconstituted with Cu (2Cu) or Co (2Co), and the half copper depleted protein reconstituted with Co (1Cu1Co) were examined (Table I).

While one TPQ carbonyl group per dimer reacts with phenylhydrazine in the native enzyme, this value is only 0.2 in the half copper depleted protein and less than 0.01 the fully copper depleted protein, reflecting the reduction state of the organic cofactor (Suzuki et al., 1983). By addition of copper or cobalt the amount of titratable carbonyl groups increased to values near 0.7 mol per dimer in good agreement with the recovery of catalytic activity in copper reconstituted species. It must be noticed that the reaction with cobalt containing species is slower but gives the same values of titratable carbonyl groups.

Table I: Recovered activity, TPQ reactivity, Cu and Co content of metal reconstituted amine oxidase

	Specific activity%	Carbonyl groups/dimer	Cu/dimer	Co/dimer	E_{480} nm (M^{-1} cm^{-1})
2Cu	68	0.68	1.7 ± 0.2		3300
1Cu1Co	27	0.66	1.0 ± 0.1	1.1 ± 0.1	2900
2Co	15	0.62	0.05 ± 0.01	2.1 ± 0.2	2600

The specific activity of the native enzyme (0.32 micromol $min^{-1}mg^{-1}$) was reduced to 16-19% in the half copper depleted enzyme and to less than 2% in the fully copper depleted protein. The intensity of the absorption band at 480 nm, attributed to the oxidized carbonyl cofactor was proportionally decreased .

After reconstitution with Cu(II), the fully copper depleted protein was 68% reactivated. Similar results were obtained upon reconstitution of the half copper depleted protein. Both reconstituted enzymes exhibited the characteristic 480 nm band.

Reconstitution with Co(II) of half copper depleted and fully copper depleted proteins lead to recovery of 27% and 15% of the native enzyme activity respectively and of 60-70% of the 480 nm absorption band intensity.

Enzyme activity, spectral features, and reactivity with phenylhydrazine were thus in part restored by incorporation of cobalt into half copper depleted and fully copper depleted species. Since this treatment did not increase the copper content of the samples (Table I), the recovery of catalytic activity, although low, cannot be attributed to adventitious Cu(II), but demonstrates that cobalt reconstituted species are catalytically competent although less efficient.

The characteristic trimodal thermogram of native amine oxidase was completely altered by removal of copper, the same broad featureless peak being obtained in the absence of only one or both copper atoms (Agostinelli et al., 1994). By addition of either copper or cobalt very similar thermograms were obtained, all of which show a trimodal profile (Fig.1) resembling that of the native enzyme. In agreement with the incomplete recovery of enzymatic activity (Table I), cooperativity was not fully restored in the thermogram of reconstituted copper enzymes. However, the thermal profiles of copper or cobalt reconstituted enzymes were always described by the same pattern of five independent two-state transitions, peculiar to the native protein (Agostinelli et al., 1994). The very limited changes in the calorimetric profile induced by substitution of copper with cobalt suggest that the cobalt atom fits the metal binding site with a small distortion of the protein architecture.

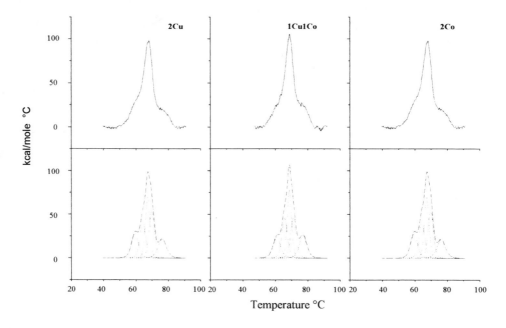

Transition	Tm °C	ΔH kcal/mol	Tm °C	ΔH kcal/mol	Tm °C	ΔH kcal/mol
I	60.7	146	58.3	128	59.3	157
II	65.6	204	66.0	198	64.1	199
III	68.5	269	69.0	288	67.2	255
IV	71.0	209	72.3	189	69.7	228
V	77.0	160	77.1	175	76.1	144

Figure 1.Thermograms, deconvolution in two-state transitions and thermodynamic parameters of reconstituted amine oxidases.

These findings have an interesting implication: since the redox properties of copper and cobalt are substantially different, it seems unlikely that the metal is involved in the redox process of the enzyme. The results reported here demonstrate that the spectral properties, the enzymatic activity and the calorimetric pattern of the copper depleted enzyme are restored only by metal addition, copper or cobalt indifferently. It should be pointed out that the original color due to oxidized TPQ in the copper depleted enzyme cannot be restored even under oxygen atmosphere and is only partially and very slowly recovered by reaction with ferricyanide (Suzuki et al., 1983).

These data as a whole lead us to conclude that the main role of the metal ions in the enzyme is that of maintaining the active site in a suitable conformation in order to allow TPQ to be reduced and reoxidized by substrates.

Acknowledgements

This work was partially supported by funds from C.N.R. Contract N° 94.00510.CT11, C.N.R. Special Project CF II N° 93.02810.72 and MURST (Ministero per l'università e la ricerca scientifica e tecnologica).

References

Agostinelli, E., Morpurgo, L., Wang, C., Giartosio, A. & Mondovì, B. (1994) Properties of cobalt-substituted bovine serum amine oxidase. *Eur.J.Biochem.* in press

Giartosio, A., Agostinelli, E. & Mondovì, B. (1988) Domains in bovine serum amine oxidase. *Biochem. Biophys. Res. Comm. 154*, 66-72.

Janes, S. M., Mu, D., Wemmer, D., Smith, A. J., Kaur, S., Maltby, D., Burlingame, A. L. & Klinman, J. P. (1990) A new redox cofactor in eukaryotic enzymes: 6-hydroxydopa at the active site of bovine serum amine oxidase. *Science 248*, 981-987.

Janes, S. M., Palcic, M. M., Scaman, C. H., Smith, A. J., Brown, D. E., Dooley, D. M., Mure, M. & Klinman, J. P. (1992) Identification of topaquinone and its consensus sequence in copper amine oxidases, *Biochemistry 31*, 12147-12154.

Morpurgo, L., Agostinelli, E., Befani, O. & Mondovì, B. (1987) Reactions of bovine serum amine oxidase with NN-diethyldithiocarbamate, *Biochem. J. 248*, 865-870.

Morpurgo, L., Agostinelli, E., Muccigrosso, J., Martini, F., Mondovì, B. & Avigliano, L. (1989) Benzylhydrazine as a pseudo- substrate of bovine serum amine oxidase, *Biochem. J. 260*, 19-25.

Morpurgo, L., Agostinelli, E., Mondovì, B. & Avigliano, L. (1990) The role of copper in bovine serum amine oxidase, *Biol Metals 3*, 114-117.

Morpurgo, L., Agostinelli, E., Mondovì, B., Avigliano, L., Silvestri, R., Stefancich, G. & Artico, M. (1992) Bovine serum amine oxidase: half-site reactivity with phenylhydrazine, semicarbazide, and aromatic hydrazides, *Biochemistry 31*, 2615-2621.

Privalov , P.L., & Potekhin, S.A. (1986) Scanning microcalorimetry in studying temperature-induced changes in protein, *Methods Enzymol. 131*, 4-51.

Suzuki, S., Sakurai, T., Nakahara, A., Oda, O., Manabe, T. & Okuyama, T. (1981) Preparation and characterization of cobalt(II) substituted bovine serum amine oxidase, *J. Biochem. 90*, 905-908.

Suzuki, S., Sakurai, T., Nakahara, A., Manabe, T. & Okuyama, T. (1983) Effect of metal substitution on the chromophore of bovine serum amine oxidase, *Biochemistry 22*, 1630-1635.

Suzuki, S., Sakurai, T., Nakahara, A., Manabe , T. & Okuyama, T. (1986) Roles of the two copper ions in bovine serum amine oxidase, *Biochemistry 25*, 338-341.

Biochemistry of Vitamin B$_6$ and PQQ
G. Marino, G. Sannia and F. Bossa (eds.)
© 1994 Birkhäuser Verlag Basel/Switzerland

Mechanistic Studies of Copper/Topa Amine Oxidases

David M. Dooley, Doreen E. Brown, Michele A. McGuirl and L. J. Sears

Department of Chemistry and Biochemistry, Montana State University, Bozeman, Montana, 59717, USA

Summary

The oxidation of benzylhydrazine by bovine plasma amine oxidase proceeds through several spectroscopically detectable intermediates, as reported previously (Morpurgo, *et al.* 1989). Here we report optical and EPR data that indicate a Cu(I)-semiquinone state may be involved in benzylhydrazine oxidation, similar to its involvement in the turnover of amine substrates.

Introduction

Evidence for a Cu(I)-semiquinone intermediate in the oxidation of primary amine substrates by copper-containing amine oxidases has been growing (Dooley, *et al.* 1991; Turowski, *et al.* 1993; Bellelli, *et al.* 1991; Pedersen, *et al.* 1992). The Cu(I)-semiquinone is generated via rapid intramolecular electron transfer from a reduced form of topa, probably the aminocatechol, and Cu(II). The Cu(I)-semiquinone and Cu(II)-reduced topa are in equilibrium (in the absence of oxygen) and the equilibrium is temperature dependent, with the Cu(II) form favored at lower temperatures. We have suggested that the Cu(I)-semiquinone state is the intermediate that reacts with oxygen during turnover (Dooley, *et al.* 1991). The mechanism by which amine substrates are oxidized to aldehydes, with the concomitant reduction of the topa quinone cofactor, has been substantially defined (see: Hartmann, *et al.* 1993; Hartmann and Klinman, 1991; Hartmann and Klinman, 1987; Janes and Klinman, 1991). Topa quinone mediates a series of addition/elimination reactions to generate the product aldehyde in the absence of oxygen; key steps are proton abstraction to generate a carbanionic intermediate, and subsequent hydrolysis of the imine to liberate the aldehyde. A very different mechanism was proposed by Morpurgo and co-workers (Morpurgo, *et al.* 1989) for the oxidation of benzylhydrazine to benzaldehyde and hydrazine (detected as the adduct with topa quinone). No spectral features attributable to a semiquinone state were observed and the reaction of oxygen appeared to precede benzaldehyde release. A hydroperoxy intermediate, generated via the addition of dioxygen to the methylene carbon of topa-bound benzylhydrazine, was suggested to break down to give benzaldehyde and a reduced hydrazinoquinone. We have reexamined the reaction of benzylhydrazine with bovine plasma amine oxidase (BPAO); a semiquinone state is observed that appears to be an intermediate in the reaction. In addition, benzaldehyde is produced under anaerobic conditions. On the basis of these observations an alternative mechanism for benzylhydrazine oxidation is suggested, which is similar to the mechanism of oxidation of amine substrates.

Materials and Methods

Anaerobic manipulations, EPR spectroscopy, and absorption spectroscopy were carried out as described previously (Dooley, *et al.* 1991). BPAO was purified by a method similar to that reported by Janes and Klinman, 1991. Benzaldehyde was detected by single ion monitoring GC/MS in the Montana State University Mass Spectrometry Laboratory using an HP 5890 GC and 5970 MS. Benzaldehyde was quantified by comparison to a standard curve generated with a *p*-xylene as an internal standard. The reaction of BPAO with benzylhydrazine under anaerobic conditions (0.650 ml of 25 µM enzyme in 0.1 M KPO$_4$ buffer, pH 7.2, with two equivalents of benzylhydrazine/protein molecule) was monitored optically and 100 µl aliquots withdrawn via gas-tight syringe for analysis by GC/MS. The aliquots were added to 100 µl of anaerobic chloroform, mixed vigorously, and then centrifuged. The aqueous layer was removed and the chloroform layer was dried, centrifuged, pipetted into a clean tube and then removed from the argon atmosphere for analysis. Control experiments confirmed that this procedure quantitatively recovered (± 10 %) benzaldehyde from aqueous protein solutions.

Results and Discussion

Absorption spectral changes accompanying the anaerobic reaction of BPAO with benzylhydrazine are shown in Figure 1A. As reported previously (Morpurgo, *et al.* 1989) the initial adduct, with λ$_{max}$ at 405 nm, decays into another species with λ$_{max}$ at 355 nm. However, new features are also observed at 484 and ~ 464 nm, these bands correspond to transitions of a topa semiquinone (Dooley, *et al.* 1987; Dooley, *et al.* 1991; Pederson, *et al.* 1992). These bands are not observed in the presence of oxygen and decrease in intensity at higher benzylhydrazine/protein ratios. Addition of oxygen-containing buffer induces the spectral changes shown in Figure 1B. As shown in Figure 1B, the final spectrum is essentially identical

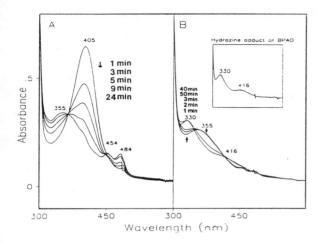

Figure 1. Time dependence of the reaction of BPAO with Bhyd. (A) Anaerobic reaction, (B) Final reaction mixture from (A), after addition of oxygen.

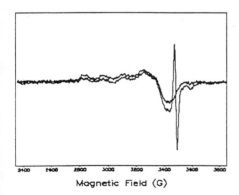

Figure 2. Room temperature EPR spectra of native BPAO and the BPAO-Bhyd adduct.

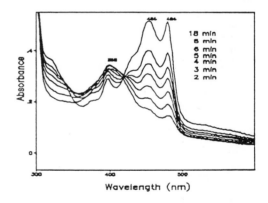

Figure 3. Visible absorption spectra showing of the reaction of BPAO with Bhyd in the presence of cyanide.

to that of the hydrazine adduct of BPAO. Room temperature EPR spectra clearly show the formation of a semiquinone signal (Figure 2); the Cu(II) EPR signal appears to be reduced, although this is difficult to quantify. Cyanide dramatically increases the intensity of the semiquinone absorption and EPR features (Figures 3 and 4). This behavior is very similar to that of the Cu(I)-semiquinone state generated via the reaction with amine substrates (Dooley, *et al.* 1990; Dooley, *et al.* 1991). Comparison of the absorption and EPR spectra indicate that the semiquinones are *not* identical, i.e. the semiquinone generated via the reaction with benzylhydrazine has a different structure from the semiquinone produced by reaction with amine substrates. Benzaldehyde is released anaerobically concomitant with the transformation of the 355 nm intermediate into another species (Table I). A mechanism consistent with the results reported here and previously (Morpurgo, *et al.* 1989) is shown in Scheme 1. This mechanism is analogous to mechanism proposed for the oxidation of amine substrates by copper-containing amine oxidases.

Table I. Time Course of Anaerobic Benzaldehyde (BAld) Release from the Reaction of 25 µM BPAO with 50 µM Benzylhydrazine.

Time (min)	Eq. BAld*	A_{355}
0	0.0	0.12
9	0.09	0.45
20	0.23	0.46
48	0.30	0.41
126	0.66	0.26
130 (open to air)	0.74	n.d.

*per active quinone (1.8 per dimer, as determined with anaerobic benzylamine).

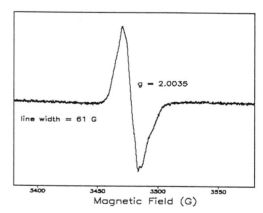

Figure 4. EPR spectra @ 77 K of the semiquinone formed from the reaction of BPAO with Bhyd in the presence of cyanide. Spectra at room temperature were identical.

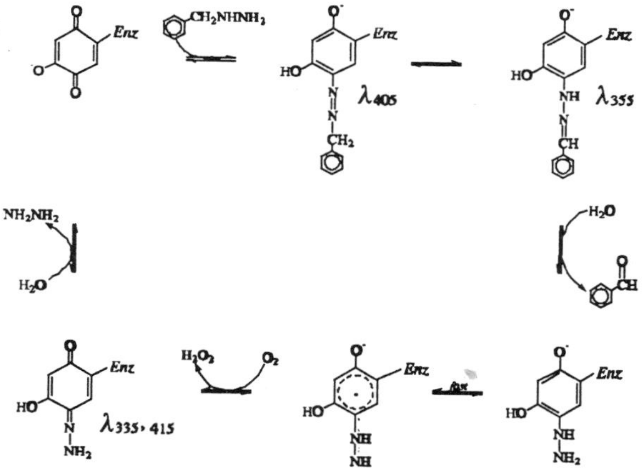

Scheme 1.

Acknowledgements

This research was supported by the NIH (grant GM 27659).

References

Bellelli, A., Finazzi-Agro, A., Floris, G., and Brunori, M. (1991) *J. Biol. Chem.* 266: 20654-20657.

Dooley, D. M., McGuirl, M. A., Peisach, J., and McCracken, J. (1987) *FEBS Lett.* 214: 274-278.

Dooley, D. M., McIntire, W. S., McGuirl, M. A., Cote, C. E., and Bates, J. L. (1990) *J. Am. Chem. Soc.* 112: 2782-2789.

Dooley, D. M., McGuirl, M. A., Brown, D. E., Turowski, P. N., McIntire, W. S., and Knowles, P. F. (1991) *Nature* 349: 262-264.

Hartmann, C. and Klinman, J. P. (1987) *J. Biol. Chem.* 262: 962-965.

Hartmann, C. and Klinman, J. P. (1991) *Biochemistry* 30: 4605-4611.

Hartmann, C., Brzovic, P., and Klinman, J. P. *Biochemistry* 32: 2234-2241.

Janes, S. M. and Klinman, J. P. *Biochemistry* 30: 4599-4604.

Morpurgo, L., Agostinelli, E., Muccigrosso, J., Martini, F., Mondovi, B. and Avigliano, L. (1989) *Biochem. J.* 260: 19-25.

Pedersen, J. Z., El-Sherbini, S., Finazzi-Agro, A., and Rotilo, G. (1992) *Biochemistry* 31:8-12.

Biochemistry of Vitamin B$_6$ and PQQ
G. Marino, G. Sannia and F. Bossa (eds.)
© 1994 Birkhäuser Verlag Basel/Switzerland

Design, synthesis and evaluation of mechanism-based inhibitors of copper amine oxidases

Lawrence M. Sayre, Fengjiang Wang, Younghee Lee, He Huang, Frederick T. Greenaway,[1] Zuwen He,[1] Alex Lightning,[1] and Herbert M. Kagan[2]

Department of Chemistry, Case Western Reserve University, Cleveland, OH 44106, USA
[1]*Department of Chemistry, Clark University, Worcester, MA 01610, USA*
[2]*Department of Biochemistry, Boston University School of Medicine, Boston, MA 02118, USA*

Summary

Structure-extended propargylic, allylic, 2-chloroallylic, and β-chloro primary amines exhibit time-dependent but only partially selective inhibition of plasma amine oxidase, diamine oxidase, and lysyl oxidase.

Introduction

The recent identification of the quinone cofactor of copper amine oxidases sets the stage for rational design of selective inhibitors of plasma amine oxidase (PAO), diamine oxidase (DAO), and lysyl oxidase (LO). Propargylamine, 2-chloroallylamine, and β-haloamines were previously shown to inactivate PAO (Hevey et al., 1973; Neumann et al., 1975), whereas β-substituted ethylamines ($BrCH_2CH_2NH_2$, $H_2NCH_2CH_2NH_2$) were shown to inactivate LO (Tang et al., 1984). In the former cases, inactivation can be rationalized on the basis of PLP-like reactive electrophile generation; for ethylenediamine, the proposed O_2-dependent formation of a cyclic (aromatized) cofactor adduct for LO is supported by a model study (Wang et al., 1994).

The three different mammalian enzymes have different substrate structure requirements. In particular, DAO prefers to deaminate four carbons away from a cationic group, whereas LO processes the aminobutyl side-chain of peptidyl lysine. Here described are our initial efforts to develop selective inhibitors by incorporating the "generic" inactivating moieties listed above into the various consensus substrate structure motifs.

Materials and Methods

Cis- and *trans-*1,4-diamino-2-butene (cDABE and tDABE) were prepared via Gabriel synthesis from the corresponding dichlorides. Hydrazinolysis of the diphthalimide derived from 1,4-dichloro-2-butyne afforded 1,4-diamino-2-butyne (DABY), whereas heating in $HCl/H_2O/HOAc$ gave *trans-*2-chloro-1,4-diamino-2-butene (CHLORDABE). Acetylation of the mono-*t*-BOC derivative of DABY and subsequent deprotection afforded N-acetyl-1,4-diamino-2-butyne (AcDABY). Conversion of 2,5-dichloroamylamine to the N-CBZ derivative and then to the corresponding diazide, followed by $H_2/Pd/C$ yielded 1,2,5-pentanetriamine (PTA). Alternatively, treatment of the initial N-CBZ derivative with 1 equiv of $C_6H_4(CO)_2NK$, followed by $H_2/Pd/C$, yielded 2-chloro-5-phthalimidopentylamine (CHLORPENA). Reaction of N^1-CBZ-CHLOR-PENA with NaN_3 and subsequent hydrazinolysis, followed either by acetylation or dimethylation (HCHO, HCOOH), and ultimately $H_2/Pd/C$, gave the N^5-acetyl (AcPTA) or N^5,N^5-dimethyl (Me_2PTA) derivatives, respectively, of PTA. Details will be described elsewhere.

Inhibitor studies on bovine plasma amine oxidase BPAO (Sigma), pH 7.2, 30°C (Wang et al., 1992), pig kidney diamine oxidase PKDAO, pH 7.2, 25°C (Castellano et al., 1993), and bovine aorta lysyl oxidase LO, pH 8.0, 37°C (Tang et al., 1984) were performed as described.

Results and Discussion

All three enzymes underwent time-dependent inactivation by the *trans-*allylamine- and 2-chloroallylamine-based inhibitors tDABE and CHLORDABE, the latter being more potent. IC_{50} and/or kinetic parameters are given below. The *cis-*allylamine compound cDABE behaved as a substrate (some inactivation was seen for PKDAO), consistent with rapid cyclization of the electrophilic *cis-*4-amino-2-butenal turnover product (giving pyrrole, see Pec et al., 1991) affording protection of the enzyme in a manner not possible in the *trans* case.

Potent inactivation of pea seedling DAO by the propargylamine-based inhibitor DABY was recently reported (Pec and Frebort, 1992). In our hands, DABY was the most potent inhibitor of BPAO. For both CHLORDABE and DABY, the plateau of initial activity loss seen for BPAO was followed at longer time by a partial regain of activity; two IC_{50} values are listed below. No activity recovery is seen upon exposure to higher concentrations of the inhibitors. Compared to DABY, AcDABY exhibits a much weaker inactivation of BPAO ($IC_{50} \sim 350$ μM), and at this concentration, the enzyme eventually recovers 90% of its activity. The β-chloroamine inhibitor CHLORPENA was a potent inactivator of BPAO ($IC_{50} = 8$ μM; $k_{inact}/K_i = 2.5$ mM^{-1}min^{-1}).

Enzyme	tDABE	CHLORDABE	DABY
BPAO	$k_{inact}/K_i = 0.01$ mM^{-1}min^{-1}	$IC_{50} = 26 \to 29$ μM	$IC_{50} = 0.8 \to 1.2$ μM
PKDAO	$k_{inact}/K_i = 0.50$ mM^{-1}min^{-1}	$k_{inact}/K_i = 10.9$ mM^{-1}min^{-1}	
LO	$IC_{50} = 0.5$ mM	$IC_{50} = 16$ μM; $K_i = 2$ μM	

The extended ethylenediamine-based inhibitors were weaker than the unsaturated amine inhibitors described above, and so far only reversible inhibition has been observed. For PKDAO, $K_i = 0.18$ mM for PTA; for LO, AcPTA exhibited $IC_{50} = 63$ μM. For BPAO, 2.5 mM PTA, AcPTA, and Me$_2$PTA exhibited 22%, 35%, and 20% inhibition, respectively.

Our results indicate that incorporation of generic inactivating moieties into the preferred diamine-based DAO substrate structure provides very potent inactivators of PKDAO, but strong inhibition is also seen for BPAO and LO. In fact, acylation of one "end" of DABY weakened rather than strengthened the inhibition of BPAO. Careful manipulation of binding and reactivity preferences will be needed to obtain highly selective inhibitors for the various copper amine oxidases.

Acknowledgements

This work was supported by NIH grants GM 48812 (LMS), GM 42104 (FTG), and AR 18880 (HMK).

References

Castellano, F.N., He, Z. and Greenaway, F.T. (1993) Hydroxyl radical production in the reactions of copper-containing amine oxidases with substrates. *Biochim Biophys Acta* 1157: 162-166.

Hevey, R.C., Babson, J., Maycock, A.L. and Abeles, R.H. (1973) Highly specific enzyme inhibitors. Inhibition of plasma amine oxidase. *J Am Chem Soc* 95: 6125-6127.

Neumann, R., Hevey, R. and Abeles, R.H. (1975) The action of plasma amine oxidase on β-haloamines. *J Biol Chem* 250: 6362-6367.

Pec, P., Chudy, J. and Macholan, L. (1991) Determination of the activity of diamine oxidase from pea with Z-1,4-diamino-2-butene as a substrate. *Biologia (Bratisl.)* 46: 665-672.

Pec, P. and Frebort, I. (1992) 1,4-Diamino-2-butyne as the mechanism-based pea diamine oxidase inhibitor. *Eur J Biochem* 209: 661-665.

Tang, S.-S., Simpson, D.E. and Kagan, H.M. (1984) β-Substituted ethylamine derivatives as suicide inhibitors of lysyl oxidase. *J Biol Chem* 259: 975-979.

Wang, F., Venkataraman, B., Klein, M.E. and Sayre, L.M. (1992) Transaminative desilylation of (aminomethyl)-trimethylsilane and transitory inactivation of plasma amine oxidase. *J Org Chem* 57: 6687-6689.

Wang, F., Bae, J.-Y., Jacobson, A.R., Lee, Y. and Sayre, L.M. (1994) Synthesis and characterization of models for the 2,4,5-trihydroxyphenylalanine (TOPA)-derived cofactor of mammalian copper amine oxidases, and initial amine reactivity studies. *J Org Chem* 59: 2409-2417.

Biochemistry of Vitamin B_6 and PQQ
G. Marino, G. Sannia and F. Bossa (eds.)
© 1994 Birkhäuser Verlag Basel/Switzerland

Copper ion-dependent biogenesis of topa quinone cofactor covalently bound to bacterial monoamine oxidase

Katsuyuki Tanizawa, Ryuichi Matsuzaki and Toshio Fukui

Institute of Scientific and Industrial Research, Osaka University, Ibaraki, Osaka 567, Japan

Summary

The gene of a Gram-positive Coryneform bacterium *Arthrobacter globiformis* encoding a copper-containing quinoprotein, phenylethylamine oxidase, has been cloned and sequenced. In the deduced amino acid sequence comprising 638 residues was found a tetrapeptide sequence, Asn-Tyr-Asp-Tyr, which is highly conserved in this class of enzymes. The former Tyr (Tyr-382) in the consensus sequence is supposed to be the precursor to the covalently-bound 2,4,5-trihydroxyphenylalanine (topa) quinone cofactor. To elucidate the mechanism of the quinone cofactor formation, an expression plasmid has been constructed for the cloned phenylethylamine oxidase gene, and the recombinant enzyme was overproduced in a Cu^{2+}-depleted medium. The Cu^{2+}-deficient inactive enzyme purified to homogeneity was dramatically activated upon incubation with Cu^{2+} under aerobic conditions, concomitantly with the formation of the topa quinone at the position corresponding to Tyr-382. The topa quinone formation was accelerated by hydrogen peroxide and retarded by catalase, but required no external enzymatic systems. The purified mutant enzyme, in which the precursor Tyr-382 to the topa quinone is replaced by Phe, had neither activity nor the topa quinone cofactor even after reconstitution with Cu^{2+}. These results demonstrate the Cu^{2+}-dependent autooxidation of a specific tyrosyl residue into the topa quinone cofactor. A possible mechanism of the topa quinone formation is discussed here, which represents a novel type of posttranslational modification of proteins to generate a covalently bound catalytic group.

Introduction

Copper-containing amine oxidases (EC 1.4.3.6), occurring widely in microorganisms, plants, and animals, catalyze the oxidative deamination of various biogenic primary amines to produce the corresponding aldehydes, ammonia, and hydrogen peroxide. The covalently-bound cofactor of the copper amine oxidase from bovine plasma was recently identified as the quinone of 3-(2,4,5-trihydroxyphenyl)-L-alanine (6-hydroxydopa; topa) by Klinman and her co-workers (1990). The novel quinone cofactor of topa has subsequently been shown to be ubiquitous in the enzymes of both eukaryotes and prokaryotes (Brown et al., 1991). Comparison of the quinone-containing peptide sequences with those of the enzymes deduced from the coding genes (cDNAs) revealed that the precursor to the covalently bound topa quinone is a specific tyrosyl residue (Mu et al., 1992), occurring in a highly conserved sequence, Asn-Tyr(topa quinone)-Asp/Glu-Tyr (Janes et al., 1992). Thus, it became evident that the tyrosyl residue is converted co- or post-translationally into the topa quinone cofactor, although the mechanism of this conversion is yet unknown.

Aiming at elucidation of the generation mechanism of the topa quinone cofactor in copper-containing amine oxidases, we have cloned and sequenced the gene encoding phenylethylamine oxidase from a Gram-positive Coryneform bacterium, *Arthrobacter globiformis* (Tanizawa et al., 1994). In the deduced amino acid sequence was found the consensus tetrapeptide sequence (Janes et al., 1992), containing a tyrosyl residue (Tyr-382) supposed to be the precursor to the topa quinone cofactor. Furthermore, we have constructed an overexpression plasmid for the recombinant phenylethylamine oxidase. Interestingly, the expression of the active, quinone-containing enzyme in *Escherichia coli* was markedly dependent on the presence of Cu^{2+} in the culture medium. The inactive, Cu^{2+}-deficient enzyme produced in the absence of Cu^{2+} could be converted *in vitro* into the active, quinone-containing form by subsequent reconstitution with Cu^{2+} of the crude extract (Tanizawa et al., 1994). We thus purified the overproduced enzyme in a Cu^{2+}-deficient precursor form and obtained unequivocal evidence for the Cu^{2+}-dependent autooxidation of Tyr-382 to the topa quinone cofactor.

Cu^{2+}-Dependent Autooxidation of Tyr-382 to Topa Quinone

The *E. coli* BL21(DE3) cells carrying the overexpression plasmid (pPEAO2) for the recombinant phenylethylamine oxidase (Tanizawa et al., 1994) were cultivated in the Cu^{2+}-depleted medium, and the inactive enzyme overproduced was purified to homogeneity in the presence of a strong Cu^{2+}-chelating agent, *N,N*-diethyldithiocarbamate. The Cu^{2+}-deficient enzyme thus purified showed very low specific activity, less than 0.5 unit/mg unless incubated with Cu^{2+}. It contained only a trace amount of Cu^{2+} (0.043 mol atom of Cu^{2+}/mol of enzyme subunit) when analyzed by atomic absorption and exhibited no absorption peak in the visible wavelength region. However, when the purified enzyme was incubated with excess Cu^{2+} (0.1-0.5 mM $CuSO_4$) at 30 °C for about 30 min, the specific activity increased to a level of 15-16 units/mg protein, which is markedly higher than those of monoamine oxidases purified from other sources (Janes et al., 1992; Cooper et al., 1992). Concomitant with the Cu^{2+}-dependent appearance of enzymatic activity, the enzyme solution colored brownish pink with an absorption maximum at 484 nm, which is ascribable to the formation of a quinone compound, most likely the topa quinone (Janes et al., 1992). The increase in absorbance at 484 nm was initiated by the addition of Cu^{2+} and reached a plateau after about 30 min. When the enzyme was anaerobically mixed with excess Cu^{2+} in an evacuated cell, there was no change in the absorption spectrum, indicating that the formation of the chromophore is strictly dependent on the presence of the dissolved oxygen. The addition of catalase to the reaction system containing 0.5 mM Cu^{2+} markedly retarded the chromophore formation, whereas the addition of hydrogen peroxide significantly accelerated the formation. However, the formation of the quinone compound required no external enzymatic systems, because the quinone was similarly formed by the *in situ* incubation with Cu^{2+} of the precursor enzyme immobilized on a polyvinylidene difluoride membrane by electroblotting.

To identify the quinone compound generated, the Cu^{2+}-activated enzyme was first treated with *p*-nitrophenylhydrazine, followed by complete digestion with thermolysin, as has been employed as the general strategy for isolation of the topa quinone-containing peptide (Janes et al., 1992). Like in the previous studies, a major yellow-colored peptide was eluted on the reversed phase liquid chromatography of the thermolysin digest. The *p*-nitrophenylhydrazone-containing peptide showed an absorption maximum at 458 nm at neutral pH and at 580 nm at alkaline pH (in 1 M KOH); the 120-nm red shift in absorption has been suggested to be unique to the topa quinone (Janes et al., 1992). Automated Edman degradation of this peptide identified its sequence as Ile-Gly-Asn-X-Asp-Tyr-Gly, where X is an unidentifiable residue. This sequence corresponds to that from Ile-379 to Gly-385, except for position 382, in the primary structure of phenylethylamine oxidase from *A. globiformis*, deduced from the nucleotide sequence (Tanizawa et al., 1994). The unidentifiable residue X is located at the position corresponding to Tyr-382. Thus the quinone compound generated by aerobic incubation with Cu^{2+} of the Cu^{2+}-deficient inactive enzyme is most likely the topa quinone, derived from Tyr-382. It has been established that resonance Raman spectroscopy is the most reliable method to identify the topa quinone in Cu^{2+}-containing amine oxidases (Brown et al., 1991; Mu et al., 1992; Janes et al., 1992). Hence we measured resonance Raman spectra of the *p*-nitrophenylhydrazine derivatives of the Cu^{2+}-activated enzyme, the quinone-containing peptide obtained by thermolysin digestion, and the topa quinone hydantoin model compound. All Raman spectra of these *p*-nitrophenylhydrazones were virtually identical, leading to the conclusion that the Cu^{2+}-generated quinone compound is the topa quinone. Furthermore, the purified Y382F mutant enzyme, in which the precursor Tyr-382 to the topa quinone is replaced by Phe (Tanizawa et al., 1994), had almost no activity (<0.05 unit/mg protein) and showed no absorption peak at 484 nm characteristic of the topa quinone, even after incubation with excess Cu^{2+}. No quinone compound was also produced by the *in situ* incubation with Cu^{2+} of the membrane-blotted mutant enzyme. These results show that the precursor to the topa quinone must be a tyrosyl residue but not a phenylalanyl residue.

Hypothetical Mechanism of Topa Quinone Generation

The results described so far demonstrate that the aerobic incubation with Cu^{2+} of the Cu^{2+}-deficient precursor form of phenylethylamine oxidase leads to the generation of its topa quinone redox cofactor. The multi-step autooxidation of a specific tyrosyl residue, as postulated for a possible pathway of the topa quinone biogenesis (Mu et al., 1992), is certainly mediated by the protein-bound copper ions, which have been well documented to present in close vicinity of the quinone cofactor (Janes and Klinman, 1991). We propose a possible mechanism of the topa quinone formation from the precursor Tyr-382, as shown in Fig. 1. Upon liganding Cu^{2+} on imidazoles from the conserved histidyl residues (Zhang et al., 1993; Novotny et al., 1994; Mu et al., 1994) and/or thiols from the conserved cysteinyl residues (Novotny et al., 1994), the precursor enzyme would then be hydroxylated at the C-3 position of Tyr-382 to 3,4-dihydroxyphenylalanine (dopa). For this initial ring hydroxylation, hydroperoxide bound to Cu^{2+} is likely formed from the dissolved oxygen, although no model reaction is known for the Cu^{2+}-catalyzed hydroperoxide formation. Oxidation of nearby thiols to disulfide may be a source of donating two electrons to produce the hypothetical Cu^{2+}-peroxide complex. Subsequent oxidation of dopa at position 382 to dopa quinone, followed by Cβ-Cγ bond rotation would place the C-2 ring carbon in close proximity to a Cu^{2+}-bound water molecule (McCracken et al., 1987). Given the high susceptibility of a dopa quinone model compound to a 1,4-addition of water at alkaline pH (Mure and Klinman, 1993), dopa hydration by Cu^{2+}-(OH_2) and the subsequent autooxidation would be expected to lead readily to topa quinone (Fig. 1).

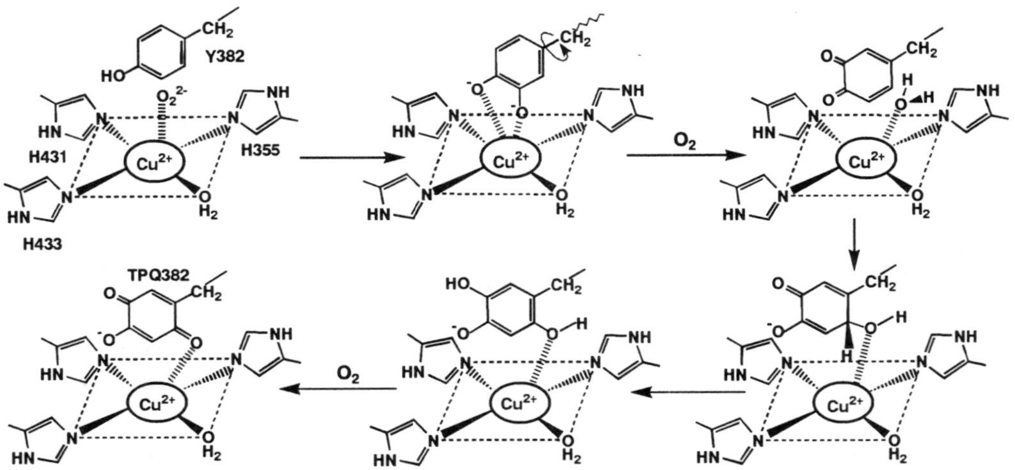

Figure 1. Hypothetical mechanism of Cu^{2+}-dependent autooxidation of Tyr-382 to topa quinone.

Conclusion

The proposed mechanism of the biogenesis of the topa quinone cofactor might represent a novel type of posttranslational modification to generate a covalently bound functional group involved in oxidoreduction. For the future it will be necessary to prove the hypothetical mechanism how the enzyme-bound Cu^{2+} converts a specific tyrosyl residue into the topa quinone cofactor through involvement of the possible formation of hydroperoxide and to examine whether the same cofactor in copper amine oxidases from eukaryotic organisms is also produced by Cu^{2+}-dependent autooxidation.

References

Brown, D.E., McGuirl, M.A., Dooley, D.M., Janes, S.M., Mu, D., and Klinman, J.P. (1991) The organic functional group in copper-containing amine oxidases. Resonance Raman spectra are consistent with the presence of topa quinone (6-hydroxydopa quinone) in the active site. *J. Biol. Chem.* 266: 4049-4051.

Cooper, R.A., Knowles, P.F., Brown, D.E., McGuirl, M.A., and Dooley, D.M. (1992) Evidence for copper and 3,4,6-trihydroxyphenylalanine quinone cofactors in an amine oxidase from the Gram-negative bacterium *Escherichia coli* K-12. *Biochem. J.* 288: 337-340.

Janes, S.M. and Klinman, J.P. (1991) An investigation of bovine serum amine oxidase active site stoichiometry: Evidence for an aminotransferase mechanism involving two carbonyl cofactors per enzyme dimer. *Biochemistry* 30: 4599-4605.

Janes, S.M., Mu, D., Wemmer, D., Smith, A.J., Kaur, S., Maltby, D., Burlingame, A.L., and Klinman, J.P. (1990) A new redox cofactor in eukaryotic enzymes: 6-Hydroxydopa at the active site of bovine serum amine oxidase. *Science* 248: 981-987.

Janes, S.M., Palcic, M.M., Scaman, C.H., Smith, A.J., Brown, D.E., Dooley, D.M., Mure, M., and Klinman, J.P. (1992) Identification of topaquinone and its consensus sequence in copper amine oxidases. *Biochemistry* 31: 12147-12154.

McCracken, Peisach, J., and Dooley, D.M. (1987) Cu(II) coordination chemistry of amine oxidases: Pulsed EPR studies of histidine imidazole, water, and exogenous ligand coordination. *J. Am. Chem. Soc.* 109: 4064-4072.

Mu, D., Janes, S.M., Smith, A.J., Brown, D.E., Dooley, D.M., and Klinman, J.P. (1992) Tyrosine codon corresponds to topa quinone at the active site of copper amine oxidases. *J. Biol. Chem.* 267: 7979-7982.

Mu, D., Medzihradszky, K.F., Adams, G.W., Mayer, P., Hines, W.M., Burlingame, A.L., Smith, A.J., Cai, D., and Klinman, J.P. (1994) Primary structures for a mammalian cellular and serum copper amine oxidase. *J. Biol. Chem.* 269: 9926-9932.

Mure, M. and Klinman, J.P. (1993) Synthesis and spectroscopic characterization of model compounds for the active site cofactor in copper amine oxidases. *J. Am. Chem. Soc.* 115: 7117-7127.

Novotny, W.F., Chassande, O., Baker, M., Lazdunski, M., and Barbry, P. (1994) Diamine oxidase is the amiloride-binding protein and is inhibited by amiloride analogues. *J. Biol. Chem.* 269: 9921-9925.

Tanizawa, K., Matsuzaki, R., Shimizu, E., Yorifuji, T., and Fukui, T. (1994) Cloning and sequencing of phenylethylamine oxidase from *Arthrobacter globiformis* and implication of Tyr-382 as the precursor to its covalently bound quinone cofactor. *Biochem. Biophys. Res. Commun.* 199: 1096-1102.

Zhang, X., Fuller, J.H., and McIntire, W.S. (1993) Cloning, sequencing, expression, and regulation of the structural gene for the copper/topa quinone-containing methylamine oxidase from *Arthrobacter* strain P1, a Gram-positive facultative methylotroph. *J. Bacteriol.* 175: 5617-5627.

Biochemistry of Vitamin B$_6$ and PQQ
G. Marino, G. Sannia and F. Bossa (eds.)
© 1994 Birkhäuser Verlag Basel/Switzerland

Modulation of lysyl oxidase activity toward peptidyl lysine by vicinal dicarboxylic amino acid residues

N. Nagan and H. M. Kagan

Department of Biochemistry, Boston University School of Medicine, Boston, MA 02118 U.S.A.

Summary

   The substrate specificity of purified lysyl oxidase has been explored with synthetic, 11-mer oligopeptides. -Glu-Lys- in Ac-Gly$_n$(Glu,Lys)Gly$_m$-NH$_2$ was a more favorable substrate than the glutamate-free control peptide and considerably more favorable than the -Lys-Glu- sequence as well as sequences in which Glu was separated from Lys by intervening Gly residues. The k$_{cat}$ for the -Asp-Glu- sequence was markedly reduced from that of the -Glu-Lys- sequence, indicating that lysyl oxidase responds to the side chain length of vicinal Asp or Glu at this position. -Asp-Glu-Lys- within an 11-mer was not oxidized, although this sequence is oxidized within the N-telopeptide of the α1(I) chain in type I collagen fibrils. Thus, lysyl oxidase exhibits distinct preferences for sequences vicinal to lysine. These results are discussed with respect to a model requiring collagen fibril formation prior to oxidation of lysine in collagen by lysyl oxidase.

Introduction

   Lysyl Oxidase initiates covalent crosslinking in collagen and elastin by oxidatively deaminating specific lysine residues to peptidyl-α-aminoadipic-δ-semialdehyde, the precursor of the crosslinkages found in these proteins. The activity of lysyl oxidase appears to be restricted to the single lysines in the N- and C-terminal non-triple helical telopeptide regions of the interstitial fibrillar collagens (Kagan, 1986). In view of the apparent preference of lysyl oxidase for lysine substrates with a net cationic charge (Kagan et al., 1984), it is noteworthy that the oxidized lysine in the N-telopeptides of types I, II, and III collagens is commonly found next or penultimate to one or two acidic amino acids, occurring within the consensus sequence -X-Asp-J-Lys-Z- where X is Tyr or Phe, J appears to be variable and Z is Ser or Gly. Surprisingly, residue Y is most commonly a glutamate in the α1(I) and α1(II) chain, potentially presenting two negative charges adjacent to the lysine residue. Similarly, the susceptible lysine in the C-terminal telopeptide of the α1(I), α1(II) and α1(III) collagen chains occurs in the -Glu-Lys-Z- sequence where Z is Ala, Ser, or Gly (Kagan, 1986). In the present study, we have explored the specificity of lysyl oxidase for collagen-like synthetic oligopeptide sequences assessing for the effects of anionic residues vicinal to lysine in an effort to clarify factors which might underlie the unusual substrate specificity of this enzyme.

Materials and Methods

Oligopeptides were synthesized as peptide amides from appropriately protected L-amino acids on a Milligen/Biosearch model 9500 solid phase peptide synthesizer using both Fmoc and *t*-Boc activation strategies (Atherton and Shepard, 1989). Lysyl oxidase was isolated from calf aortas by a modification of a previously described method (Williams and Kagan, 1985). The specific activity of lysyl oxidase ranged from 400,000 to 800,000 units mg^{-1} of protein as determined with a tritiated elastin substrate (Kagan and Sullivan, 1982). Activity toward oligopeptide substrates was determined by a peroxidase-coupled fluorescence assay for H_2O_2 production containing 0.25 mg homovanillic acid, 40 µg of horseradish peroxidase, 1.2 M urea and varying concentrations of the peptide substrate in 0.05 M sodium borate at pH 8.2 and 55°C (Trackman et al., 1981).

Results and Discussion

Glycine was chosen as the principal peptide backbone residue for the synthetic peptides used in this study. The C-terminus of each peptide was amidated while the N-terminus was acetylated. It was found that the k_{cat} increased significantly while there were lesser decreases in K_m as "n" increases from 1 to 5 in Ac-(Gly)$_n$-Lys-(Gly)$_n$-NH$_2$ (not shown), pointing toward multiple interactions between the substrate and an extended binding site in the enzyme. Further studies utilized peptides containing lysine and other selected residues within 11-mer oligopeptides.

As shown (Figure 1 and Table I), the presence of a Glu immediately C-terminal to Lys (Peptide 3) reduced the k_{cat}/K_m nearly 2-fold while Glu immediately N-terminal to Lys (Peptide 2) increased the k_{cat}/K_m nearly 5-fold relative to the control 11-mer lacking Glu (Peptide 1). Indeed, the K_m for the -KE- sequence (Peptide 3) exceeded that for the -EK- sequence (Peptide 2) by 24-fold. As shown (Figure 1), the -KE- sequence (Glu at +1 position) has the most unfavorable K_m in comparison to other positions within the peptide. The prominent maximum seen in the k_{cat}/K_m plot (Figure 1) indicates that the -EK- sequence is clearly optimal for lysyl oxidase whereas the -KE- sequence is the least efficiently oxidized. Introduction of an Asp residue immediately N-terminal to lysine (Peptide 4) decreases the K_m to a degree similar to that seen with the -EK- sequence. In marked contrast to the increase in k_{cat} seen with the -EK- sequence, k_{cat} is decreased 6.5-fold with the -DK- sequence when compared to the control (Peptide 1). The graphic representation of the effects of Asp and Glu at different residue distances from Lys reveals that the enzyme clearly discriminates between the 2- or 3-carbon sidechains of Asp and Glu, respectively, noting that the -KD- sequence is not unusually unfavorable nor is the -DK- sequence favorable, relative to the control lacking either Asp or Glu (0 distance), in marked contrast to the effects noted with the -EK- and -KE-sequences (Figure 1).

Table I. Effect of Vicinal Dicarboxylic Amino Acids on Peptidyl Lysine Oxidation

Peptide Number	Sequence	K_m, mM	k_{cat}, min^{-1}	k_{cat}/K_m, min^{-1} mM^{-1}
1.	G_5-K-G_5	2.61	1.82	0.68
2.	G_4-EK-G_5	0.69	2.29	3.34
3.	G_5-KE-G_4	16.6	6.28	0.38
4.	G_4-DK-G_5	0.71	0.28	0.40
5.	G_5-KD-G_4	2.94	1.91	0.65
6.	G_3-DEK-G_5	---	---	---
7.	ELSYGY-DEK-STG	3.64	0.44	0.12
8.	G_3-DQK-G_5	20.0	22.1	1.10
9.	G_4-QEK-G_4	0.83	1.15	1.39
10.	G_4-REK-G_4	2.66	4.26	1.60
11.	G_3-DPK-G_5	0.33	2.17	6.58

As noted, the N-terminal telopeptide of the $\alpha 1$(I) chain in type I collagen contains the sequence -Tyr-Asp-Glu-Lys-Ser-, thus combining two potentially anionic residues at the N-terminal of the lysine which is oxidized by lysyl oxidase. Remarkably, although the 11-mer oligopeptides containing -DGK- or -GEK- sequences are productive substrates for lysyl oxidase (Figure 1), the 11-mer containing the -DEK- sequence (Peptide 6) was not oxidized within the limits of detection. In addition, a 12-mer oligopeptide sequence was assembled which more closely resembled the N-terminal telopeptide of the $\alpha 1$(I) chain, differing only by the substitution of an N-acetylglutamate for the pyroglutamate occurring at the N-terminus of the natural sequence of the N-terminal telopeptide. Although this synthetic peptide was oxidized by lysyl oxidase (Peptide 7), the k_{cat}/K_m was 5.6-fold less than that of the control 11-mer (Peptide 1) and 28-fold less than that obtained with the favorable -EK- sequence (Peptide 2). Replacing Glu in the -DEK- sequence (Peptide 7) with a non-ionic but polar glutamine side chain (-DQK-, Peptide 8), results in a large increase in K_m, accompanied by a large increase in k_{cat}, with the resulting k_{cat}/K_m indicating that this is a reasonably efficient substrate, relative to the control 11-mer. Similarly, replacing the aspartate in the -DEK-with a glutamine (-QEK-, Peptide 9) restores favorable substrate properties to the 11-mer oligopeptide. Replacement of Asp by Arg in the -DEK-sequence (Peptide 10) restores favorable substrate potential. The effect of Pro in -DPK- (Peptide 11) suggests that a conformational factor influences the susceptibility to lysyl oxidase. These results reveal that the kinetic effects of a favorably positioned glutamate (-EK-) or aspartate (-DGK-) residue are not additive since their combined presence in the -DEK- sequence as in type I collagen presents a highly unfavorable substrate to lysyl oxidase. Moreover, the data argue that it is the anionic nature of the dicarboxylic amino acids in the -DEK- sequence that suppresses the efficiency of oxidation.

The specificity of the enzyme seen here with respect to vicinal anionic residues can be considered in the light of susceptible lysine sequences in the collagen substrates of lysyl oxidase. Most notably, a glutamate has not been seen immediately C-terminal to a lysine which is oxidized in collagen consistent with the present observation that the -KE- sequence is a poor substrate. Glutamate is consistently present in types I, II and III collagens in the C-telopeptide regions immediately N-terminal to the susceptible lysine, again consistent with the favorable kinetics seen here with the -EK- sequence. Given the intrinsic resistance of the -DEK- sequence to oxidation shown in the present study, it is of considerable interest that Fukae and Mechanic (1980) have shown that lysine in the -EK- sequence at the C-terminal telopeptide of type I collagen appears to be oxidized before the lysine in the N-telopeptide -DEK- sequence in vivo. Thus, the kinetic responses of purified lysyl oxidase to single anionic residues proximal to lysine seen in the present study are consistent with the distribution of anionic residues near lysine in collagen substrates of this enzyme. Although the -DEK- sequence is at best a very poor substrate for lysyl oxidase, this sequence is oxidized in the N-terminal telopeptides of $\alpha 1(I)$ and $\alpha 1(II)$ collagen chains. It is of particular interest in this regard that monomeric type I collagen molecules are very poor substrates for lysyl oxidase unless these molecules are first allowed to aggregate into quarter- (D-) staggered fibrils prior to enzyme action (Siegel, 1974). This results in the close approximation of the N- and C-telopeptide sequences with the conserved -Gly-X-Hyl-Gly-His-Arg-Gly- sequences occurring at the N- and C-terminal triple helical regions of adjacent collagen units (Siegel, 1979). Conceivably, the three basic residues in these triple helical sequences may provide a cationic environment critical to the oxidization of lysine in the adjacent telopeptide sequence (Kagan, 1986). Indeed, it has been previously noted that the guanidinium group of the arginine of this conserved, triple helical sequence could interact with the β-carboxylate of the N-telopeptide aspartate in the -DEK- sequence (Helseth et al., 1979). The effective charges vicinal to Lys 9^N in the telopeptide would then stem from the -Glu-Lys- sequence, shown in the present study to be most favorable to the expression of lysyl oxidase activity. The necessity for fibril formation prior to oxidation of lysine 9^N within the -DEK- N-telopeptide sequence could be accounted for by such charge neutralization effects.

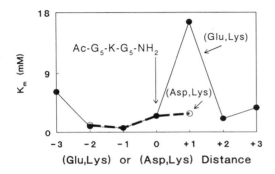 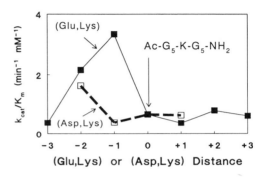

Figure 1. Effect of Glu or Asp at selected distances from Lys in 11-mer peptides. Solid lines, (Glu,Lys) peptides. Dashed lines, (Asp, Lys) peptides. (+) distance values are in the C-terminal and (−) distance values are in the N-terminal direction from peptidyl lysine.

Acknowledgements

This research received support from NIH grants R37 AR 18880, HL 13262 and HL 46902.

References

Atherton, E., and Shepard, R.C. (1989) *Solid Phase Peptide Synthesis: A Practical Approach.* IRL Press

Fukae, M., and Mechanic, G.L. (1980) Maturation of collagenous tissue. *J. Biol. Chem.* 255: 6511-6518

Helseth, D.L., Lechner, J.H., and Veis, A. (1979) Role of the amino-terminal extrahelical region of type-I collagen in directing the 4D overlap in fibrillogenesis. *Biopolymers.* 18: 3005-3014

Kagan, H.M. (1986) Characterization and regulation of Lysyl oxidase. In: Mecham, R.P. (eds): *Regulation Of Matrix Accumulation.* Academic Press Inc. (LONDON) LTD, pp. 321-397

Kagan, H.M., Williams, M.A., Williamson, P.R., and Anderson, J.M. (1984) Influence of sequence and charge on the specificity of Lysyl oxidase toward protein and synthetic peptide substrates. *J. Biol. Chem.* 259: 11203-11207

Siegel, R.C. (1974) Biosynthesis of collagen crosslinks: Increased activity of purified Lysyl oxidase with reconstituted fibrils. *Proc. Natl. Acad. Sci. U.S.A.* 71: 4826-4830

Siegel, R.C. (1979) Lysyl oxidase. *Int. Rev. Connect. Tissue. Res.* 8: 73-118

Williams, M.A., and Kagan, H.M. (1985) Assessment of Lysyl oxidase variants by urea gel electrophoresis: evidence against disulfide isomers as bases of enzyme heterogeneity. *Anal. Biochem.* 149: 430-437

QUINOPROTEIN DEHYDROGENASES

Biochemistry of Vitamin B$_6$ and PQQ
G. Marino, G. Sannia and F. Bossa (eds.)
© 1994 Birkhäuser Verlag Basel/Switzerland

The structure and function of quinoprotein dehydrogenases

C. Anthony

SERC Centre for Molecular Recognition, Department of Biochemistry, University of Southampton, UK

Introduction

Bacterial methanol dehydrogenase (MDH) and methylamine dehydrogenase are the only quinoprotein dehydrogenases whose structure has been determined by X-ray crystallography and both have an $\alpha_2\beta_2$ tetrameric structure in which the heavy subunit is a superbarrel made up of 4-stranded antiparallel β-sheet segments (Xia *et al.*, 1992; White *et al.*, 1993; Blake *et al.*, 1994; Chen *et al.*, 1992). However, this feature is the only similarity. The prosthetic group in MDH is PQQ which is located within the barrel of the α subunit, and the electron acceptor is cytochrome c_L; by contrast, the prosthetic group of methylamine dehydrogenase is TTQ, derived from two tryptophan residues in the light subunit, and the electron acceptor is the blue copper protein amicyanin. Furthermore, there is no similarity in the amino acid sequences of the two proteins and only methanol dehydrogenase has Ca^{2+} at its active site. This brief review will therefore consider only the structure of methanol dehydrogenase and discuss it in relation to two other bacterial quinoproteins; the quinohaemoprotein alcohol dehydrogenase (ADH) isolated from membranes of acetic acid bacteria and the membrane-bound glucose dehydrogenase (GDH) of many bacteria including *Acinetobacter*, *E. coli* and acetic acid bacteria. These three enzymes all have PQQ as prosthetic group and a Ca^{2+} ion at the active site, but they differ in their electron acceptors. MDH uses cytochrome c_L (Anthony, 1992a); ADH probably passes electrons from PQQ to ubiquinone by way of haem C on the same subunit and a separate cytochrome c (Matsushita *et al.*, 1994); and GDH passes electrons direct to ubiquinone (Beardmore-Gray & Anthony, 1986; Matsushita *et al.*, 1994).

The structure of methanol dehydrogenase (MDH) and comparison with the quinohaemoprotein alcohol dehydrogenase (ADH) and glucose dehydrogenase (GDH)

The basic structure of MDH from *Methylobacterium extorquens* which forms the basis of this review is very similar to that determined for MDH from *Methylophilus methylotrophus*, and organism W3A1 (Xia *et al.*, 1992). MDH has an $\alpha_2\beta_2$ tetrameric structure, each α subunit having a single molecule of PQQ and a Ca^{2+} ion. There is no interaction between the β subunits which are, as predicted from their primary structures, folded around the surface of the α subunits, bonded to them by hydrophobic interactions, which also bind the $\alpha\beta$ domains together (Blake *et al.*, 1994). This is as expected from the observation that it is not possible to reversibly dissociate the α and β subunits, or the $\alpha\beta$ subunits from each other, except by treatment with strong denaturing agents or detergents such as SDS.

Neither ADH nor GDH has any sequence corresponding to the β-subunit of MDH whose function remains obscure. Because 15 of its 74 amino acids are lysines it was suggested that it might play a role in interaction with the acidic electron acceptor cytochrome c_L (Anthony, 1990; Anthony, 1993); this now appears less likely because these lysines are not conserved in all MDHs and cross-linking studies suggest that interaction with cytochrome c_L is by way of the α-subunit (Cox *et al.*, 1992).

The peptide chain of the α subunit of MDH is organised in a very compact form as eight 4-stranded β sheet segments (or β-leaflets), arranged radially around a pseudo 8-fold axis. There are sequences in subunit I of ADH (1-594) and GDH (153-N-terminus) with sufficient similarity to MDH (1-599) to suggest that they might all have essentially the same type of structure (ADH being most similar) (Anthony, 1992b). This is perhaps supported by the observation that the sequences showing greatest similarity are the 4-stranded β-leaflets. ADH has a *C*-terminal extension that includes the haem C site and shows some similarity in sequence to cytochrome c_L (Inoue *et al.*, 1990; Anthony, 1992b), whereas the N-terminal sequence of GDH (1-152) provides 4-5 membrane-spanning helices, consistent with its membrane location (Cleton-Jansen *et al.*, 1990). It has been suggested (Friedrich *et al.*, 1994) that this N-terminal region might be the location of the ubiquinone-binding site in GDH.

In methanol dehydrogenase PQQ is buried within the α-subunit in an internal chamber, communicating with the exterior through a funnel-shaped depression in the surface which is quite narrow where it meets the chamber. The floor of the chamber is formed by Trp_{243} whose indole group is parallel to, and in contact with, the planar ring system of PQQ (Fig. 1) (Blake *et al.*, 1994).

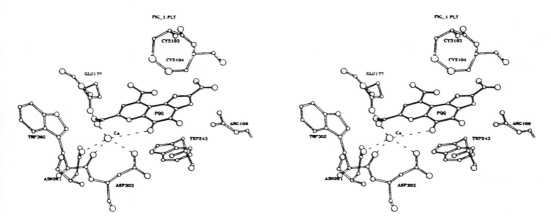

Figure 1. A stereo diagram of the active site of methanol dehydrogenase of *Methylobacterium extorquens*. This shows the PQQ prosthetic group, located between the ring structure formed from the Cys_{103}-Cys_{104} disulphide bridge in the roof of the active site chamber and the planar Trp_{243} in the floor. The proposed coordinations of the Ca^{2+} ion to active site groups are shown by dashed lines; these include coordination to the C7 carboxylate, and the oxygen of the C5 carbonyl of PQQ. The active site is contained entirely within the α subunit, some distance from the symmetry-related site and from the β chains. This Figure was provided by Dr Meenakshi Ghosh and is reproduced (with permission) from Blake *et al.* (1994).

The ceiling of the chamber is formed by a novel ring structure arising from a disulphide bridge between adjacent cysteine residues ($Cys_{103-104}$) which are joined by a *cis* peptide bond; this is the first observation of such a structure in an active enzyme (Fig. 1). When the disulphide bond is reduced all activity with cytochrome c_L is lost while activity with phenazine ethosulphate is retained, indicating that this structure may have particular importance in electron transport to cytochrome c_L. This conclusion is perhaps supported by the fact the adjacent cysteines are conserved in other MDHs and in ADHs, in which electron transfer is also probably to a haem C, whereas the disulphide bridge is not conserved in GDH in which the immediate electron acceptor is ubiquinone in the membrane (sequences from Anthony, 1992b):

Methanol dehydrogenase:	AVACCDLVNRGLAYWP
Alcohol dehydrogenase:	DKGCCDTVNRGAGYWN
Glucose dehydrogenase:	HLTC-----RGVMYYD

A second important feature seen in the active site is the Ca^{2+} ion which clearly plays a role in maintaining PQQ in the correct configuration, as predicted from spectroscopic and reconstitution studies of a mutant form of MDH that lacks Ca^{2+} and is unable to oxidise substrates (Richardson & Anthony, 1992). The ion is coordinated by 4 protein ligands, Glu_{177}, Asn_{261}, Asp_{303} and the main chain carbonyl of Trp_{302}, as well as the C7 carboxyl group of PQQ (Fig. 1). A sixth ligand to the C5 quinone oxygen of PQQ perhaps allows the Ca^{2+} to act as a Lewis acid thus facilitating nucleophilic attack of substrate at the quinone carbon. Previous proposals relating to the mechanism have involved base- or acid/base catalysis as a likely feature (for reviews see (Duine et al., 1987; Anthony, 1993), and it is probable that the Ca^{2+} ion and Aspartate 303 are involved in the catalytic mechanism. A similar function for Ca^{2+} in ADH and GDH is implied by the observation that of the four residues involved in coordinating Ca^{2+} (Glu_{177}, Asn_{261}, Asp_{303} and Trp_{302}), all are conserved in ADH, and two are conserved in GDH (Glu_{177} is replaced by Aspartate and Asn_{261} is absent).

A remarkable feature of the outer face of MDH is the entrance to the funnel leading to the active site 'chamber'; the funnel mouth is almost exclusively made up of hydrophobic residues. The sequences comprising these are summarised here with the **surface-accessible** residues in bold type; these are almost all hydrophobic residues and are identical in all MDHs:

```
MDH: 100-AVACCDL;    420-PFMLP;      430-FFV;   540-WPGVGLVFDLADPTAGL
ADH:     DKGCCDT;        NQVGG;          WNV;       I---missing--YPISM
GDH:     HLTC---;     no alignment            no alignment
```

There is clearly no similarity in GDH. In ADH the only similar hydrophobic, surface-accessible residues are the adjacent cysteines and those equivalent to F_{430}-V_{432} in MDH.

In the absence of an X-ray structure the primary sequences of proteins provide material for speculation of what might constitute their functional domains. In previous discussions of the sequences of these three proteins it has been suggested that the region with the highest degree of similarity between the three proteins (residues 477-539 in MDH) must constitute the PQQ domain (Cleton-Jansen *et al.*, 1990; Inoue *et al.*, 1990; Anthony, 1992b). This conclusion appears, however, to be unfounded. This region forms 3 well-defined loops which have no direct relationship to binding PQQ or Ca^{2+}. One small part is important in the interface between the α subunits of MDH (509-512) and this perhaps suggests that ADH and GDH also have an α_2 structure. The only part of this region that approaches the position of PQQ is at the end where the (unconserved) Trp_{540} is in the active site region. This example perhaps offers an appropriate warning against the dangers of speculation, to conclude this brief review of the structure and function of quinoprotein dehydrogenases.

Acknowledgements

I should like to thank my colleagues (M. Ghosh, K. Harlos and C.C.F. Blake) for valuable discussions, and the SERC (UK), Zeneca Bio-Products and The Wellcome Trust for financial support.

References

Anthony, C.(1990). The oxidation of methanol in Gram-negative bacteria. *FEMS.Microbiol.Rev.* **87**, 209-214.

Anthony, C.(1992a). The *c*-type cytochromes of methylotrophic bacteria. *Biochim.Biophys.Acta* **1099**, 1-15.

Anthony, C.(1992b). The structure of bacterial quinoprotein dehydrogenases. *Int.J.Biochem.* **24**, 29-39.

Anthony, C. (1993) Methanol dehydrogenase in Gram-negative bacteria. In: V.L. Davidson (ed.): *Principles and applications of quinoproteins*, Marcel Dekker, New York, pp. 17-45.

Beardmore-Gray, M. and Anthony, C. (1986) The oxidation of glucose by *Acinetobacter calcoaceticus*: Interaction of the quinoprotein glucose dehydrogenase with the electron transport chain. *J.Gen.Microbiol.* **132**, 1257-1268.

Blake, C.C.F., Ghosh, M., Harlos, K., Avezoux, A. and Anthony, C. (1994) The active site of methanol dehydrogenase contains disulphide bridge between adjacent cysteine residues. *Nature Struct.Biol.* **1**, 102-105.

Chen, L.Y., Mathews, F.S., Davidson, V.L., Huizinga, E.G., Vellieux, F.M.D. and Hol, W.G.J. (1992) 3-Dimensional structure of the quinoprotein methylamine dehydrogenase from *Paracoccus denitrificans* determined by molecular replacement at 2.8 Å resolution. *Protein-Struct.Funct.Genet.* **14**, 288-299.

Cleton-Jansen, A-M., Goosen, N., Fayet, O. and van de Putte, P. (1990) Cloning, mapping, and sequencing of the gene encoding *Escherichia coli* quinoprotein glucose dehydrogenase. *J.Bacteriol.* **172**, 6308-6315.

Cox, J.M., Day, D.J. and Anthony, C. (1992) The interaction of methanol dehydrogenase and its electron acceptor, cytochrome c_L, in the facultative methylotroph *Methylobacterium extorquens* AM1 and in the obligate methylotroph *Methylophilus methylotrophus*. *Biochim.Biophys.Acta* **1119**, 97-106.

Duine, J.A., Frank, J. and Jongejan, J.A. (1987) Enzymology of quinoproteins. *Advances in Enzymology*, **59**, 169-212.

Friedrich,,T., Van Heek, P., Leif, H., Ohnishi, T., Forche, E., Kunze, B., Jansen, R., Trowitzsch-Kienast, W., Hofle, G., Reichenbach, H. and Weiss, H. (1994) Two binding sites of inhibitors in NADH:ubiquinone oxidoreductase (complex I). Relationship of one site with the ubiquinone-binding site of bacterial glucose:ubiquinone oxidoreductase. *Eur. J. Biochem.* **219**, 691-698.

Inoue, T., Sunagawa, M., Mori, A., Imai, C., Fukuda, M., Takagi, M. and Yano, K. (1990) Possible functional domains in a Quinoprotein Alcohol dehydrogenase from *Acetobacter aceti*. *J.Ferment.Bioeng.* **70**, 58-60.

Matsushita, K., Toyama, H. and Adachi, O. (1994) Respiratory chains and bioenergetics of acetic acid bacteria. *Adv.Microbial.Physiol.* **36**, 247-301.

Richardson, I.W. and Anthony, C. (1992) Characterization of mutant forms of the quinoprotein methanol dehydrogenase lacking an essential calcium ion. *Biochem.J.* **287**, 709-715.

White, S., Boyd, G., Mathews, F.S., Xia, Z.X., Dai, W.W., Zhang, Y.F. and Davidson, V.L. (1993) The active site structure of the calcium-containing quinoprotein methanol dehydrogenase. *Biochemistry* **32**, 12955-12958.

Xia, Z.X., Dai, W.W., Xiong, J.P., Hao, Z.P., Davidson, V.L., White, S. and Mathews, F.S. (1992) The 3-dimensional structures of methanol dehydrogenase from 2 methylotrophic bacteria at 2.6 Å resolution. *J.Biol.Chem.* **267**, 22289-22297.

Biochemistry of Vitamin B$_6$ and PQQ
G. Marino, G. Sannia and F. Bossa (eds.)
© 1994 Birkhäuser Verlag Basel/Switzerland

Quinoprotein oxidoreductases for the oxidation of alcohols, sugars and amines

J.A. Duine, J.A. Jongejan and S. de Vries

Delft University of Technology, Dept. of Microbiology & Enzymology, Julianalaan 67, 2628 BC Delft, The Netherlands

Summary

Quinoproteins are enzymes containing a quinone cofactor, that is the non-covalently bound PQQ or the protein-chain-integrated TPQ or TTQ. Quinoprotein dehydrogenases play a role in non-phosphorylative degradation of sugars, alcohols, aldehydes, ketones, and amines by Gram-negative bacteria, providing useful energy to the organism by their capacity to transfer electrons to the respiratory chain. Since the quinoprotein dehydrogenase mostly occurs in high quantity or has a high turnover number, very efficient substrate conversions can be achieved with it, as observed in *Pseudomonads, Acetobacters* and *Gluconobacters*. However, since the quinoprotein dehydrogenase always catalyzes the first step and subsequent steps in the route are sometimes lacking or are less efficient, in these cases incomplete oxidation or overproduction occurs, as exemplified by the production of vinegar or gluconic acid. Progress in the enzymology and bioenergetics of these quinoproteins as well as applicational aspects related to enantioselective kinetic resolutions and electrode-directed electron transfer are discussed.

TPQ-containing amine oxidases are widely distributed among prokaryotes and eukaryotes. An efficient method for the isolation of TPQ or hydrazine-derivatizatable cofactors is described.

Introduction

During the past 15 years, three novel cofactors (Fig. 1) have been discovered, pyrroloquinoline quinone (PQQ), tryptophyl tryptophanquinone (TTQ), and topaquinone (TPQ) (Duine, 1991). As compared to the well known cofactors and coenzymes, these novel ones have a high redox potential and a quinone moiety, providing unique properties to the enzymes having such a cofactor (quinoproteins). In addition, based on primary structures, it appears that the quinoenzymes form a\ distinct family of proteins (vide infra) and some features of the tertiary structure are unique as well.

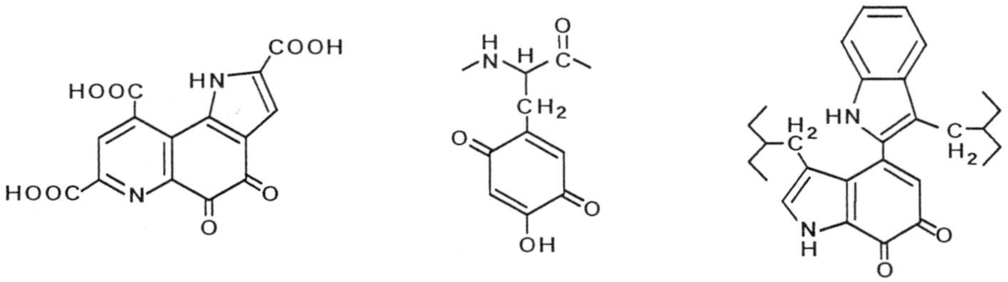

Figure 1. The structures of PQQ, TPQ and TTQ.

The exclusive structural properties indicated above could be related to special catalytic features required by the microbes in which quinoproteins fulfill a physiological role (as far is known, only in oxidation of substrates). This could form an explanation for the fact that an enormous variety of different oxidoreductases exists catalyzing one and the same reaction. For instance, microbial oxidation of ethanol can occur via NAD(P)-dependent dehydrogenases (of which many isoenzymes exist in mammals), nicotinoprotein dehydrogenases, quinoprotein and quinohaemoprotein dehydrogenases, and flavoprotein dehydrogenases as well as oxidases (van Ophem and Duine, 1993). Thus, is this enormous diversity due to the accidental emergence in evolutionary history of different enzymes for a certain reaction or is it related to the need for unique catalysts tailored to the special constraints (which are presently obscure) imposed by the respective organisms? Placed in this context, elucidation of structure/function relationships in quinoproteins might contribute to understand the biochemical meaning of cofactor-diversity in enzymes catalyzing one and the same reaction. In addition, exploration of these enzymes might also be rewarding in the field of biotechnology as the special properties could circumvent bottlenecks presently hampering the application of oxidoreductases with respect to kinetic resolution of racemates or electron transfer processes. It will be tried to discuss the progress made by our research group in the light of these two main leads.

Quinoprotein alcohol dehydrogenases

Ethanol dehydrogenase (EDH). EDH from *Pseudomonas aeruginosa* appears to have similar structural properties as methanol dehydrogenase (MDH, EC 1.1.99.8) from Gram-negative methylotrophic bacteria, except that the Ca^{2+} and the PQQ are less firmly bound (Schrover et al., 1993). In a search for the natural electron acceptor for this enzyme, a novel cytochrome c was discovered in this organism when grown on ethanol. This so-called cytochrome c_{EDH} seems to function as in vivo electron acceptor for EDH since no other compound with such a property was found in the cell-free extract and electron transfer rates between the two components was sufficiently high to assign physiological significance to it. In the meantime, a further search for the next electron acceptor revealed a blue copper protein able to mediate electron transfer between reduced cytochrome c_{EDH} and the respiratory chain, and which appears to be identical to azurin. Subsequently, the electrons are transferred to a "co"-type oxidase, as judged from the changes in the absorption spectrum of membrane particles upon addition of reduced azurin. Since MDH transfers its electrons to the respiratory chain via two soluble cytochromes c, the pathway for EDH appears to be different. In addition, besides the generally accepted role in (anaerobic) nitrate respiration, the discovery of this novel chain shows that azurin also has a role in aerobic respiration. Further work is in progress on characterization of the co-type oxidase and structural comparison of the anaerobically and aerobically induced azurins.

Quinohaemoprotein ethanol dehydrogenase (QH-EDH). All strains of *Comamonas testosteroni* tested from the LMD culture collection contain QH-EDH (in the apo-form, i.e. without PQQ) but not *C. acidovorans* and *C. terrigena* strains (Geerlof et al., 1994[a]). The enzyme (in the holo-form) oxidizes primary alcohols as well as aldehydes. Kinetical investigations as well as product analysis revealed the following: conversion of ethanol in a pH-stat requires addition of 4 equivalents of potassium ferricyanide as electron acceptor and consumes 5 equivalents of NaOH (due to the protons formed and the dissociation of acetic acid at the pH maintained); acetaldehyde is observed as a transient in the conversion, in line with a ping pong mechanism in which the produced aldehyde is released and the enzyme is reoxidized (in two steps) before a next round of oxidation of either ethanol or acetaldehyde starts. Screening of many alcohol oxidoreductases for kinetic resolution of racemic solketal (2,2-dimethyl-4-(hydroxymethyl)-1,3-dioxolane) and glycidol (2,3-epoxy-1-propanol), of which the enantiomers are interesting building blocks for synthesis of homochiral pharmaceuticals, revealed a high activity and enantioselectivity of QH-EDH's for these compounds (Geerlof et al, 1994[b]), as shown for solketal (Fig. 2). Investigations with whole organisms using such enzymes for the primary step in alcohol conversion (e.g. *Acetobacter* bacteria) (Geerlof et al., 1994[a,c]) show that besides hydrolases, oxidoreductases are also suited as biocatalysts in production of fine chemicals.

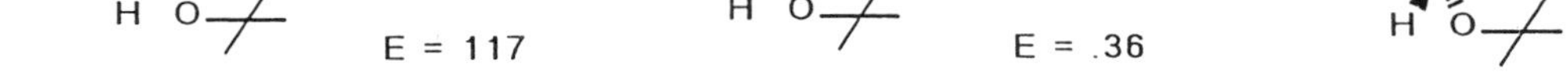

Figure 2. Kinetic resolution of racemic solketal by QH-EDH.

Quinoprotein glucose dehydrogenases

Soluble glucose dehydrogenase (EC 1.1.99.17) (s-GDH). s-GDH has sofar only been found in *Acinetobacter calcoaceticus* strains. Just as other quinoprotein dehydrogenases which have PQQ as the sole cofactor, certain cationic, artificial dyes function as electron acceptor for s-GDH. However, the enzyme can also be assayed with nitrosoanilines (Fig. 3). This latter property and the insensitivity to O_2 by definition, make this enzyme suited for application in diagnostic strips for glucose estimations.

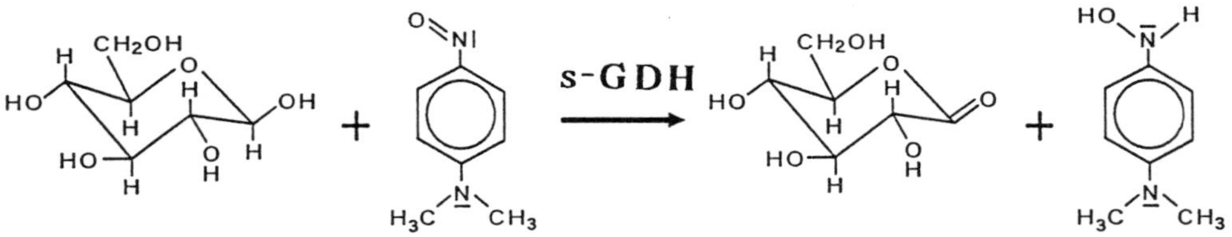

Figure 3. Assay reaction of s-GDH with ß-D-glucose and N,N-dimethyl-4-nitrosoaniline.

The enzyme has also excellent properties for another approach in glucose analysis, namely the amperometric biosensor: it has a high turnover number; the redox potential is high so that equilibria due to back reaction do not complicate analysis. Preliminary investigations (Ye et al., 1993) have shown indeed that: s-GDH is able to transfer electrons to an electron-conducting polymeric network and that the current density is the highest ever achieved in such systems; in contrast to an electrode based on the commonly used glucose oxidase (EC 1.1.3.4), no effects of changing the O_2 tension from that in air to "anaerobic conditions" are observed. Although it may appear that the enzyme is not perfect for this, the present status of knowledge warrants that improvements can be made: the gene has been cloned and the enzyme can be easily purified from an *Escherichia coli* recombinant strain (van der Meer et al., 1990); the 3-dimensional structure is coming (Schlunegger et al., 1993).

Membrane-bound glucose dehydrogenase (m-GDH). m-GDH occurs in many Gram-negative bacteria, including *E. coli*. It is a hydrophobic, membrane-spanning enzyme which transfers its electrons to ubiquinone (Yamada et al., 1993). Surprisingly, most of these bacteria produce the enzyme but not PQQ. Although it has been suggested (Biville et al., 1991) that *E. coli* contains silent genes for PQQ biosynthesis, this has not been confirmed sofar and controversial observations exist: production of GDH activity by *E. coli* (and thus probably of PQQ) requires introduction of 5 genes from *A. calcoaceticus* (Goosen et al., 1989); production of PQQ by *E. coli* requires introduction of 6 genes from *Klebsiella pneumoniae* (Meulenberg et al., 1990); production of gluconic acid by *E. coli* requires introduction of a small piece of DNA from *Erwinia herbicola* (Liu et al., 1992). Thus, another explanation, namely the possibility that other Gram-negative bacteria provide these apo-m-GDH-producing ones with PQQ, cannot be excluded. Complementation of two different PQQ⁻-mutants has been achieved and elucidation of the structure of the intermediate is in progress (J. Velterop, this symposium).

Table 1. Substrate specificities of m-GDH and s-GDH, both from *A. calcoaceticus* LMD 79.41. Both enzymes were assayed with various sugars and phenazine methosulphate, coupled to dichlorophenol indophenol, as electron acceptor

Substrate Activity (in %, related to the k'_{sp} value of glucose)

Substrate	m-GDH	s-GDH
D-glucose	100	100
D-xylose	31	3
L-xylose	22	0
D-fucose	51	26
2-deoxy-glucose	46	0.2
L-arabinose	6	85
D-ribose	2	0.6
D-mannose	3	3
D-galactose	5	9
Lactose	2	46
Maltose	3	47
Cellobiose	0.2	63

m-GDH and s-GDH have a quite different structure and substrate specificity (Table I), although the PQQ-binding sites as shown in the 3-dimensional structure of MDH, are present in both enzymes.

Efficient electron transfer occurs from m-GDH to the respiratory chain, as exemplified by *Gluconobacter oxidans* strains which are used in the industrial production of gluconic acid. Attempts have already been made by protein engineering to modify the substrate specificity of this enzyme (Cleton-Jansen et al., 1991).

Quinoprotein amine oxidoreductases

Methylamine dehydrogenase (EC 1.4.99.3) (MADH). The TTQ-containing MADH catalyzes oxidation of primary amines and is found in several Gram-negative methylotrophic bacteria. It was the first quinoprotein dehydrogenase of which the 3-dimensional structure was obtained and recent refinement shows much detail, including the angle between the planes of the two tryptophan moieties in TTQ (Huizinga et al., 1992). The genes for MADH synthesis have been isolated and sequenced for *Methylobacterium extorquens* (Chistoserdov et al., 1991), *Paracoccus denitrificans* (C. van der Palen, this symposium), and a few for *Thiobacillus versutus* (Huitema et al., 1993). Strong indications exist that gene products are involved (a.o. a protein having sequence similarity to cytochrome c peroxidase) in the processing of the two tryptophans to TTQ.

Quinoprotein amine oxidases (EC 1.4.3.6). This copper- and TPQ-containing type of amine oxidase is widespread, the distribution ranging from man to bacteria. First results presented on this symposium by K. Tanizawa, indicate that spontaneous formation of TPQ occurs when Cu_2^+ is added to the apo-enzyme under aerobic condition. Apparently, the specific tyrosine precursor in the protein chain becomes easily oxidized in the presence of the metal ion, a conversion which may also take place in vivo.

To enable identification of TPQ in amine oxidases of several bacteria (V. Steinebach, A. Hasisalihoglu, J.A. Jongejan and J.A. Duine, this symposium), the following method was developed: the cofactor in the enzyme is derivatized with a hydrazine; the adduct is liberated in an easy way and in good yield by proteolysis with pronase; the adduct is purified and structure elucidation carried out with NMR and MS (Fig. 4).

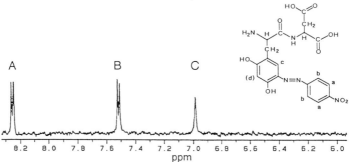

Figure 4.
^{1}H-NMR spectrum of the TPQ-4-nitrophenylhydrazine adduct (azo-form) isolated from pig kidney diamine oxidase.

Acknowledgements

We thank A. Olsthoorn, A. Dewanti, J. Schrover, A. de Jong, and Dr. J. Stoorvogel for providing us unpublished information.

References

Biville, F., Turlin, E. and Gasser, F. (1991) *J. Gen. Microbiol.* 137: 1775-1782.

Chistoserdov, A.Y., Tsygankov, Y.D. and Lidstrom, M.E. (1991) *J. Bacteriol.* 173: 5901-5908.

Duine, J.A. (1991) *Eur. J. Biochem.* 200: 271-284.

Geerlof, A., Stoorvogel, J., Jongejan, J.A., Leenen, E.J.T.M., van Dooren, T.G.M., van den Tweel, W.J.J. and Duine, J.A. (1994)[a] *Appl. Microbiol. Biotechnol.*, in press.

Geerlof, A., van Tol, J.B.A., Jongejan, J.A. and Duine, J.A. (1994)[b] *Biosci. Biotech. Biochem.* 58: 1028-1036.

Geerlof, A., Jongejan, J.A., van Dooren, T.G.M., Raemakers-Franken, P.C., van den Tweel, W.J.J. and Duine, J.A. (1994)[c] *Enzyme Microbial Technol.*, in press.

Goosen, N., Horsman, H.P., Huinen, R.G. and van de Putte, P. (1989) *J. Bacteriol.* 171: 447-455.

Huitema, F., van Beeumen, J., van Driessche, G., Duine, J.A. and Canters, G.W. (1993) *J. Bacteriol.* 175: 6254-6259.

Huizinga, E.G., van Zanten, B.A.M., Duine, J.A., Jongejan, J.A., Huitema, F., Wilson, K. and Hol, W.G. (1992) *Biochemistry* 31: 9789-9759.

Liu, S-T., Lee, L-Y., Tai, C-Y., Hung, C-H., Chang, Y-S., Wolfram, J.H., Rogers, R. and Goldstein, A.H. (1992) *J. Bacteriol.* 174: 5814-5819.

Meulenberg, J.J.M., Sellink, E., Loenen, W.A.M., Riegman, N.H., van Kleef, M.A.G. and Postma, P.W. (1990) *FEMS Microbiol. Lett.* 71: 337-344.

Schlunegger, M.P., Gruetter, M.G., Streiff, M.B., Olsthoorn, A.J.J. and Duine, J.A. (1993) *J. Mol. Biol.* 233: 784-786.

Schrover, J.M.J., Frank, J., van Wielink, J.E. and Duine, J.A. (1993) *Biochem. J.* 290: 123-127.

Van Ophem, P.W. and Duine, J.A. (1993) In: H. Weiner et al., (eds): *Enzymology of carbonyl metabolism 4*, Plenum Press, New York, pp. 605-620.

Yamada, M., Sumi, K., Matsushita, K., Adachi, O. and Yamada, Y. (1993) *J. Biol. Chem.* 268: 12812-12817.

Ye, L., Haemmerle, M., Olsthoorn, A.J.J., Schuhmann, W., Schmidt, H-L., Duine, J.A. and Heller, A. (1993) *Anal Chem.* 65: 238-241.

Biochemistry of Vitamin B₆ and PQQ
G. Marino, G. Sannia and F. Bossa (eds.)
© 1994 Birkhäuser Verlag Basel/Switzerland

The ternary complex between methylamine dehydrogenase, amicyanin and cytochrome c_{551i}

F.S. Mathews, L. Chen, R.C.E. Durley and V. L. Davidson[1]

Washington University School of Medicine, Dept. of Biochemistry and Molecular Biophysics, St. Louis, MO, USA
[1]*University of Mississippi Medical Center, Dept. of Biochemistry, Jackson MS, USA*

Summary

The structure of a ternary complex between methylamine dehydrogenase (MADH), amicyanin and cytochrome c_{551i}, all from *Paracoccus denitrificans* has been determined at 2.4 Å resolution. MADH and amicyanin associate so that the exposed edges of Trp 108 of TTQ and the His 95 ligand of copper are juxtaposed. Amicyanin and cytochrome c_{551i} associate so that one edge of the β-sandwich of amicyanin is in contact with a chain segment of the cytochrome close to the heme propionates. The distance from the catalytically active quinone oxygen of TTQ to the copper is 16.8 Å and from the copper to the iron is 24.8 Å, respectively. Two efficient paths for electron flow from TTQ to copper were found, one passing through Trp 108 of MADH. Two paths from copper to iron were also found, one through the cysteine and one through the methionine ligand to copper, which converge at Tyr 30 of amicyanin.

Introduction

Oxidation of methylamine in methylotrophic bacteria is catalyzed by methylamine dehydrogenase (MADH), an inducible, periplasmic enzyme. This enzyme is a quinoprotein and contains the novel cofactor tryptophan tryptophylquinone (TTQ), which is derived from two tryptophan side chains (McIntire et. al., 1991). Subsequently, electrons are transferred to the membrane bound terminal oxidases, via a series of soluble electron carrier proteins (Davidson and Kumar, 1989). In facultative autotrophs, such as *Paracoccus denitrificans*, the initial electron acceptor in this chain is amicyanin, a blue copper protein (Husain and Davidson, 1985). *In vitro* studies indicate that the next acceptor along the chain is cytochrome c_{551i} (Husain and Davidson, 1986). All three proteins are induced when the bacteria are grown on methylamine as the sole carbon source. MADH is a hetero-tetramer consisting of two identical pairs of heavy (H) and light (L) subunits. The H and L subunits from *Paracoccus denitrificans* have molecular weights 46.7 kDa and 15.5 kDa, respectively (Husain and Davidson, 1987). Amicyanin is a cupredoxin of 11.5 kDa with two His, one Met and one Cys serving as ligands to the copper (Durley et. al., 1993). Cytochrome c_{551i} is an acidic protein, with a pI of 3.3, and has a molecular weight of 17.5 kDa (Gary et. al., 1986).

Materials and Methods

Crystals of the ternary complex were obtained by vapor difussion of a mixture of MADH, amicyanin and cytochrome c_{551i} in the molar ratio 1:3:3 against 2.5 M phosphate buffer (NaH_2PO_4/K_2HPO_4), pH 5.5, as described previously (Chen et. al., 1992). The structure was solved by molecular replacement using the MADH/amicyanin binary complex (Chen et. al., 1991) as a search probe. The cytochrome c_{551i} structure was traced in a $2F_o$-F_c electron density map in which 147 of the 155 amino acid residues could be located. The structure has been refined using the program X-PLOR. The current model of the apoamicyanin ternary complex has an R-factor of 0.179 (12.0 to 2.4 Å) with root mean squared deviation from ideal bond lengths and angles of 0.017 Å and 3.58°, respectively and consists of 5805 protein atoms and 128 solvent molecules in each asymmetric unit.

Results and Discussion

The relationship of the cytochrome, amicyanin and the light subunit of MADH in the

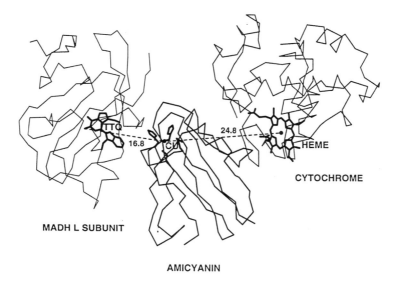

Figure 1. Cα diagram of the L-subunit of MADH, amicyanin and cytochrome c_{551i} in the ternary complex. The redox cofactors, TTQ, Cu^{++} and heme and the distances between them are shown.

ternary complex is shown in Fig. 1. The exposed edge of L:Trp 108 of TTQ (where A and C refer to amicyanin and cytochrome) is juxtaposed to the exposed copper ligand, A:His 95. The distance fro m the copper atom to O6 of TTQ is 16.8 Å and is 9.3 Å to the closest atom of

TTQ. β-Strand 3 of amicyanin, which is shared between the two sheets of the β-sandwich, is in contact with a peptide segment of the cytochrome which lies close to the two heme propionates. The copper to iron distance is 24.8 Å and the distance from copper to the nearest atom of the heme is about 21 Å. The MADH-amicyanin interface is largely hydrophobic and covers an area of approximately 750 Å². About 40% of the residues in the interface are hydrophilic, but most of these are pointing into solution at the edge of the interface. There are two salt bridges and 3 water molecules connecting the two molecules. The amicyanin-cytochrome interface is smaller, covering approximately 425 A², and more polar, with approximately 65% hydrophilic residues. The amicyanin and cytochrome are joined by 1 salt bridge, 4 hydrogen bonds and two solvent molecules. One of the solvent molecules may be a cation such as sodium or potassium. It is coordinated to 2 acidic side chains, A:Glu 31 and C:Asp 75, which also interact with each other, and to the carbonyls of C:Gly 72 and C:Tyr 77 (Fig. 2). It corresponded to the highest peak of the difference map and

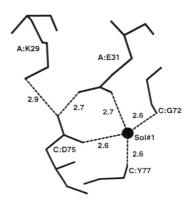

Figure 2. Coordination of solvent #1 in the amicyanin-cytochrome interface.

refined to a very low temperature factor. Presence of a cation would help explain the interaction between A:Glu 31 and C:Asp 75 through partial neutralization of their negative charges.

Possible pathways for electron flow were analyzed using the program PATHWAYS-II (Regan, 1992) as a guide, two paths, leading from the quinone-containing indole ring of TTQ to the copper atom, were predicted to be the most efficient ones (Fig. 3a). One of these goes through L:Trp 108 then on to residue A:Pro 94 and to the copper via A:His 95. The other path follows the side and main chain of L:Trp 57 to L:Ser 56 and to the side chain of A:His95 via hydrogen bonds to an intra-complex water molecule. The electronic coupling of this path is about 3-fold more efficient than the former. However, the pathway depends critically on the presence of a water molecule, which corresponds to an intermediate level density value, and might be only partially occupied, thereby reducing the relative efficiency of this pathway. The efficiency of the former path is limited by a through-space jump of 3.5 Å from L:Trp 108 of

TTQ to A:Pro 94. If electron delocalization extends throughout TTQ, then electron transfer directly from L:Trp108 to A:His95 might also be feasible. In the case of the electron transfer from copper to iron, the two most likely paths partially overlap (Fig. 3b). The common portion involves main chains of A:Tyr 30, A:Glu 31, C:Gly 72 and C:Pro 71 and the side chain of C:His 61, an iron ligand.

This part includes passage through 2 hydrogen bonds, one from A:Glu 31 O to C:Gly 72 N and the other from C:Pro 71 O to C:His 61 ND1. The two paths differ in their routing from the copper to the main chain of A:Tyr 30. In one case transfer is via the side chain of A:Cys 92, a copper ligand, through the side chain of A:Tyr 30 and onto the main chain. In the other, the path goes through A:Met 98 CE, another copper ligand, and onto the main chain of A:Tyr 30. Both of these paths include a through space jump, 3.4 Å between A:Cys 92 CB and A:Tyr 30 OH in the first case, and 4.1 Å between A:Met 98 CB to A:Lys 29 C in the other. Both branches have approximately equal efficiency. However, the route through Cys 92 may be favored by the electronic structure of the copper (Lowery et. al., 1993).

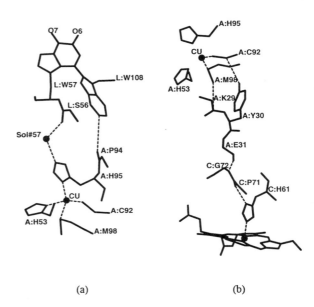

(a)   (b)

Figure 3. Electron transfer pathways between TTQ and copper (a) and between copper and the heme iron (b) in the ternary complex.

Conclusions

This study provides the first detailed analysis of a crystalline complex of 3 sequential components of an electron transport chain and the first description of an acidic c_L class cytochrome. Kinetic and thermodynamic studies of the electron transfer reaction between amicyanin and cytochrome c_{551i} are planned. Eventually, by using site directed mutagenesis it should be possible to elucidate the importance of specific amino acids in the binding and electron transfer reactions between these three proteins.

Acknowledgements
This work has been supported by NSF Grant No. MCB-9119789 (F.S.M.) and by USPHS Grant No. GM41574 (V.L.D.).

References

Chen, L., Durley, R., Poliks, B. J., Hamada, K., Chen, Z.-w., Mathews, F. S., Davidson, V. L., Satow, Y., Huizinga, E., Vellieux, F. M. D. and Hol, W. G. J. (1992) Crystal structure of an electron-transfer complex between methylamine dehydrogenase and amicyanin. *Biochemistry* 31: 4959-4964.

Chen, L., Mathews, F.S., Davidson, V.L., Tegoni, M., Rivetti, C., and Rossi, G.L. (1993) Preliminary crystal structure studies of a ternary electron transfer complex between a quinoprotein, a blue copper protein and a c-type cytochrome. *Protein Science* 2: 147-154 (1993).

Davidson, V.L. and Kumar, M.A. (1989) Cytochrome c-550 mediates electron transfer from inducible periplasmic c-type cytochromes to the cytoplasmic membrane of *Paracoccus denitrificans*. *FEBS Lett*. 245:271-273.

Durley, R., Chen, L., Lim, L.W., Mathews, F.S. and Davidson, V.L. (1993) Crystal structure analysis of amicyanin and apoamicyanin from *Paracoccus denitrificans* at 2.0 Å and 1.8 Å resolution *Protein Science*. 2:739-752.

Gary, K.A., Knaff, D.B., Husain, M. and Davidson, V.L. (1986) Measurement of the oxidation-reduction potentials of amicyanin and c-type cytochromes from *Paracoccus denitrificans*. *FEBS Lett*. 207:239-242.

Husain, M. & Davidson, V. L. (1985). An inducible periplasmic blue copper protein from *Paracoccus denitrificans*. *J. Biol. Chem*. 260: 14626-14629.

Husain, M. & Davidson, V. L. (1987). Purification and properties of methylamine dehydrogenase from *Paracoccus denitrificans*. *J. Bacteriol*. 169: 1712-1717.

Husain, M. and Davidson, V. L. (1986) Characterization of two inducible periplasmic c-type cytochromes from *Paracoccus denitrificans*. *J. Biol. Chem*. 261: 8577-8580.

Lowery, M.D., Guckert, J.A., Gebhard, M.S. and Solomon, E.I. (1993) Active-site electronic structure contributions to electron transfer pathways in rubredoxin and plastocyanin: direct *versus* superexchange. *J. Am. Chem. Soc*. 115: 3012-3013.

McIntire, W.S., Wemmer, D.E., Chistoserdov, A. and Lidstrom, M.E. (1991) A new cofactor in a prokaryotic enzyme: tryptophan tryptophylquinone as the redox prosthetic group in methylamine dehydrogenase. *Science* 252:817-824.

Regan, J.J. *Pathways II software v2.01*, San Diego:Jeffrey J. Regan (1993).

Biochemistry of Vitamin B$_6$ and PQQ
G. Marino, G. Sannia and F. Bossa (eds.)
© 1994 Birkhäuser Verlag Basel/Switzerland

Model studies directed toward the action of quinoprotein methanol dehydrogenase

Shinobu Itoh

Department of Applied Chemistry, Faculty of Engineering, Osaka University, 2-1 Yamada-oka, Suita, Osaka 565, Japan

Summary

Methanol addition to the trimethyl ester of cofactor PQQ (PQQTME) was investigated in detail to obtain information on the action of quinoprotein methanol dehydrogenase. The hemiacetal-type adduct was easily isolated from a methanol solution of PQQTME. The crystal structure of the adduct was determined by X-ray diffraction for the first time, showing that methanol addition occurred at the 5-position (C-5) of the quinone. On the other hand, treatment of PQQTME in methanol under acidic conditions gave the dimethyl acetal derivative as a major product for which the addition position of methanol was determined to be C-4 by X-ray crystallographic analysis. Studies of the adduct formation reactions with methanol using a series of PQQ model compounds and the molecular orbital calculations provided a clear-cut explanation for the difference in positions between the hemiacetal formation and the acetal formation. Because the C-5 hemiacetal was not very stable, it readily reverted to the quinone in solution, while the C-4 acetal was reduced to the quinol derivative when treated with base. The biological significance (particularly in the enzymatic alcohol oxidation mechanism) of the C-4 and C-5 adducts of cofactor PQQ are discussed.

Introduction

PQQ is a novel cofactor that was first isolated and identified from methanol dehydrogenase (MDH) of methylotrophic bacteria in 1979 (Salisubury *et al.*). However little was known about the mechanistic details of the methanol oxidation by MDH (Anthony). In the present study, reaction of the trimethyl ester of cofactor PQQ (PQQTME) and methanol was investigated in detail to obtain information on the action of quinoprotein methanol dehydrogenase.

Results and Discussion

Hemiacetal derivative **1** of cofactor PQQ was isolated and characterized for the first time (Eq 1). The crystal structure of the methanol adduct clearly indicated that the addition position is C-5 (Figure 1). Considering the electron-withdrawing nature of the pyridine nucleus having two carbomethoxy groups, this tendency to add at the C-5 position in the adduct formation is very reasonable. In general, hydration or alcohol addition to carbonyl compounds is largely enhanced when the carbonyl compounds have a highly electron-withdrawing substituent. The pyrrole ring, on the other hand, showed an opposite effect, which can be attributed to its electron-releasing nature.

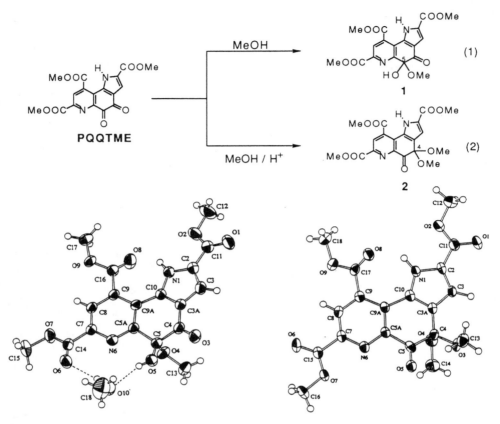

Figure 1. ORTEP drawing of hemiacetal **1**   Figure 2. ORTEP drawing of acetal **2**

Surprisingly, PQQTME was mainly converted into the C-4 acetal derivatives **2** in the reaction with methanol under acidic conditions (Eq 2). In order to discuss the mechanism, we performed semiempirical molecular orbital calculations on hemiacetals **1** and **1'**. The calculated values of the heat of formation clearly indicate that the C-5 hemiacetal is more stable than the C-4 counterpart by about a few kcal/mol (1-3 kcal/mol, depending on the method used). Since hemiacetal **1** is readily converted into the original quinone in solution (*vide infra*), the *hemiacetal formation step* is considered to be completely reversible. Under such circumstances, the reaction can be regarded as thermodynamically controlled. Thus, it is reasonable that hemiacetal **1** is formed as a solo isolable product under the neutral conditions (Eq 1). In the presence of acid, elimination of water from the protonated intermediate **1'H+** may proceed much faster than that from protonated hemiacetal **1H+**, because the generated carbocationic intermediate can be stabilized by simultaneous release of the pyrrole proton (H-1) (**1'H+** to **3**; Scheme 1). Attack by the second molecule of the solvent gives C-4 acetal **2**. Once C-4 acetal **2** is formed, it cannot revert to C-4 hemiacetal **1'** in the presence of excess methanol ([MeOH >> [H$_2$O]). Therefore C-4 acetal **2** is gradually accumulated under acidic conditions.

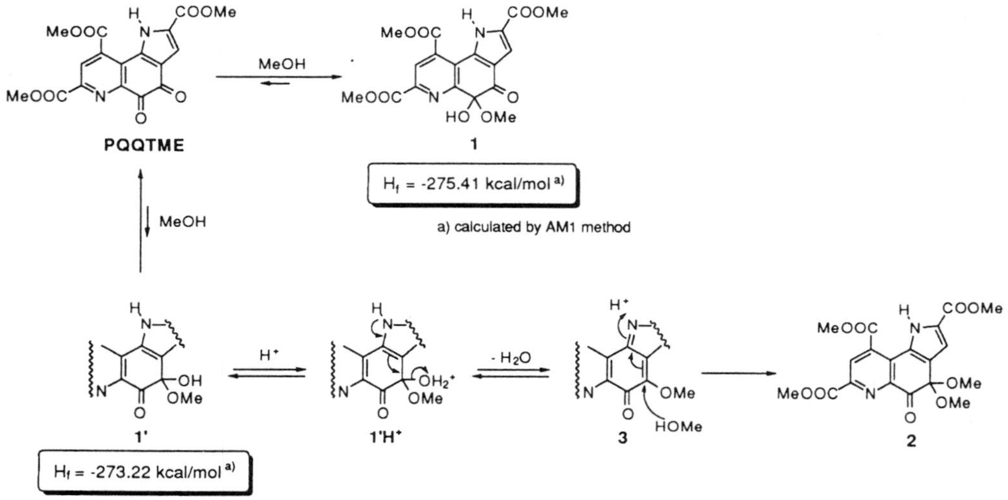

$$H_f = -275.41 \text{ kcal/mol} \text{ a)}$$

a) calculated by AM1 method

$$H_f = -273.22 \text{ kcal/mol} \text{ a)}$$

Scheme 1

This mechanism is supported by the results of acetal formation reactions of other quinones. C-4 acetal **5** was also obtained in the case of benzindolequinone **4** (Eq 3), which has the same indole-4,5-quinone skeleton in the molecule, but the acetal formation occurred at the opposite site of the quinone, C-5 and C-10, in the cases of 1-methyl PQQTME **6** and benzoquinolinequinone **8**, respectively (Eqs 4 and 5). Acetals **7** and **9** were derived from the corresponding C-5 and C-10 hemiacetals, which must be more stable than the corresponding C-4 and C-9 adducts, as discussed above.

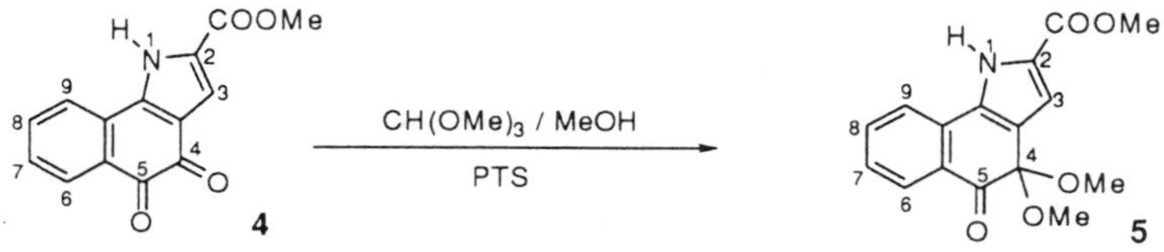

(3)

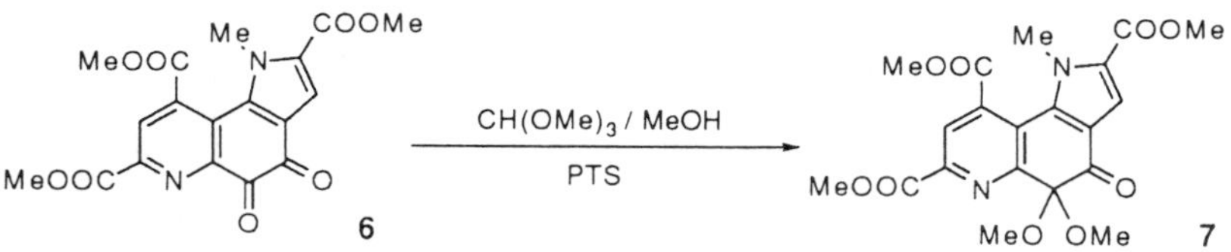

(4)

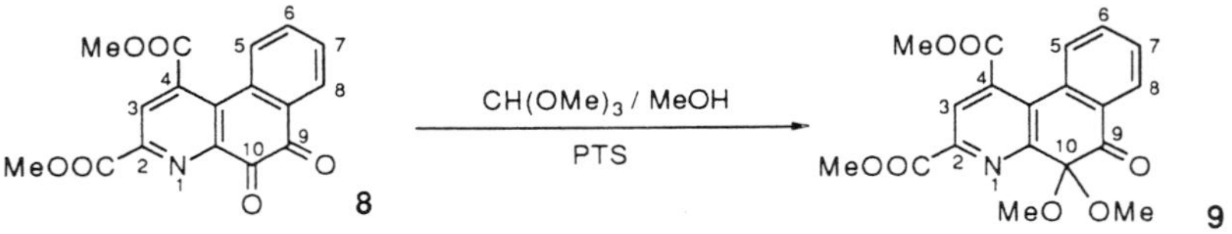

$$CH(OMe)_3 / MeOH \xrightarrow{PTS}$$ (5)

Little was known about the mechanistic details of the enzymatic reaction of quinoprotein alcohol dehydrogenases. So far, oxidation of alcohols by PQQ in enzymatic systems proceeds via an addition-elimination mechanism through the C-5 hemiacetal intermediate (Anthony). This mechanism seems to be plausible, because the quinone was easily converted into hemiacetal 1 by treatment with methanol under neutral conditions. However, hemiacetal 1 itself is not very stable in solution, and it reverts to the original quinone immediately when treated with acid or base. If the enzyme operated according to this mechanism, it should have a special device to stabilize the hemiacetal intermediate.

On the other hand, treatment of acetal 2 with excess triethylamine in CH3CN gave reduced compound 10 in a 29% isolated yield (Eq 6). This result indicates that some kind of redox reaction occurred from the C-4 adduct, although the attempt to detect formaldehyde, the oxidation product of methanol, failed. In order to confirm the formation of aldehyde, the same reaction was carried out by using diethyl acetal derivative 2' and tripropylamine as a base. In this case, a relative amount of acetaldehyde (35%), the oxidation product of the ethanol moiety, was obtained together with the corresponding reduced compound 10' (57 %) (Eq 7). In this case, however, a relative amount of propionaldehyde, derived from the added amine, was obtained in addition to acetaldehyde (Eq 7). These interesting results could be explained as follows.

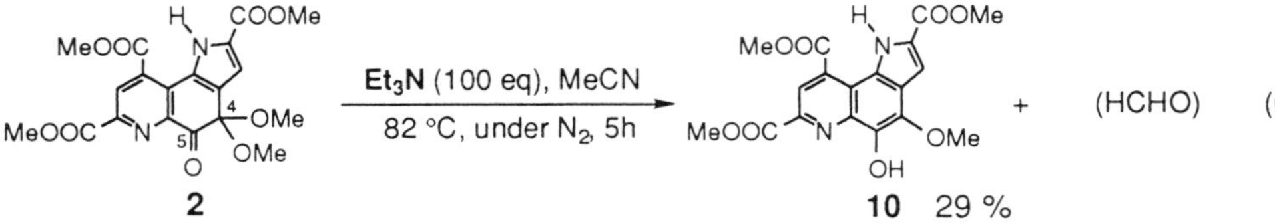

$$\xrightarrow[\text{82 °C, under N}_2, \text{ 5h}]{\text{Et}_3\text{N (100 eq), MeCN}}$$ + (HCHO) (6)

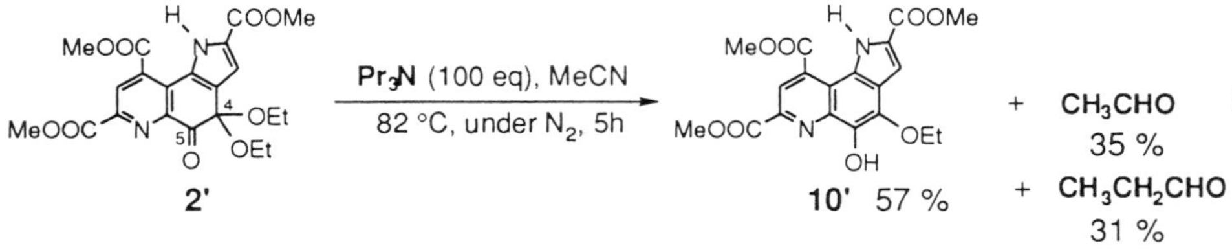

10   29 %

$$\xrightarrow[\text{82 °C, under N}_2, \text{ 5h}]{\text{Pr}_3\text{N (100 eq), MeCN}}$$ + CH$_3$CHO (7)

10' 57 %   35 %

+ CH$_3$CH$_2$CHO

31 %

There are two possible mechanisms for the production of aldehyde from the C-4 acetal (Scheme 2). The first possibility is the oxidative elimination of the alcohol moiety, providing the aldehyde and the reduced PQQ. In this case, the amine acts as a base to abstract the α-proton of the substrate.

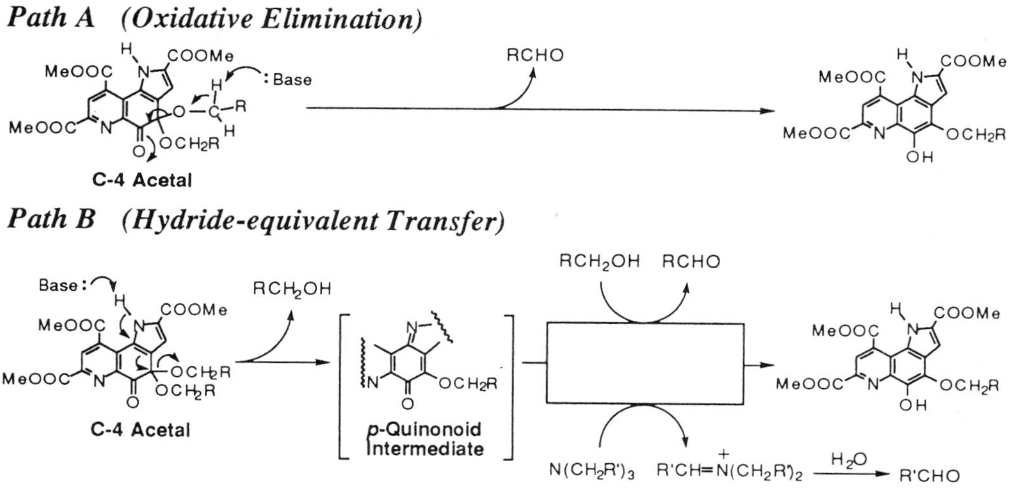

Path A (Oxidative Elimination)

C-4 Acetal

Path B (Hydride-equivalent Transfer)

C-4 Acetal   p-Quinonoid Intermediate

Scheme 2

The second one is the hydride-transfer mechanism from the substrate to the *p-quinonoid intermediate*, which can be formed from the C-4 acetal derivative via 1,4-alcohol elimination. In this mechanism, the amine abstracts the pyrrole proton to enhance the alcohol-elimination. At this moment, it's not clear which one is an actual reaction pathway for the alcohol-oxidation, but the oxidation of added amine could be only explained by the hydride transfer mechanism. Based on these results, we propose a new enzymatic mechanism involving the *p*-quinonoid compound as a key intermediate.

There are still several problems to be solved in the mechanism of oxidation by quinoprotein methanol dehydrogenase. But the present results give us possible implications for the mechanism of PQQ-containing alcohol dehydrogenases. Further investigations of the enzyme active site and model studies of alcohol oxidation by PQQ will provide a more precise picture of the enzymatic oxidation mechanism.

References

Anthony, C. (1993) Davidson V. L. (ed.): *Principles and Applications of Quinoproteins*, Marcel Dekker, Inc.: New York, pp. 17-45.

Salisubury, S. A., Forrest, H. S., Cruse, W. B. T., and Kennard, O. (1979) A novel coenzyme from bacterial primary alcohol dehydrogenases. *Nature* 280: 843-844.

MOLECULAR PHYSIOLOGY

Nutritional aspects of vitamin B$_6$: requirements, recommendations and intake

David A. Bender

Dept of Biochemistry & Molecular Biology, University College London, Gower Street, London WC1E 6BT, UK

Summary

There is general agreement that the Reference Intake of vitamin B$_6$ should be calculated on the basis of 15-16µg /gram protein intake. However, this figure is derived from a very limited number of depletion / repletion studies, on a small number of subjects, and cannot be considered to be a reliable reflection of requirements. Studies of the turnover of whole body vitamin B$_6$ have so far failed to give useful information on requirements to replace metabolic losses. Clinical deficiency in adults is unknown, and dietary surveys suggest that average intakes are more than adequate. Nevertheless, a significant proportion of the population show biochemical evidence of inadequacy. In view of the role of pyridoxal phosphate in modulating the actions of steroid hormones, there is a clear need for further studies to establish vitamin B$_6$ requirements more firmly than present estimates.

Reference intakes and estimates of vitamin B$_6$ requirements

Many national and international authorities publish tables of reference intakes of nutrients. These are calculated by adding 2 SD to the mean observed requirement in experimental studies, and thus represent a level of intake greater than the requirements of 97.5% of the population. The consensus view is that vitamin B$_6$ requirements are related to protein intake, and there is agreement between the three most recently published tables of reference intakes: the US RDA is 16 µg /g protein intake (National Research Council, 1989), the British RNI (Department of Health, 1991) and the European Union PRI (Scientific Committee for Food, 1993) are both 15µg /g protein intake. Despite this agreement, reference intakes cannot be considered to be soundly based; they have been extrapolated from a few depletion / repletion studies, involving small numbers of subjects, and using only a limited range of intakes of vitamin B$_6$ and protein.

Dependence of requirements on protein intake; depletion / repletion studies

Kelsay *et al* (1968) showed that during depletion whole blood vitamin B$_6$ fell more rapidly in young men receiving 150g protein /day than those receiving a marginally adequate intake of 54g /day. The increase on repletion was greater in those receiving the lower protein intake. These results suggest a relationship between protein intake and vitamin B$_6$ requirements, but the results cannot be interpreted with confidence. Subjects were adapted to the protein intakes (with 1.66 mg/d vitamin B_6) for different periods; at the beginning of the depletion period plasma vitamin B_6 was lower in those receiving the high protein diet. There was a rapid fall in blood vitamin B_6 in both groups; concentrations were first measured after 8d (high protein) or 10d (low protein); the high protein subjects were more severely depleted, but it is not possible to determine rates of depletion from the published data. After 16d the high protein subjects were repleted with 0.6 mg vitamin B_6 /d for 16d; the low protein group were depleted for 39d, then repleted for 7d; at the end of the repletion period the blood vitamin B_6 was higher in the low protein group than those receiving the high protein diet, although still only 50% of that seen prior to depletion.

Miller and Linkswiler (1967) reported studies of the metabolism of a 2g test dose of L-tryptophan in the same subjects. After 14d depletion there was a considerable increase in urinary tryptophan metabolites in the high protein group, which was partially corrected by repletion with an additional 0.6 mg/d vitamin B_6. After 23d, 4 of the 5 subjects receiving the low protein diet showed modest impairment of tryptophan metabolism; two of these continued for 40d, by which time there was a significant impairment of tryptophan metabolism, although less marked than at 14d in the high protein group. Repletion resulted in normalisation of tryptophan metabolism in these two subjects. The results suggest that 14µg vitamin B_6 /g protein is adequate to normalise tryptophan metabolism, whereas 5µg/g protein is not.

Baker et al (1964) studied xanthurenic acid excretion after a 10g test dose of DL-tryptophan in subjects receiving 30 or 100g protein /day; after an initial adaptation period of 1w at 4mg vitamin B_6 /day they were fed an essentially vitamin B_6 free diet. Xanthurenic acid excretion increased more rapidly in the high protein group, and at the end of the third week was greater than in the low protein group after 6w depletion. Five of the 6 subjects receiving the high protein diet showed abnormal electro-encephalograms, suggesting functional deficiency (Canham et al, 1969). Each subject was repleted with varying levels of vitamin B_6 (0.5-1.0mg/d for those receiving 30g protein and 0.75-1.75mg/d for those receiving 100g protein). At the high protein intake 1.25mg vitamin B_6 (= 12.5µg/g protein) was not adequate to normalise xanthurenic acid excretion, while 1.5mg/day (15µg/g protein) was. This is the main experimental evidence for a reference intake of 15-16µg/g protein intake. However, for those subjects receiving 30g protein, 1.0mg/d (33µg/g protein) was inadequate, and 1.25mg/d (42µg/g protein) adequate to normalise tryptophan metabolism. Interpretation is confounded by the fact that 30g/d protein is insufficient to meet requirements, and the subjects were in negative nitrogen balance throughout the study.

Miller et al (1985) fed 8 men a diet providing 1.6mg vitamin B_6 /d, with 0.5, 1.0 and 2.0g protein /kg bw. They were in negative nitrogen balance at 0.5 and positive balance at 1 and 2g protein /kg body weight. Urine 4-pyridoxic acid and plasma PLP and total vitamin B_6 were highest in the subjects receiving the low protein diet and lowest in those receiving 2 g/kg bw. In none was there any abnormality of the metabolism of a test dose of 2g L-tryptophan, suggesting that all were receiving an adequate intake of vitamin B_6. From their body weights, it appears that 9.5-13µg vitamin B_6 /g protein was adequate to meet metabolic requirements, despite the difference in blood vitamin B_6 and urine 4-pyridoxic acid.

David and Kalyankar (1983) showed a fall in liver PLP in rats after adrenalectomy, and restoration following cortisol administration, associated with changes in liver aminotransferases. It is likely that the apparent dependence of vitamin B_6 requirements on protein intake discussed above reflects changes in the amount of PLP bound to (inducible) enzymes of amino acid metabolism and changes in muscle mass (and hence glycogen phosphorylase) with changing nitrogen balance. Apparent vitamin B_6 requirements during adaptation to changed protein intake may not reflect dependence of vitamin B_6 requirement on habitual protein intake

Estimates of requirement based on metabolic turnover

An alternative approach to determining requirements is determination of the total body pool of vitamin B_6 and the fractional rate of turnover using isotopically labelled vitamin; to estimate the minimum requirement to replace metabolic losses. Coburn *et al* (1988) calculated that the total body pool of vitamin B_6 is approximately 1000µmol, by determination of PLP in muscle biopsy samples, estimation of muscle mass by determination of urinary excretion of creatinine and the assumption that 80% of total body vitamin B_6 is in muscle. A single sample of muscle was taken from each subject; citing animal studies, the authors suggest that the vitamin B_6 content estimated from one muscle *probably does not differ by > 20% from the overall average muscle value.*

Using [^{2}H]pyridoxine, Coburn (1990) showed an average turnover of 0.13%/d suggesting a requirement for replacement of metabolic losses of 350µg/day for a 70kg adult - considerably lower requirements estimated in depletion / repletion studies. However, muscle pyridoxal phosphate responds considerably more slowly to repletion after a period of deficiency than does that in other tissues. Bender *et al* (1989) showed that in rats that had been maintained on a vitamin B_6 free diet for 3w, then given a single oral dose of 1mg pyridoxine HCl /kg bw, the pyridoxal phosphate content of liver was restored to control levels within 2h, and that of kidney within 5h, while that of skeletal muscle increased from 25 to 45% of control within 30min of repletion, and only reached 65% of control after 5h. This suggests that pools of vitamin B_6 associated with amino acid metabolism turn over relatively rapidly, while a separate pool in muscle (presumably associated with glycogen phosphorylase) has a considerably slower turnover.

Beynon *et al* (1993) determined the isotope enrichment of urinary 4-pyridoxic acid after [^{2}H]pyridoxine as a means of estimating turnover in mice. They showed that there are two clearly distinct pools of the vitamin in the body: a small pool with a rapid turnover ($k=1.2$ d^{-1}) and a larger pool with a slow turnover ($k=0.13$ d^{-1}). The situation may be considerably more complex, with multiple small pools of pyridoxal phosphate with different relatively fast turnover (Coburn, 1990). There is clearly a need for more studies of vitamin B$_6$ metabolic turnover before the results can be used to estimate requirements.

The adequacy of average intakes of vitamin B$_6$

Clinical deficiency of vitamin B$_6$ is unknown in adults except in deliberate depletion studies, and most dietary surveys suggest that intakes are adequate when compared with reference intakes. In Britain the 95% range for men is 25.5-34.6µg/g protein and for women 22.4-28.4 - considerably greater than reference intakes (Gregory et al, 1990). However, in various plant foods which are apparently good sources of the vitamin between 15-50% is present as pyridoxine glucoside, which is only 20-30% available. Overall, 70-80% of the vitamin B$_6$ in the average diet is biologically available (Tarr et al, 1981).

Marginally inadequate vitamin B$_6$ status may be relatively common. A number of studies have suggested, on the basis of determination of either plasma PLP or erythrocyte aminotransferase activation, that 10-30% of the population are inadequately supplied with vitamin B$_6$, although relatively few people show inadequacy when both criteria are assessed (Bender, 1989; 1993).

The implications of marginal vitamin B$_6$ inadequacy

Marginal vitamin B$_6$ inadequacy may be important. Cidlowski and Thanassi (1981) proposed that pyridoxal phosphate has a role in modulating the actions of steroid (and other nuclear acting) hormones, displacing the hormone-receptor complex from tight nuclear binding, and terminating its action. More recently, Allgood and Cidlowski (1992) demonstrated that the expression of hormone-responsive gene constructs in a variety of cell lines in culture is affected by PLP: deficient cells show higher gene expression, and vitamin B$_6$ supplemented cells lower expression, than those cultured with control concentrations of the vitamin.

Vitamin B$_6$ deficiency affects steroid hormone responsiveness under physiological conditions. Symes et al (1984) and Bowden et al (1986) showed that in vitamin B$_6$ deficient animals there is greater uptake and more prolonged nuclear retention of oestradiol in the uterus and testosterone in the prostate. This was associated with enhanced sensitivity of target organs to hormone stimulation, including increased stimulation of uterine growth by low doses of ethynyl-oestradiol in ovariectomised female animals and increased growth and mitotic index in the prostate of castrated male rats after low doses of testosterone. It is likely that marginal vitamin B$_6$

inadequacy may be a factor in the development of hormone-dependent cancer of the breast, uterus and prostate (for review see Bender, 1987; 1994).

References

Allgood V. A. and Cidlowski J.A. (1992) Vitamin B_6 modulates transcriptional activation by multiple members of the steroid hormone receptor superfamily. *Journal of Biological Chemistry* 267: 3819-3824.

Baker, E.M., Canham, J.E., Nunes, W.T., Sauberlich, H.E. and McDowell, M.E. (1964). Vitamin B_6 requirement for adult men. *American Journal of Clinical Nutrition* 15: 59-66.

Bender, D.A. (1987) Oestrogens and vitamin B_6: actions and interactions. *World Review of Nutrition and Dietetics* 51: 140-188.

Bender, D.A. (1989) Vitamin B_6 requirements and recommendations. *European Journal of Clinical Nutrition* 43: 289-309.

Bender, D.A. (1993) Lack of concordance between two biochemical indices of vitamin B_6 nutritional status. *Proceedings of the Nutrition Society* 52: 315A.

Bender, D.A. (1994) Novel functions of vitamin B_6. *Proceedings of the Nutrition Society - in press*.

Bender, D.A., Gartey-Sam, K. and Singh, A. (1989) Effects of vitamin B_6 deficiency and repletion on the uptake of steroid hormones into uterus slices and isolated liver cells of rats. *British Journal of Nutrition* 61: 619-628.

Beynon, R.J., Flannery, A.V., Edwards, R.H.T., Evershed, R.P. and Leyland, D.M. (1993) Protein degradation in skeletal muscle: a study of glycogen phosphorylase, in *Proteolysis and protein turnover*, Portland Press, London, pp 157-162.

Bowden, J-F., Bender, D.A., Symes, E.K. and Coulson, W.F. (1986) Increased uterine uptake and nuclear retention of [3H]oestradiol through the oestrous cycle and enhanced end-organ sensitivity to oestrogen stimulation in vitamin B_6 deficient rats. *Journal of Steroid Biochemistry* 25: 359-365.

Canham, J.E., Baker, E.M., Harding, R.S., Sauberlich, H.E. and Plough, I.C. (1969). Dietary protein - its relationship to vitamin B_6 requirements and function. *Annals of the New York Academy of Sciences* 166: 16-29.

Cidlowski, J.A. and Thanassi, J.W. (1981) Pyridoxal phosphate, a possible cofactor role in steroid hormone action. *Journal of Steroid Biochemistry* 15: 11-16.

Coburn, S.P. (1990) Location and turnover of vitamin B_6 pools and vitamin B_6 requirements of humans. *Annals of the New York Academy of Sciences* 585: 76-85.

Coburn, S.P., Lewis, D.L.N., Fink, W.J., Mahuren, J.D., Schaltenbrand, W.E. and Costill, D.L. (1988) Human vitamin B-6 pools estimated through muscle biopsies. *American Journal of Clinical Nutrition* 48: 291-294.

David, S. and Kalyankar, G.D. (1983) Influence of adrenalectomy on vitamin B_6 status. *Experientia* 39: 329.

Department of Health / Ministry of Agriculture, Fisheries and Food. (1991) *Dietary Reference Values for Food Energy and Nutrients in the United Kingdom*, HMSO, London.

Gregory, J., Foster, K., Tyler, H. and Wiseman, M. (1990) *The Dietary and Nutritional Survey of British Adults*, Office of Population Censuses and Surveys, HMSO, London.

Kelsay J., Baysal, A. and Linkswiler, H. (1968) Effects of vitamin B_6 depletion on the pyridoxal, pyridoxamine and pyridoxine content of the blood and urine of man. *Journal of Nutrition* 94: 490-494.

Miller, L.T., Leklem, J.T. and Schultz, T.D. (1985). The effect of dietary protein on the metabolism of vitamin B-6 in humans. *Journal of Nutrition* 115: 1663-1672.

Miller, L.T. and Linkswiler, H. (1967) Effect of protein intake on the development of abnormal tryptophan metabolism by men during vitamin B_6 depletion. *Journal of Nutrition* 93: 53-59.

National Research Council / National Academy of Sciences. (1989) *Recommended Dietary Allowances, 10th Edition*. National Academy Press, Washington DC.

Scientific Committee for Food. (1993) *Nutrient and Energy Intakes for the European Community*. Reports of the Scientific Committee for Food (thirty-first series), Directorate-General Industry, Commission of the European Communities, Luxembourg.

Symes, E.K., Bender, D.A., Bowden, J-F. and Coulson, W.F. (1984) Increased target tissue uptake of, and sensitivity to, testosterone in the vitamin B_6 deficient rat. *Journal of Steroid Biochemistry* 20: 1089-1093.

Tarr, J.B., Tamura, T. and Stokstad, E.L.R. (1981) Availability of vitamin B-6 and pantothenate in average American diet. *American Journal of Clinical Nutrition* 34: 1328-1337.

Biochemistry of Vitamin B$_6$ and PQQ
G. Marino, G. Sannia and F. Bossa (eds.)
© 1994 Birkhäuser Verlag Basel/Switzerland

Vitamin B$_6$ transport and metabolism: Clues for delivery of bioactive compounds

Donald B. McCormick

Department of Biochemistry, Emory University,
Atlanta, GA 30322-3050, U.S.A.

Summary

The transport of vitamin B$_6$ into mammalian cells is facilitated and exhibits relative specificity that permits the 4' linkage of diverse amines. The latter thereby gain enhanced transport into cells followed by metabolic release.

Introduction

The cellular assimilation of vitamins requires both transport and metabolic events that are connectedly related. When these processes are thoroughly understood, possibilities for biomedical utilization become apparent. The knowledge we have gained from our studies with vitamin B$_6$ may serve to conceptualize a general principle for delivery of bioactive compounds.

Transport

As with most water-soluble vitamins, the entry of B$_6$ into mammalian cells is facilitated within physiologic levels (McCormick and Zhang, 1993). Characteristics that distinguish such mediated transport from passive diffusion, which also occurs, are the greater initial rate and saturation kinetics evident in the process of uptake. Kinetic constants relating to uptake of pyridoxine measured in freshly isolated cells from the livers (Kozik and McCormick, 1984) and kidneys (Bowman and McCormick, 1989) of normal male rats are given in Table I.

Table I. [^{3}H]Pyridoxine uptake in mammalian cells

Cells	v_0	V_{max}	K_t
	(pmol/10^6 cells·min)		(μmol/liter)
Liver	2	106	28
Kidney	6	14	1.3

Saturation occurs reasonably above the level of total B$_6$ vitamers found in the plasma of mammalian species.

A further characteristic that distinguishes mediated transport, expected when carrier proteins are involved, is the relative specificity. That for the cellular transporters of B_6 measured in liver (Kozik and McCormick,1984) and kidney (Bowman and McCormick, 1989) is noted from data in Table II.

Table II. Relative specificity of B_6 uptake

[³H]Pyridoxine (concentration as control)	Liver	Kidney
	100 (0.5 µM)	100 (0.3 µM)
+ Pyridoxamine		64 (5 µM)
+ Pyridoxal		102 (5 µM)
+ 5'-Deoxypyridoxal		57 (5 µM)
+ 5'-Deoxypyridoxine	85 (0.5 µM)	76 (5 µM)
+ 4'-Deoxypyridoxine	65 (0.5 µM)	60 (5 µM)

Pyridoxamine, as one vitaminic form of B_6, competes fairly effectively against pyridoxine for uptake, but pyridoxal does not. Synthetic analogs with methyl groups replacing the hydroxymethyls at position 4 or 5 are also fairly effective competitive inhibitors against B_6 uptake.

The ability of simple 4'-substituted B_6 analogs to compete for entry into cells suggested our synthesis and use of a 4'-N-alkyl-pyridoxamino-affinose to purify B_6-binding proteins from renal brush-border membranes solubilized with n-octyl-ß-D-glucoside, as reported in the last International Symposium on Vitamin B_6 and Carbonyl Catalysis (McCormick et al.,1991). Since then we have amplified our understanding of the considerable capacity of the B_6 transport system for handling other 4'(N)-substituted pyridoxamines, structures for which are summarized in Table III.

In tests with renal proximal tubular epithelial cells, it was found that both initial rate and extent of [³H]pyridoxine uptake was inhibited by the unlabeled analogs (Zhang and McCormick,1992a; Zhang and McCormick, 1991), as illustrated in Fig. 1.

Table III. Synthetic N-(4'-pyridoxyl)amines

Original amine	Derived B_6 analog	R
Methylamine		CH_3
Benzylamine		CH_2-⟨⟩
Tryptamine		CH_2CH_2-indole
Ethylenediamine		$CH_2CH_2NH_3^{\oplus}$
ß-Alanine		$CH_2CH_2CO_2^{\ominus}$

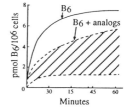

Fig. 1. Kidney cell uptake of µM [³H]pyridoxine ± µM N-(4'-pyridoxyl)amines.

That this apparent inhibition, shown to be competitive, was actually the result of uptake of the analogs via the same transporter system that facilitates entry of B_6, was demonstrated by measuring the uptake of 4'-[^{3}H] analogs by kidney (Zhang and McCormick, 1992a; Zhang and McCormick, 1991) and liver (Zhang and McCormick, 1991; Zhang and McCormick, 1992b) cells. Though the initial velocities for uptake of N-(4'-pyridoxyl)amines range somewhat lower (10 to 75%) than for pyridoxine (at100%), values for both maximal velocity and the transport constant are modestly higher, as summarized in Table IV.

Table IV. Uptake of N-(4'-pyrixoxyl)amines

[^{3}H]Compound	V_{max} (pmol/10^{6}cells·min)		$K_t(\mu M)$	
	Liver	Kidney	Liver	Kidney
Pyridoxine	28	6.4	6.3	4.3
NP-methylamine	78	7.6	8.4	6.7
NP-benzylamine	126	6.6	9.0	4.0
NP-tryptamine	32	5.6	7.6	6.7
NP-ethylenediamine	50	6.6	13	5.0
NP-ß-alanine	22	6.6	15	10

Within these relatively water-soluble analogs, the size of the substituted amine seems to have less effect on the uptake than net anionic or cationic charge.

An extension of hydrophobic structure, such that the 4'-(N)-alkyl substituent confers lipid solubility, changes the character of transport. This is seen with N-(4'-pyridoxyl)-D-sphingosine synthesized as a potential delivery-modified form of a signal transducer (Zhang et al., 1993). The liver cell uptake of [4'-^{3}H]pyridoxamine is compared with that of N-([4'-^{3}H]pyridoxyl)sphingosine in Fig. 2 and 3, respectively.

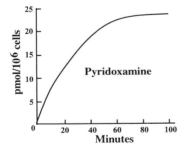

Fig. 2. Liver cell uptake of 0.5 μM [^{3}H]pyridoxamine.

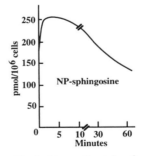

Fig. 3. Liver cell uptake of 0.5 μM N-[^{3}H]P-sphingosine.

314

The uptake of B_6-sphingosine reaches a maximum very quickly (~3 min) and then decreases. This reflects the rapid partitioning of the compound into cell membranes, at least some of which are internalized.

Pyridoxine 5'-ß-D-glucoside, a major form of B_6 in plant-derived foods, is among natural derivatives that use the transporter with relative specificity for water-soluble forms (Zhang et al., 1993). The unlabeled glucoside competitively inhibits the uptake of [3H]pyridoxine presented to liver cells, as shown in Fig. 4. The Ki for the glucoside was calculated to be 1.4 µM. That the glucoside can in fact enter the cell is shown in Fig. 5.

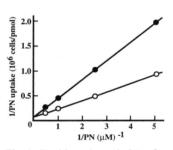

Fig. 4. Double-reciprocal plots of the initial liver cell uptake of [3H]PN in the absence ($\circ$) and presence ($\bullet$) of 2 µM PN-5'-ß-D-glucoside.

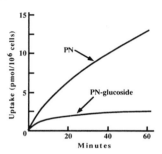

Fig. 5. Liver cell uptake of 0.5 µM [3H]PN or [3H]PN-5'-ß-D-glucoside.

The amount of glucoside transported was about 20% that of pyridoxine. Analyses of concentration dependence of [3H]PN-glucoside uptake gave an apparent $K_t=13.8$ µM and a $V_{max} = 82$ pmol/10^6 cells·min (Zhang et al., 1993).

It should be obvious from the foregoing that the systems for B_6 transport in mammalian cells can facilitate the entry of a fair range of analogs that bear the essential B_6 structure to which compounds can be attached with the potential for metabolic release.

Metabolism

Upon entry of B_6 into cells, metabolic trapping occurs as a result of phosphorylation catalyzed by pyridoxal kinase. In earlier years, we had circumscribed specificity of this kinase (McCormick and Snell,1959; McCormick et al., 1961; McCormick and Snell, 1961) and more recently demonstrated that it tolerated considerable variation in size and charge of amines borne as 4'-substituents on the B_6 structure (Zhang and McCormick, 1992a; Zhang and McCormick, 1991; Zhang and McCormick, 1992b; Zhang et al., 1993). The 5'-phosphates resulting from the kinase reaction are substrates for pyridoxamine (pyridoxine) 5'-phosphate oxidase, which we had shown can act upon diverse 4' secondary amine derivatives of B_6 phosphate (Kazarinoff and McCormick, 1973; Kazarinoff and McCormick, 1975; DePecol and McCormick, 1980; Bowers-Komro and McCormick, 1987), including those selected to determine limits for uptake and metabolism (Zhang and McCormick, 1992a; Zhang and McCormick, 1991; Zhang and McCormick, 1992b; Zhang et al., 1993). The extent of release of pyridoxal 5'-phosphate following the transport and metabolism of diverse N-(4'-pyridoxyl)amines, which we first quantitated in the kidney cortical cells (Zhang and McCormick, 1991), is quite similar to what was found with the more active liver cells (Zhang and McCormick, 1992b). Data from 50-min incubations of NP-amines with the liver cells prior to extraction and chromatographic resolution of [^{3}H]PLP are presented in Table V.

Table V. Release of PLP following uptake of NP-amines by liver cells

[^{3}H]Compound	Uptake (pmol/10^6 cells)	[^{3}H]PLP (after 50 min)
Pyridoxine	26	23
NP-methylamine	69	12
NP-benzylamine	47	21
NP-tryptamine	29	13
NP-ethylenediamine	24	23
NP-ß-alanine	29	10

The concomitant release of amines used to synthesize N-(4'-pyridoxyl)amine 5'-phosphates had been directly shown by us with examples of ^{14}C-amino acids (Kazarinoff and McCormick, 1973) and fluorescent conjugates (DePecol and McCormick, 1980) tested as substrates with pyridoxamine (pyridoxine) 5'-phosphate oxidase in vitro.

An extension of this knowledge explains the bioavailability of B_6 from the cellular release of PLP and L-lysine from N-(4'-pyridoxyl)-L-lysine. The latter results from hydrolysis of N-(5'-phospho-4'-pyridoxyl)-L-lysyl peptides formed during the thermal and partially anaerobic process of canning meats.

The enzymatic release of PLP and the original amine is quite limited from the bulky lipophilic structure of N-(4'-pyridoxyl)sphingosine (Zhang et al., 1993), which is taken in more like a lipid and is less readily presented to the cytosolic kinase and oxidase systems, as seen by data in Table VI.

Table VI. Results of 50-min uptake, cellular metabolism, or cytosolic enzyme treatment of B_6 or B_6-sphingosine

[^{3}H]Compound (0.5 µM)	Uptake (pmol/10^6 cells)	Cellular metabolism (pmol PLP/10^6 cells)	Cytosolic metabolism (pmol PLP/mg protein)
B_6 (-ine or -amine)	26	23	43 to 78
B_6-sphingosine	126	2.5	8

Though pyridoxine 5'-ß-D-glucoside is quite water-soluble and enters the cell via the B_6 transporter with modest efficiency, release of PLP is quite limited, as noted from data in Table VII.

Table VII. Results of 50-min uptake, cellular metabolism, or enzymatic treatments of pyridoxine or pyridoxine 5'-ß-D-glucoside

Compound (0.5 mM)	Uptake (pmol/10^6 cells)	Cellular metabolism (pmol PLP/10^6 cells)	Homogenate	Supernatant
			(pmol PLP/mg protein/min)	
Pyridoxine	12	23	0.56	1.78
PN-glucoside	2.6	0.044	0.018	0.034

The cellular metabolism of the glucoside is only 0.2% that of pyridoxine. Also formation of PLP is much lower from the glucoside than free vitamin with homogenate or supernatant solution enriched with cytosolic kinase and oxidase. The hydrolytic release of pyridoxine from the glucoside depends upon a broad-specificity ß-glucosidase, which must act to unfetter the 5'-hydroxymethyl group that becomes phosphorylated prior to oxidation of the 4'-hydroxymethyl to generate PLP.

Enhancing effector delivery

Overall, it is clear that a range of bioactive amines can be delivered into cells by condensing them with pyridoxal followed by reduction of the aldimine to form 4'-(N)-substituted pyridoxamines. These gain facilitated transport across the plasma membrane to be successively phosphorylated and then oxidized at cytosolic level to release the original amine plus pyridoxal phosphate and H_2O_2. The general principle of enhancing effector transport may be widely applicable. As we have stated previously (Zhang and McCormick, 1991), by selection of the types of transporters and levels of activities of cleavage enzymes within various cells, it should be possible to design compounds that are somewhat selective in their ultimate targets.

Acknowledgements

This work was supported by grants from the N.I.H. (DK 43005) and The Coca-Cola Foundation. Acquisition of data was assisted by those noted in references.

References

Bowers-Komro, D.M. and McCormick, D.B. (1987) Single- and double-headed analogs of pyridoxamine 5'-phosphate as probes for pyridoxamine 5'-phosphate utilizing enzymes. *Bioorg. Chem.* 15, 224-236.

Bowman, B.B. and McCormick, D.B. (1989) Pyridoxine uptake by isolated rat liver cells. *J. Nutr.* 119, 745-749.

DePecol, M. and McCormick, D.B. (1980) Syntheses, properties, and use of fluorescent N-(5'-phospho-4'-pyridoxyl)amines in assay of pyridoxamine (pyridoxine) 5'-phosphate oxidase. *Anal. Biochem.* 101, 435-441.

Kazarinoff, M.N. and McCormick, D.B. (1973) N-(5'-Phospho-4'-pyridoxyl)amines as substrates for pyridoxine (pyridoxamine) 5'-phosphate oxidase. *Biochem. Biophys. Res. Commun.* 52, 440-446.

Kazarinoff, M.N. and McCormick, D.B. (1975) Rabbit liver pyridoxamine (pyridoxine) 5'-phosphate oxidase: purification and properties. *J. Biol. Chem.* 250, 3436-3442.

Kozik, A. and McCormick, D.B. (1984) Mechanism of pyridoxine uptake by isolated rat liver cells. *Arch. Biochem. Biophys.* 229, 187-193.

McCormick, D.B., et al. (1991) Characteristics of a transporter for uptake of vitamin B$_6$ into mammalian cells: Isolation of B$_6$-binding proteins from brush-border membranes of rat renal proximal tubular epithelial cells. In: Fukui, T., Kagamiyama, H., Soda, K. & Wada, H., (eds.) *Enzymes Dependent on Pyridoxal Phosphate and Other Carbonyl Compounds as Cofactors,* Pergamon Press, pp. 609-611.

McCormick, D.B., Gregory, M.E. and Snell, E.E. (1961) Pyridoxal phosphokinases. I. Assay, distribution, purification, and properties. *J. Biol. Chem.* 236, 2076-2084.

McCormick, D.B., and Snell, E.E. (1961) Pyridoxal phosphokinases. II. Effects of inhibitors. *J. Biol. Chem.* 236, 2085-2088.

McCormick, D.B. and Snell, E.E. (1959) Pyridoxal kinase of human brain and its inhibition by hydrazine reagents. *Proc. Natl. Acad. Sci. USA* 45, 1371-1379.

McCormick, D.B. and Zhang, Z. (1993) Cellular assimilation of water-soluble vitamins in the mammal: Riboflavin, B$_6$, biotin, and C. *Proc. Soc. Exp. Biol. Med.* 202, 265-270.

Zhang, Z., Gregory III, J.F. and McCormick, D.B. (1993) Pyridoxine-5'-ß-D-glucoside competitively inhibits uptake of vitamin B-6 into isolated rat liver cells. *J. Nutr.* 123, 85-89.

Zhang, Z. and McCormick, D.B. (1991) Uptake of N-(4'-pyridoxyl)amines and release of amines by renal cells: A model for transporter-enhanced delivery of bioactive compounds. *Proc. Natl. Acad. Sci. USA* 88, 10407-10410.

Zhang, Z. and McCormick, D.B. (1992a) Uptake and metabolism of 4'(N)-substituted pyridoxamines by cells from the liver and kidneys of rats. In: Kobayashi, T., (ed.) *Proceedings of the 1st International Congress on Vitamins and Biofactors in Life Sciences,* Center for Academic Publications, Japan, pp. 208-211.

Zhang, Z. and McCormick, D.B. (1992b) Uptake and metabolism of N-(4'-pyridoxyl)amines by isolated rat liver cells. *Arch. Biochem. Biophys.* 294, 394-397.

Zhang, Z., Smith, E., Surowiec, S.M., Merrill, Jr., A.H. and McCormick, D.B. (1993) Synthesis of N-(4'-pyridoxyl)sphingosine and its uptake and metabolism by isolated cells. *Membrane Biochem.* 10, 53-59.

Biochemistry of Vitamin B$_6$ and PQQ
G. Marino, G. Sannia and F. Bossa (eds.)
© 1994 Birkhäuser Verlag Basel/Switzerland

Vitamin B$_6$ Modulation of Steroid Receptor-mediated Gene Expression

Douglas B. Tully, Alyson B. Scoltock and John A. Cidlowski

Department of Physiology and the Lineberger Comprehensive Cancer Center
University of North Carolina at Chapel Hill, Chapel Hill, N.C. 27599-7545, USA

Summary

Steroid hormones regulate many physiological processes in tissues and cell types throughout the body, including such fundamental biological processes as growth, development, reproduction, regulation of metabolic state, and maintenance of homeostasis. Steroid hormones elicit their biological effects at the single cell level by regulating the expression of distinct target genes. Each type of steroid hormone binds specifically to a unique intracellular receptor protein, and this binding initiates transformation of the receptor into a form which is capable of selective interaction with DNA regulatory sequences that typically reside within or near the promoter regions of hormone-responsive genes. Interactions of the steroid-receptor complex with these DNA regulatory sites results in modulation of target gene expression that ultimately alters the phenotype of steroid-responsive cells. Because steroid receptors are critically involved in so many biological processes, there has been considerable interest in determining both the mechanisms through which steroid hormone action is mediated and related regulatory mechanisms which control the degree of cellular responsiveness to steroid hormones. We have recently shown that vitamin B$_6$ modulates transcriptional activation of gene expression by glucocorticoid, progesterone, estrogen and androgen receptors in a variety of cell lines. In each case elevated intracellular pyridoxal phosphate concentrations inhibit steroid responses, whereas vitamin B$_6$ deficiency enhances cellular responses to steroid administration. We have further shown that modulation of receptor-mediated gene expression by vitamin B$_6$ occurs only on complex promoters containing a binding site for Nuclear Factor 1 in addition to the appropriate steroid hormone response element. This new finding suggests that pyridoxal phosphate modulates the ability of steroid receptors to communicate with other transcription factors.

Introduction

The steroid hormone receptors belong to a superfamily of ligand-activated transcription factors which share extensive amino acid sequence and structural homology. These receptors also share many common features in their overall mechanism of action and all exert their biological effects through regulation of target gene expression. As illustrated for glucocorticoid-regulated gene expression in Figure 1, steroid hormones readily diffuse across target cell membranes and are subsequently bound by their specific intracellular receptor. Once the glucocorticoid receptor (GR) binds its specific steroid ligand, the receptor undergoes a poorly understood process termed transformation or activation (Currie & Cidlowski, 1982; Holbrook et al. 1982). Activation, which may involve dissociation of GR from an oligomeric complex with heat shock proteins and likely also involves a conformational change in the receptor protein itself, yields a new receptor form

320

which exhibits high affinity for specific DNA regulatory sites termed hormone response elements (HRE) that typically reside within or near the promoter regions of hormonally responsive genes. Binding of activated steroid receptors to these HREs results in modulation of target gene expression (Burnstein & Cidlowski, 1993).

While this model describes many features of the general mechanisms by which steroid hormones elicit their regulatory effects on gene expression,

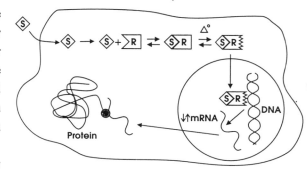

Figure 1. Model of the general mechanism of glucocorticoid receptor-mediated regulation of gene expression in a prototypical glucocorticoid responsive cell.

it is becoming apparent that a number of other factors also play important roles (Beato, 1991; Burnstein & Cidlowski, 1993; Schule et al., 1988). For example, *in vivo* binding of GR to HREs in the mouse mammary tumor virus promoter is thought to alter chromatin structure to facilitate binding of nuclear factor 1 (NF1) as well as the ubiquitous octamer transcription factor, OTF-1 (Truss et al., 1992). Thus, interactions between steroid receptors and various cell-specific and/or ubiquitous transcription factors may affect the degree of transcriptional enhancement elicited by steroid hormones. Numerous other factors also affect the magnitude of cellular response to steroid hormones. For example, the capacity of cells to respond to steroid hormone stimulation is directly affected by the number of intracellular receptors (Gehring, 1984; Vanderbilt et al., 1987), the state of cellular differentiation (Kalinyak et al., 1989; Littlefield & Cidlowski, 1984), the stage of the cell cycle (Cidlowski & Michaels, 1977; Griffin & Ber, 1969), and the nutritional status of the cell (Allgood & Cidlowski, 1991;Tully et al., 1994; Tully et al., 1993). Recently characterized interactions between vitamin B_6, and steroid hormone action are the subject of this paper.

Materials and Methods

Details of cell culture and recombinant plasmids have been previously described (Allgood et al., 1993; Allgood et al., 1990)] The transfection strategy employed in these experiments is illustrated in Figure 2. Briefly, cells were transfected by calcium phosphate precipitation using 5 μg per 100 mm culture dish of a reporter plasmid containing the coding sequence for bacterial chloramphenicol acetyltransferase (CAT) enzyme (Allgood, et al., 1990). Sixteen hours after transfection, the cell culture media were supplemented with either 1 mM pyridoxine (PYR),

5 mM 4-deoxypyridoxine (4-DXY), or vehicle (H$_2$O). After incubation for 48 h under these conditions, cells were exposed to hormone as detailed in the figure legends prior to determination of CAT activity.

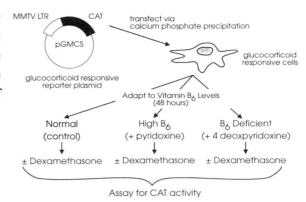

Figure 2. Outline of transfection strategy used to study the effects of changes in intracellular pyridoxal phosphate concentration on glucocorticoid-regulated gene expression.

Results

To investigate the effects of changes in intracellular PLP concentration on glucocorticoid-regulated gene expression, we first determined conditions which would allow us to manipulate intracellular PLP levels. These studies showed that supplementation of cell culture media with the PLP synthesis precursor pyridoxine caused an increase in intracellular PLP concentration. By contrast, removing vitamin B$_6$ from culture medium failed to decrease intracellular PLP concentration, suggesting that cells must be able to recycle intracellular PLP metabolites to maintain adequate levels of this essential micronutrient. We therefore used the pyridoxal kinase inhibitor 4-deoxypyridoxine (4-DXY) to achieve vitamin B$_6$ deficiency states. As shown in the left panel of Figure 3, HeLa cells transfected with the glucocorticoid-responsive CAT reporter plasmid pGMCS and grown in the

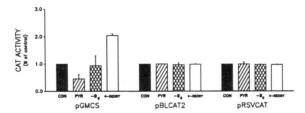

Figure 3. Effect of alterations in intracellular pyridoxal phosphate concentration on CAT activity derived from glucocorticoid-responsive and non-responsive plasmids in transfected HeLa cells. Following transfection with either the glucocorticoid-responsive plasmid pGMCS or a glucocorticoid-insensitive plasmid, pBLCAT2 or pRSVCAT, HeLa cells were cultured in unaltered medium (CON), pyridoxine-deficient medium (-B$_6$), or medium supplemented with either 1 mM pyridoxine (PYR) or 5 mM 4-deoxypyridoxine (4-DEOXY) for 48 hours. Cells were then stimulated with 100 nM dexamethasone for 8 h and assayed for CAT activity. The values shown are representative of the mean +/- standard error from two independent transfections, with CAT activity from cells grown in unaltered medium assigned a value of 1.0, and CAT activity from cells grown in other media expressed as a percentage of this value. The first 4 lanes are from cells transfected with pGMCS, lanes 5-8 from cells transfected with pBLCAT2, and lanes 9-12 from cells transfected with pRSVCAT. (From (Allgood & Cidlowski, 1992) Allgood, V. E., Powell-Oliver, F. E., and Cidlowski, J. A. (1990) *J. Biol. Chem.*, **265**, 12424-33. Reproduced by permission of ASBMB.)

presence of pyridoxine (PYR) exhibited a decrease in glucocorticoid-induced CAT activity compared with cells grown in control medium. Glucocorticoid-induced CAT activity was essentially unaffected in cells grown in vitamin B_6 deficient medium, but was enhanced approximately 2-fold over controls in cells grown in medium containing 4-DXY. By contrast with results obtained with the glucocorticoid-responsive CAT reporter plasmid, variations in intracellular PLP concentration had virtually no effect on CAT gene expression regulated by two constitutive, hormone-independent promoters, pBLCAT2 and pRSVCAT. These results demonstrate that variations in intracellular PLP concentration selectively affect glucocorticoid-regulated gene expression.

Because the glucocorticoid and other steroid hormone receptors share extensive amino acid sequence homology and many functional similarities, we wondered if alterations in intracellular PLP concentration might also affect the transcriptional activation capacity of other steroid receptors. As shown in Figure 4, the effects of altered intracellular PLP concentration on the levels of androgen-, progesterone- and estrogen-induced gene expression (panels A, B, and C, respectively) were qualitatively analogous in all three cell types to the PLP effects observed with endogenous GR in HeLa cells. That is, the levels of androgen-, progesterone- or estrogen-

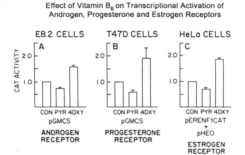

Figure 4. Effect of variations in vitamin B_6 concentration on the level of gene expression induced by androgen, progesterone or estrogen. (A.) Sixteen hours after transfection with pGMCS CAT reporter plasmid, E8.2 cells containing endogenous androgen receptor were cultured for 48 hours in unaltered control medium (CON), medium supplemented with 2 mM pyridoxine (PYR), or medium supplemented with 3 mM 4-deoxypyridoxine (4DXY). Cells were then treated with 10 nM R1881 or vehicle for 12 hours prior to CAT activity determination. (B.) Sixteen hours after transfection with pGMCS, T47D cells containing endogenous progesterone receptor were cultured for 48 hours in control medium (CON), medium supplemented with 3 mM pyridoxine (PYR), or medium supplemented with 2 mM 4-deoxypyridoxine (4DXY) prior to 24 hour treatment with 1 nM progesterone or vehicle and CAT activity determination. (C.) HeLa cells were cotransfected with the estrogen receptor expression vector pHEO and the estrogen-regulated CAT reporter plasmid pERENF1CAT. Sixteen hours after transfection, cells were exposed to control medium (CON), medium supplemented with 1 mM pyridoxine (PYR), or medium supplemented with 5 mM 4-deoxypyridoxine (4DXY) prior to 24 hour treatment with 17β-estradiol or vehicle and CAT activity determination. The data shown are representative of at least 3 individual transfection experiments. (Adapted from Allgood, V. E. and Cidlowski, J. A. (1992) *J. Biol. Chem.* **267**, 3819-24. Reproduced by permission of ASBMB.)

induced CAT gene expression were suppressed when cells were cultured under conditions that elevate intracellular PLP concentration, and hormone-induced gene expression was enhanced under conditions which produced PLP deficiency. Thus, the effects of variations in intracellular PLP concentration are not restricted to the GR, but extend to at least three other members of the steroid hormone receptor superfamily, including the androgen, progesterone and estrogen receptors. It is also important to note that these effects of PLP are not limited to the MMTV LTR promoter, since variation of intracellular pyridoxal phosphate concentration also affects transcription mediated through the estrogen-regulated promoter. These studies provide direct evidence that PLP acts to affect the transcriptional activation function of four classes of steroid hormone receptors.

Reports from several labs had shown that steroid-dependent enhancement of gene expression could be obtained using simple promoters containing only one or two copies of a small HRE and a TATA box (Klock et al., 1987; Schule, et al., 1988). Natural promoters for many hormonally responsive genes are complex and contain binding sites for other transcription factors in addition to steroid hormone receptors (Cordingley & Hager, 1988; Schule, et al., 1988; Strahle et al., 1988). For example, the glucocorticoid-responsive MMTV LTR promoter and the estrogen-inducible vitellogenin gene promoter both contain binding sites for nuclear factor 1 (NF1), and mutations of the NF1 site have been shown to affect the ability of these promoters to respond to steroid hormones (Corthesy et al., 1989; Toohey et al., 1990). These reports prompted us to wonder if the transcriptional modulatory effects PLP exerts on steroid-induced gene expression might affect the ability of receptors to interact with other transcription factors.

To investigate this possibility, we prepared simplified recombinant reporter plasmids containing or lacking binding sites for GR and/or NF1 (Allgood, et al., 1993). Transfection experiments demonstrating the effects of altered intracellular PLP concentration on glucocorticoid-induced gene expression from these simplified promoter constructs are shown in Figure 5. As we had seen before, variations in intracellular PLP concentration modulated glucocorticoid-induced CAT gene expression from the complex MMTV LTR promoter in pGMCS, but had no effect on CAT activity expressed by the constitutively active, glucocorticoid-insensitive thymidine kinase promoter in pBLCAT2 in panel B. Surprisingly, however, as shown in panels C and D, alteration of intracellular PLP concentration had virtually no effect on glucocorticoid-mediated gene expression regulated by CAT reporter plasmids containing either two or three GREs. This occurred regardless of the fact that glucocorticoids clearly induced CAT gene expression well above basal levels of CAT activity observed in cells grown in control medium. These results suggest that PLP may exert these transcriptional modulatory effects by inhibiting functional interactions between GR and NF1.

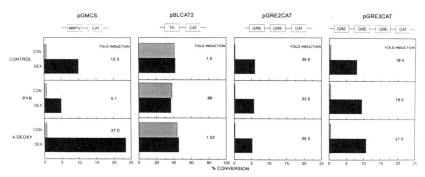

Figure 5. Effect of vitamin B_6 concentration of the level of glucocorticoid-induced gene expression from complex and simple promoters. HeLa cells were transfected with pGMCS, pBLCAT2, pGRE2CAT, or pGRE3CAT. Sixteen hours after transfection, the culture media were supplemented with either pyridoxine (PYR), 4-deoxypyridoxine (4DEOXY), or left unaltered (CONTROL). After incubation under these conditions for 48 h, cells were exposed to 100 nM dexamethasone (DEX), or vehicle control (CON) for 8 h and then harvested and assayed for CAT activity. The data shown are from one experiment, representative of at least three independent experiments. TK, thymidine kinase. (From Allgood, V.E., Oakley, R.H. and Cidlowski, J.A. (1993) *J. Biol. Chem.* **268**, 20870-20876. Reproduced by permission of ASBMB.)

Further examination of this possibility, as shown in Figure 6, indicated that PLP mediated transcriptional modulatory effects on glucocorticoid-induced gene expression were restored when an NF1 binding site was re-introduced into the pGRE2CAT reporter construct. However, these

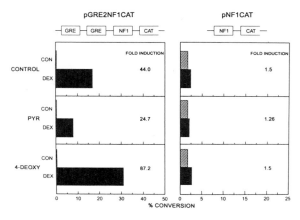

Figure 6. Transcription factor NF1 is important for modulation of glucocorticoid-induced gene expression. HeLa cells were transfected with (left panel) pGRE2NF1CAT or (right panel) pNF1CAT. Sixteen hours after transfection, the culture media were supplemented with either pyridoxine (PYR), 4-deoxypyridoxine (4DEOXY), or left unaltered (CONTROL). After 48 h under these conditions, cells were exposed to 100 nM dexamethasone (DEX), or vehicle control (CON), for 8 h and then harvested and assayed for CAT activity. The data shown are from one experiment, representative of at least three independent experiments. (From Allgood, V.E., Oakley, R.H. and Cidlowski, J.A. (1993) *J. Biol. Chem.* **268**, 20870-20876. Reproduced by permission of ASBMB.)

transcriptional modulatory effects of PLP could not be attributed solely to the presence of the NF1 site, since alteration of intracellular PLP concentration elicited virtually no effect on CAT activity induced by a CAT reporter construct which contained only an NF1 binding site and a TATA box, pNF1CAT (Allgood, et al., 1993). These results further suggest that the transcriptional modulatory effects PLP exerts on glucocorticoid-induced gene expression may occur through binding of the vitamin at a site on GR that interferes with its ability to communicate with NF1.

CONCLUSION

The results of our experiments demonstrate that moderate changes in the intracellular concentration of PLP can alter the capacity of various cells to respond to steroid hormone stimulation. Our recent data strongly suggests that the mechanism by which these effects occur may involve binding of the vitamin at a site on the receptor that inhibits its ability to form a functional interaction with NF1, as modeled in Figure 7. It is generally agreed that glucocorticoid receptors bind their specific DNA regulatory sites as dimer forms, and it is thought that these homodimers adopt a conformation that enables their transcriptional activation capacity. This transcriptionally active, homodimer form of GR is further thought to interact directly with NF1 to enhance target gene expression, as illustrated schematically in the top panel of Figure 7 ($-B_6$). Elevated intracellular PLP levels could potentiate interaction of the vitamin at a site on the receptor that blocks homodimer formation and consequently leads to receptor conformations which are unable to achieve optimal interactions with NF1 (middle panel). Alternatively, PLP may bind receptor sites that directly inhibit interaction with NF1 (bottom panel). The possibility that PLP may interact with NF1 instead of GR has not been included in these

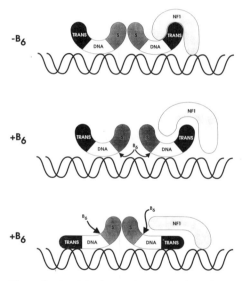

Figure 7. Model of potential mechanisms by which pyridoxal-5'-phosphate may repress glucocorticoid receptor-induced gene transcription

models because there is a large body of *in vitro* evidence demonstrating direct interactions of PLP with GR, reviewed in (Tully, et al., 1994). Efforts are currently underway to localize the site(s) of interaction of PLP with GR in order to improve to our understanding of the mechanisms by which this vitamin modulates steroid hormone-induced gene transcription.

The demonstration that moderate variations in intracellular PLP concentration can have large effects on hormonally-regulated target gene expression suggests that this vitamin may act as an important physiologic modulator of steroid hormone action. Variations in the vitamin B_6 microenvironment maintained in particular cells could provide a novel mechanism allowing cells to govern the magnitude of their response to steroid hormones. Characteristically different intracellular PLP levels have been found to occur in the tissues and cell types for which they have been measured (Ebadi & Bifano, 1978; Leklem, 1991; Merrill et al., 1964). Thus specific concentrations of this essential micronutrient, characteristic of particular cells or tissue types, could allow selected cells or tissues to respond differently to the same concentration of steroid hormone.

Acknowledgments

Supported by DK 32459 from the U. S. National Institutes of Health. We thank Christopher P. Tully for design and implementation of figures 1, 2 and 7.

References

Allgood, V.E., & Cidlowski, J.A. (1991) Novel role for vitamin B_6 in steroid hormone action: a link between nutrition and the endocrine system. *J. Nutr. Biochem.*, 2: 523-534.

Allgood, V.E., & Cidlowski, J.A. (1992) Vitamin B_6 modulates transcriptional activation by multiple members of the steroid hormone receptor superfamily. *J. Biol. Chem.*, 267: 3819-3824.

Allgood, V.E., Oakley, R.H., & Cidlowski, J.A. (1993) Modulation by vitamin B_6 of glucocorticoid receptor-mediated gene expression requires transcription factors in addition to the glucocorticoid receptor. *J. Biol. Chem.*, 268: 20870-20876.

Allgood, V.E., Powell, O.F.E., & Cidlowski, J.A. (1990) The influence of vitamin B_6 on the structure and function of the glucocorticoid receptor. *Ann. N. Y. Acad. Sci.*, 585: 452-465.

Beato, M. (1991) Transcriptional control by nuclear receptors. *FASEB J.*, 5: 2044-2051.

Burnstein, K.L., & Cidlowski, J.A. (1993) Multiple mechanisms for regulation of steroid hormone action. *J. Cell. Biochem.*, 51: 130-134.

Cidlowski, J.A., & Michaels, C.A. (1977) Alteration in glucocorticoid binding site number during the cell cycle in HeLa cells. *Nature (London)*, 266: 643-645.

Cordingley, M.G., & Hager, G.L. (1988) Binding of multiple factors to the MMTV promoter in crude and fractionated nuclear extracts. *Nucleic Acids Res.*, 16: 609-628.

Corthesy, B., Cardinaux, J.R., Claret, F.X., & Wahli, W. (1989) A nuclear factor I-like activity and a liver-specific repressor govern estrogen-regulated in vitro transcription from the Xenopus laevis vitellogenin B1 promoter. *Mol. Cell. Biol.*, 9: 5548-5562.

Currie, R.A., & Cidlowski, J.A. (1982) Physicochemical properties of the cytoplasmic glucocorticoid receptor in HeLa S_3 cells. *J Steroid Biochem*, 16: 419-428.

Ebadi, M., & Bifano, J. (1978) The synthesis of pyridoxal phosphate in rat brain regions. *Int. J. Biochem.*, 9: 607-611.

Gehring, U. (1984) Cellular receptor levels and glucocorticoid responsiveness of lymphoma cells. *J. Mol. Endocrionl.*, 36: 107-113.

Griffin, M.J., & Ber, R. (1969) Cell cycle events in the hydrocortisone regulation of alkaline phosphatase in HeLa cells. *J. Cell. Biol.*, 40: 297-304.

Holbrook, N.J., Bodwell, J.E., Jeffries, M., & Munck, A. (1982) Characterization of nonactivated and activated glucocorticoid receptors from intact rat thymus cells. *J Biol Chem*, 258: 6477-6485.

Kalinyak, J.E., Griffin, C.A., Hamilton, R.W., Bradshaw, J.G., Perlman, A.J., & Hoffman, A.R. (1989) Developmental and hormonal regulation of glucocorticoid receptor messenger RNA in the rat. *J. Clin. Invest.*, 84: 1843-1848.

Klock, G., Strahle, U., & Schutz, G. (1987) Oestrogen and glucocorticoid responsive elements are closely related but distinct. *Nature*, 329: 734-736.

Leklem, J.E. (1991) Vitamin B_6. In: *Handbook of Vitamins*, Marcel Dekker, New York, NY, pp. 341-392

Littlefield, B.A., & Cidlowski, J.A. (1984) Increased steroid responsiveness during sodium butyrate-induced "differentiation" of HeLa S3 cells. *Endocrinology*, 114: 566-575.

Merrill, A.H., Henderson, J.M., Wang, E., McDonald, B.W., & Millikan, W.J. (1964) Metabolism of vitamin B_6 by human liver. *J. Nutr.*, 114: 1664-1674.

Schule, R., Muller, M., Kaltschmidt, C., & Renkawitz, R. (1988) Many transcription factors interact synergistically with steroid receptors. *Science*, 242: 1418-1420.

Strahle, U., Schmid, W., & Schutz, G. (1988) Synergistic action of the glucocorticoid receptor with transcription factors. *EMBO J.*, 7: 3389-3395.

Toohey, M.G., Lee, J.W., Huang, M., & Peterson, D.O. (1990) Functional elements of the steroid hormone-responsive promoter of mouse mammary tumor virus. *J. Virol.*, 64: 4477-4488.

Truss, M., Chalepakis, G., & Beato, M. (1992) Interplay of steroid hormone receptors and transcription factors on the mouse mammary tumor virus promoter. *J. Steroid Biochem. Mol. Biol.*, 43: 365-378.

Tully, D.B., Allgood, V.E., & Cidlowski, J.A. (1994) Modulation of steroid receptor-mediated gene expression by vitamin B_6. *FASEB J*, 8: 343-349.

Tully, D.B., E., A.V., & Cidlowski, J.A. (1993) Vitamin B_6 modulation of steroid-induced gene expression. In: (Eds.), *Nutrition and Gene Expression*, CRC Press, Boca Raton, Florida, pp. 547-567

Vanderbilt, J.N., Miesfeld, R., Maler, B.A., & Yamamoto, K.R. (1987) Intracellular receptor concentration limits glucocorticoid-dependent enhancer activity. *Mol. Endocrinol.*, 1: 68-74.

MOLECULAR PATHOLOGY

Biochemistry of Vitamin B$_6$ and PQQ
G. Marino, G. Sannia and F. Bossa (eds.)
© 1994 Birkhäuser Verlag Basel/Switzerland

Pyridoxine (vitamin B$_6$), neurotransmitters and hypertension

K. Dakshinamurti, K.J. Lal and S.K. Sharma

Department of Biochemistry and Molecular Biology, Faculty of Medicine, University of Manitoba, Winnipeg, Canada R3E 0W3

In the past decade nontraditional functions for various vitamins which are not necessarily secondary arising out of cofactor function, have been recognized. From the notion of vitamin depletion and deficiency syndromes the newer concept that vitamins as chemicals do regulate or alter the rate of some metabolic reactions has found acceptance.

The putative neurotransmitters, dopamine, norepinephrine, serotonin and γ-aminobutyric acid (GABA) are the products of pyridoxal phosphate (PLP)-dependent decarboxylases. There is a rank order in the affinity of PLP for the various apoproteins of the PLP-dependent enzymes. Hence, during the course of the progressive depletion of tissue PLP, the activities of the various PLP-dependent enzymes are decreased to different extents. Significant decrease in the contents of GABA and serotonin with no change in the contents of the catecholamine neurotransmitters in various brain areas is the central feature of moderate pyridoxine deficiency (1). The decarboxylation of serotonin (5 HT) precursor 5-hydroxytryptophan (5-HTP) is catalyzed by an isoenzyme with a low affinity for PLP as compared with dihydroxyphenylalanine (DOPA) decarboxylase which has a high affinity for PLP.

We have examined the physiological consequences of the decrease in serotonin. Serotonin is implicated in various physiological processes such as body temperature regulation, sleep, nociception, regulation of the hypothalamo-pituitary-end organ systems, regulation of blood pressure, secretion of melatonin and behaviour.

The secretion by the anterior pituitary of adrenocorticotrophic hormone, growth hormone, prolactin, thyroid stimulating hormone (TSH) and the gonadotropins is governed by releasing factors and in some instances by release-inhibiting factors from the hypothalamus. Both dopamine and serotonin are present in high concentration in the hypothalamus and are essentially antagonistic in their effects on pituitary hormone release (2,3).

We found that the concentrations of T_4 and T_3 in serum of pyridoxine-deficient rats were significantly lower in comparison with controls (4). Pituitary content of TSH was significantly lowered. The increased pituitary TRH-receptor content, response to TRH administration and the fact that regulation at the level of the pituitary was not affected in the pyridoxine-deficient rat indicates the hypothalamic origin for the hypothyroidism of the pyridoxine-deficient rat (5).

The reduction in plasma prolactin in pyridoxine-deficient rats corresponds with the significantly reduced hypothalamic contents of PLP and serotonin. Administration of pyridoxine or the serotonin $5HT_{1A}$ agonist, 8-hydroxy 2-n-dipropylamino tetralin (8-OH-DPAT) to deficient rats resulted in a significant increase in plasma prolactin. The specific $5HT_{1A}$ antagonist spiroxatrine had the opposite effect suggesting that the hypothalamic serotonergic regulation of prolactin release is impaired in moderate pyridoxine deficiency (6).

We have examined the effect of pyridoxine deficiency on indoleamine metabolism in the pineal gland. Our results indicate that the decreased availability of 5HT is an important factor in the regulation of the synthesis of pineal melatonin (7).

The role of pyridoxine in neuronal development was earlier studied in congenitally pyridoxine-deficient rat pups (8) and in young rats subjected to pyridoxine deficiency during lactation (9). The seizure proclivity of these rats was related to the decreased GABA levels in brain areas. In more recent work (10) we have observed the spontaneous generation of tonic-clonic seizure in pyridoxine-deficient adult rats after 10 weeks of dietary pyridoxine depletion. Moderately pyridoxine-deficient rats had reduced seizure thresholds to local thalamic ventrolateral posterior (VPL) application of either picrotoxin or pentylenetetrazole. Cerebral GABA levels were reduced and glutamate increased in the deficient rats. Local (VPL) GABA or pyridoxine induced neuronal recovery in convulsant-treated normal or pyridoxine deficient rats (11). Glutamate decarboxylase (12) may be the site of regulation of GABA synthesis as the activity of this isoenzyme depends on the availability in situ of PLP. This is in keeping with our earlier (9) and other (13,14) reports that indicated that even in pyridoxine-replete animals, brain GAD is only partially saturated with respect to the cofactor PLP.

In other work we have examined domoic acid-induced seizure activity in the rat (15) as well as hippocampal changes in developing postnatal mice following intrauterine exposure to domoic acid (16). In more recent work we found that a single subconvulsive dose of domoic acid (0.6 mg/kg, i.v.) given to adult male mice resulted in electrical seizure activity. Prophylactic or therapeutic administration of antiepileptic drugs such as sodium valproate, pyridoxine, nimodipine or 5α-pregnan 3α-ol-20-one provided partial protection against domoic acid-induced excitotoxicity. ^{1}H-NMR spectra revealed increased accumulation of glutamate and reduction in GABA levels in the hippocampus. The protective action of the antiepileptic drugs are related to the increased GABA ergic neurotransmission (17).

Pyridoxine deficient hypertension

We have earlier shown (18) that the systolic blood pressure (SBP) of pyridoxine deficient rats is triphasic-prehypertensive, hypertensive and post hypertensive. The hypertension of the B6DHT rats was returned to normal within 12-24 h by a single injection of pyridoxine (10 mg/kg body weight), precluding permanent structural damage to the vessel wall. We have also established that the hypertension is related to increased peripheral sympathetic activity in the B6DHT rats (19,20).

Functional activity of serotonin (5HT) receptors in B6DHT rats was assessed. $5HT_{1A}$ receptor agonists were all effective in reducing the SBP of the B6DHT rats (21). The putative $5HT_{1A}$ receptor antagonist spiroxatrine, dose-dependently antagonized the hypotensive effect of $5HT_A$ agonists. The affinity and B_{max} of $5HT_{1A}$ receptors were increased in B6DHT rats. Activity in central sympathetic pathways can be modified by stimulating central α_2 adrenoreceptors (22). α_2 adrenergic output to the brain stem is reduced in the pyridoxine-deficient rat (20). Serotonergic neurons participate in regulation of sympathetic nervous activity. Stimulation of $5HT_{1A}$ receptors causes central sympatho inhibition and an increase in cardiac vagal drive which results in a fall in blood pressure (23,24).

Peripheral effects of pyridoxine deficiency

Increased peripheral resistance resulting from increased permeability of vascular smooth muscle (VASM) plasma membrane to Ca^{2+} is thought to be one of the mechanisms of hypertension (25). ^{45}Ca influx into the intracellular compartment of VASM of the caudal artery was significantly increased in B6DHT rats. This increased influx was attenuated by nifedipine. Arterial segments from B6DHT rats maintained a higher resting tone (26).

In more recent work, we have shown that pyridoxine vitamers blocked the in vitro calcium influx into the caudal artery of B6DHT rats as well as the calcium channel agonist, BAY K 8644-mediated influx into the caudal artery segments from pyridoxine replete normotensive control rats (27). In corresponding in vivo work all the calcium channel antagonists were effective in lowering the SBP of B6DHT rats (28).

Pyridoxine-calcium relationship

Rats fed the pyridoxine deficient diet containing less than 1.0% calcium in the diet developed hypertension. We investigated the relationship between low calcium (0.1%)-induced hypertension and the vitamin B_6 status of the rat. The effect of varying dietary levels of calcium on the SBP of vitamin B_6-sufficient or vitamin B_6-deficient rats was studied. Lowering calcium to 0.1% in the vitamin B_6-sufficient diet of rats resulted in a significant increase in their SBP. Low levels of calcium in the diet potentiated the hypertension induced by vitamin B_6 deficiency when both deficiencies were present from the start of the experiment. Feeding a low calcium diet during the hypertensive or post-hypertensive phases failed to increase the SBP of these rats. Normalizing the vitamin B_6 status of post-hypertensive vitamin B_6 deficient rats restored the ability of low dietary calcium to induce hypertension in these rats. Increasing the dietary levels of vitamin B_6 also attenuated the low dietary calcium-induced hypertension. A similar effect of attenuation of the SBP of the Zucker obese rat by increasing the vitamin B_6 content of the diet to 2.5 times the normal was also seen.

The Ca^{2+} abnormalities underlying hypertension in the B6DHT rats appear to be similar to that seen in other models of hypertension. Low calcium in the diet decreases ionic serum calcium resulting in enhanced Ca^{2+} influx through defective membrane of VASM (29). In the post hypertensive phase of vitamin B_6 deficiency this membrane defect is probably complete (27). In addition, it is possible that in this condition there is uncoupling between increased intracellular calcium influx and the contractile mechanisms of the VASM. Hence,

335

lowering the calcium content of the diet had no effect on the SBP of these rats. Vitamin B$_6$ may correct the membrane abnormality by a mechanism similar to that of the calcium channel blockers (30) and so, could be an important part of the mechanisms regulating the flux of calcium across the plasma membrane.

This work was supported by grants from the Medical Research Council of Canada and the Heart and Stroke Foundation of Canada.

References

1. Dakshinamurti, K., LeBlancq, W.D., Hercht, R. and Harbicek, V. (1976) Exp. Brain Res. 26, 355-366.
2. Krulich, L. (1979) Ann. Rev. Physiol. 41, 603-615.
3. Dakshinamurti, K., Paulose, C.A., Viswanathan, M. and Siow, Y.O. (1988) Neuroscience and Biobehavioural Reviews 12, 189-193.
4. Dakshinamurti, K., Paulose, C.S., Thliveris, J.A. and Vriend, J. (1985) J. Endocrinol. 104, 339-344.
5. Dakshinamurti, K., Paulose, C.S. and Vriend, J. (1986) J. Endocrinol. 109, 345-349.
6. Sharma, S.K. and Dakshinamurti, K. (1994) Neurochem. Res. 19, 687-692.
7. Viswanathan, M., Siow, Y.L., Paulose, C.S. and Dakshinamurti, K. (1988) Brain Research 473, 37-42.
8. Dakshinamurti, K. and Stephens, M.C. (1969) J. Neurochem. 16, 1515-1522.
9. Stephens, M.C., Havlicek, V. and Dakshinamurti, K. (1971) J. Neurochem. 18, 2407-2416.
10. Sharma, S.K. and Dakshinamurti, K. (1992) Epilepsia 32, 235-247.
11. Sharma, S.K., Bolster, B. and Dakshinamurti, K. (1993) J. Neurological Sciences 121, 1-9.
12. Denner, L.A. and Wu, J.Y. (1985) J. Neurochem. 44, 957-65.
13. Nitsch, C. (1980) J. Neurochem. 34, 822-30.
14. Martin, D.L., Martin, S.B., Wu, S.J. and Espina, S. (1991) Neurochem. Res. 16, 243-249.
15. Dakshinamurti, K., Sharma, S.K. and Sundaram, M. (1991) Neuroscience Letters 127, 193-197.
16. Dakshinamurti, K., Sharma, S.K., Sundaram, M. and Watanabe, T. (1993) J. Neuroscience 13, 4486-4495.
17. Sharma, S.K., Dakshinamurti, K., Pillay, N., Peeling, J., Buist, R. and Marat, R.K. (1994) Manuscript submitted.
18. Paulose, C.S., Dakshinamurti, K., Packer, S. and Stephens, N. (1988) Sympathetic stimulation and hypertension in pyridoxine-deficient adult rat. Hypertension 11, 387-391.
19. Paulose, C.S. and Dakshinamurti, K. (1987) J. Neurosci. Methods 22, 141-146.
20. Viswanathan, M., Paulose, C.S., Lal, K.J., Sharma, S.K. and Dakshinamurti, K. (1990) Neuroscience Letters 111, 201-205.
21. Lal, K.J. and Dakshinamurti, K. (1993) Eur. J. Pharmacol. 234, 183-189.
22. Kobinger, W. and Pichler, L. (1980) Naumyn-Schmiedbergs Arch. Pharmacol. 315, 21-27.
23. Saxena, P.R. and Willalon, C.M. (1990) Pharmacol. 15 (Suppl. 7), S17-S34.
24. Ramage, A.C. (1990) J. Cardiovasc. Pharmacol. 15 (Suppl. 7), S75-S85.
25. Rapp, J.P., Nghiem, C.X. and Oniwachei, M.O. (1986) J. Hypertens. 4, 493-499.
26. Viswanathan, M., Bose, R. and Dakshinamurti, K. (1991) Am. J. Hypertens. 4, 252-255.
27. Lal, K.J., Sharma, S.K. and Dakshinamurti, K. (1993) Clin. Exp. Hypertens. 15, 489-500.
28. Lal, K.J. and Dakshinamurti, K. (1993) J. Hypertens. 11, 1357-1362.
29. McCarron, D.A. (1985) Hypertension 7, 607-627.
30. Dominiczak, A.F. and Bohr, D.F. (1990) Clin. Sci. 79, 415-423.

Biochemistry of Vitamin B$_6$ and PQQ
G. Marino, G. Sannia and F. Bossa (eds.)
© 1994 Birkhäuser Verlag Basel/Switzerland

A liver enzyme, serine:pyruvate/alanine:glyoxylate aminotransferase and its mutant in a primary hyperoxaluria type 1 case

K. Ishikawa, T. Suzuki, T. Funai, K. Nishiyama, C. Uchida and A. Ichiyama

Dept. of Biochemistry, Hamamatsu University School of Medicine, 3600 Handa-cho, Hamamatsu, Shizuoka, 431-31, Japan

Summary

In the liver of herbivorous animals and man, serine:pyruvate/alanine:glyoxylate aminotransferase (SPT/AGT) locates in peroxisomes, and plays an important role of removing glyoxylate by transamination to Gly. Primary hyperoxaluria type 1 (PH1), a congenital metabolic disease characterized by increased oxalate production and precipitation of calcium oxalate crystals in many tissues, is caused by a defect in SPT/AGT. In a PH1 case we are studying, there is a point mutation of T to C in exon 6 of the SPT/AGT gene, encoding a Ser to Pro substitution at residue 205. A remarkable feature of the SPT/AGT deficiency in the PH1 case was that the mutant SPT/AGT appeared to be actively synthesized in the patient's liver, but the enzyme was very low with respect to not only the activity but also the protein detectable on Western blot analysis. This discrepancy was explained by the finding that the mutant enzyme is decomposed much faster than normal in transfected cells and *in vitro*, and the degradation *in vitro* with a reticulocyte lysate system is ATP-dependent. The mutant SPT/AGT was purified as a fusion with maltose-binding protein (MBP), followed by cleavage with factor Xa protease. The mutant enzyme thus purified did not show the enzyme activity under the assay conditions used. However, it was not possible to conclude that the mutant enzyme is inactive, because the mutant enzyme or its fusion with MBP aggregated considerably rapidly, and after the aggregation, even normal SPT/AGT did not exibit the enzyme activity. We then attempted to determine whether or not the mutation site (Ser-205) is in a neighborhood of the pyridoxal phosphate (PLP)-binding Lys. Comparison of the predicted secondary structures of SPT/AGT with those of three other aminotransferases suggested that Lys-209 is the PLP-binding residue. Upon BrCN cleavage of the NaBH$_4$-reduced and pyridylethylated recombinant rat SPT/AGT, a 22-23 kd fragment was recovered as main product as expected, but most products with a molecular weight over 10 kd, including the 22-23 kd product, showed pairs of bands on SDS-PAGE. Amino acid sequences of the 22-23 kd pair were determined to be the same, except that Lys was released from only one of the pair on the 14th cycle corresponding to Lys-209, suggesting that the paired bands are derived from apo- and holo-SPT/AGT. These results in turn suggested that Lys-209 is indeed the PLP-binding residue. Based on these data, we are inclined to think that mutant SPT/AGT in the PH1 case is not only susceptible to the ATP-dependent intracellular degradation but also enzymically inactive.

Introduction

Serine:pyruvate/alanine:glyoxylate aminotransferase (SPT/AGT) of animal liver is an enzyme of dual organelle localization and presumably of dual function. In carnivores, this enzyme locates mostly in mitochondria (Takada & Noguchi, 1982; Noguchi, 1987; Danpure *et al.*, 1990) and is probably involved in serine metabolism. In herbivores and man, this enzyme locates in peroxisomes (Noguchi & Takada, 1978; Takada & Noguchi, 1982; Noguchi, 1987; Danpure *et al.*, 1990), where glyoxylate, an immediate precursor of oxalate, is mainly produced. It is well known that calcium salt of oxalate is hardly soluble in aqueous solutions and frequently forms calucli in urinary and other tissues. Since plants are rich in oxalate, precursors of oxalate may also be included in this staple food of herbivores. Therefore, the peroxisomal localization of SPT/AGT is essential, especially for herbivores, to remove glyoxylate by transamination to glycine and to keep animals from harmful overproduction of oxalate. In fact, primary hyperoxaluria type 1 (PH1), a congenital metabolic disease characterized by increased oxalate production and precipitation of calcium oxalate crystals in many tissues, is caused by a defect in SPT/AGT. The PH1 case we are studying had had recurrent urinary calculi since the age of 6, and reached the end-stage renal failure at age 38 which necessitated hemodialysis. His parents are consanguineous to each other, and many of his relatives also suffered from juvenile-onset urolithiasis. The patient suddenly died at age 45. We assume that calcium oxalate calculi in the heart may have blocked the conduction system.

We cloned SPT/AGT-cDNA from the patient's liver, and demonstrated a point mutation of T to C in exon 6 encoding a Ser to Pro subsitution at residue 205. The T to C conversion created a new *Sma*I site, which enabled us to demonstrate that the mutation occurs in the patient's gene and that the patient is homozygous with respect to this mutation (Fig. 1-A) (Nishiyama *et al.*, 1991). In this paper, biosynthesis, degradation and properties of mutant SPT/AGT in the PH1 case are summarized.

Materials and Methods

Methods for RNA blot analysis, *in vitro* translation, expression of cDNA in COS and other cells, Western blot analysis, pulse-chase experiments and *in vitro* protein degradation with reticulocyte lysate have been described previously (Nishiyama *et al.,* 1993) Expression and purification of normal and mutant SPT/AGT as MBP fusions were carried out essentially according to Riggs (1989). Human and recombinant rat SPT/AGT were purified and the SPT activity was determined as described previously (Oda *et al.*,1982; Oda *et al.*, 1989; Nishiyama *et al.*, 1990). Cleavage of peptide chain by BrCN and reductive cleavage of disulfides were performed according to Gross (1967) and Rüegg and Rudinger (1977), respectively. N-Terminal amino acid sequence was determined with the aid of an ABI protein sequencer, model 476A.

Results and Discussions

A remarkable feature of the SPT/AGT deficiency in this PH1 case was that the mutant SPT/AGT

(A) Mutation of Ser-205 to Pro

Normal human
SPT/AGT

                          ★

\- GAC ATC CTG TAC TCG GGC TCC CAG AAG -

Asp Ile Leu Tyr Ser Gly Ser Gln Lys

201   205   209

                              <u>_SmaI_</u>

Mutant SPT/AGT
in the PH1 Case

                          ★

\- GAC ATC CTG TAC CCG GGC TCC CAG AAG -

Asp Ile Leu Tyr Pro Gly Ser Gln Lys

201   205   209

(B) Cleavage of SPT/AGT with BrCN (●:M)

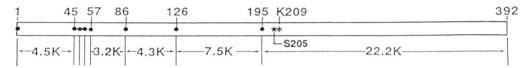

Figure 1. Amino acid sequence around the mutation site in the primary hyperoxaluria type 1 case. The nucleotide numbers in (A) are relative to the 5'-ends of cDNAs. The deduced amino acid residues are numbered from the initiation Met.

appeared to be actively synthesized in the patient's liver but the enzyme was very low with respect to not only the activity but also the protein detectable on Western blot analysis. Upon RNA blot analysis, a single band of SPT/AGT-mRNA was observed in both control and patient's liver, and the level of the mRNA in the patient's liver was even higher than normal. The size of patient's mRNA was the same as that of the 1.7 kb SPT/AGT-mRNA from control human liver. In addition, the mRNA from the patient's liver was translated as effectively as that from control liver _in vitro_ in a reticulocyte lysate system and in pulse-chase experiments with transfected COS-I cells and _E. coli._ On Western blot analysis, on the other hand, mutant SPT/AGT was barely detectable when as much as 500 mg protein of sonicated liver extrct was applied, whereas normal enzyme was clearly observed with 10 mg of the liver extract. Immunocytochemically detectable SPT/AGT labeling was also low in the patient's liver, although it was detected predominantly in peroxisomes.

    The discrepancy between the synthesis and the intracellular steady state level of mutant SPT/AGT was explained by the finding that the mutant enzyme is decomposed in transfected cells and _in vitro_ much faster than normal. In addition, the degradation _in vitro_ with a reticulocyte lysate system was ATP-dependent (Nishiyama _et al._,1993). It appears that a single amino acid substitution in mutant SPT/AGT in this PH1 case caused a mis-folded structure which is recognized in cells as that of an abnormal protein to be eliminated by degradation. Although the biological and pathological importance of intracellular degradation system to eliminate mis-folded proteins has long been suspected, this is still one of the relatively few cases in which rapid degradation of mutant protein is demonstrated in a hereditary disease.

One of major questions remained to be answered was whether or not the mutant SPT/AGT is enzymically active. In order to solve this question, the mutant enzyme was expressed and purified as a fusion with maltose-binding protein (MBP), followed by cleavage with factor Xa protease. When the purification processes were monitored by SDS-PAGE, both normal and mutant SPT/AGT were effectively expressed and purified. With respect to the enzyme activity, on the other hand, no activity was detectable in mutant SPT/AGT or its fusion with MBP under conditions used, whereas normal enzyme showed a definite SPT activity not only after but also before the factor Xa cleavage. However, we felt it too impetuous to conclude that mutant SPT/AGT is inactive, because the mutant enzyme or its fusion with MBP aggregated considerably rapidly, and after the aggregation, even normal SPT/AGT did not exhibit any enzyme activity.

Therefore, we then intended to clarify whether or not the mutation site (Ser-205) is in a neighborhood of pyridoxal phosphate (PLP)-binding Lys. We previously presumed from a comparison of the predicted secondary structures of rat SPT/AGT with those of three other aminotransferases that Lys-209 is the PLP-binding residue (Oda et al., 1987). We tentatively separated the secondary structures of the four aminotransferases into three segments, A, B, and C. Segment B consists of a cluster of b-structure, whereas segments A and C have a structure of alternative α-helix and β-structure. The PLP-binding Lys of mitochondrial asparatate aminotransferase (Lys-250) and that of ornithine aminotrnsferase (Lys-267) are located in segment B (Huynh et al., 1980; Simmaco et al.,1986), where in the four aminotransferase there is only one or two Lys residues. It is probable that the PLP-binding Lys residue of SPT/AGT is Lys-209 in segment B. If Lys-209 is indeed the PLP-binding residue, Ser-205, the amino acid residue mutated to Pro in the PH1 case, seems to be adjacent enough to the active Lys to interfere with the cofacter or substrate binding.

We have previously shown that the predicted amino acid sequence of human SPT/AGT shares with that of rat enzyme 79.3% identity and as much as 92.6% similarity including conservative amino acid substitutions (Nishiyama et al., 1990). Therefore, recombinant rat SPT/AGT was purified and subjected to BrCN cleavage after reduction with $NaBH_4$ and reductive pyridylethylation, followed by SDS-PAGE. Lys-209 was expected to be recovered in a 22.2 kd fragment (Fig. 1-B), and in fact, ^3H from NaB^3H_4 was incorporated into the 22-23 kd fragment in a preliminary experiment. We then noticed that most BrCN-cleavage products with a molecular weight over 10 kd, including the 22-23kd product, show pairs of bands on SDS-PAGE. Since the binding of PLP to SPT/AGT appears to be rather weak, we understood this result to mean that the paired bands are derived from apo- and holo-SPT/AGT. In fact, the 22-23 kd pair gave essentially the same sequence which was fully compatible with that expected. Only the difference between the 22-23 kd pair was that Lys was released only from the larger one (23 kd band) on the 14th cycle corresponding to Lys-209, suggesting that they are derived from holo- and apo-SPT/AGT. These results in turn suggested that Lys-209 is indeed the PLP-binding residue. Based on all the results mentioned above, we are inclined to think that mutant SPT/AGT in the PH1 case is not only susceptible to the ATP dependent intracellular degradation but also enzymically inactive.

References

Danpure, C.J., Guttrige, K.M., Fryer, P., Jennings, P. R., Allsop, J., and Purdue, P.E. (1990) Subcellular distribution of hepatic alanine: glyoxylate aminotransferase in various mammalian species. J. Cell Sci. 97: 184-188

Gross, E. (1967) The cyanogen bromide reaction. Methods Enzymol. 11: 238-255

Huynh, Q.K., Sakakibara, R., Watanabe, T., and Wada, H. (1980) Primary structure of mitochondrial glutamic oxaloacetic transaminase from rat liver: Comparison with that of the pig heart isozyme. Biochem. Biophys. Res. Commun. 97: 474-479

Nishiyama, K., Berstein, G., Oda, T., and Ichiyama, A. (1990) Cloning and nucleotide sequence of cDNA encoding human liver serine-pyruvate aminotransferase. Eur. J. Biochem. 194: 9-18

Nishiyama, K., Funai, T., Katafuchi, R., Hattori, F., Onoyama, K., and Ichiyama, A. (1991) Primary hyperoxaluria type 1 due to a point mutaion of T to C in the coding region of the serine:pyruvate/alanine:glyoxylate aminotransferase gene. Biochem. Biophys. Res. Commun. 176: 1093-1099

Nishiyama, K., Funai, T., Yokota, S., and Ichiyama, A. (1993) ATP-dependent degradation of mutant serine:pyruvate/alanine:glyoxylate aminotransferase in a primary hyperoxaluria type 1 case. J. Cell Biol. 123: 1237-1248

Noguchi, T. and Takada, Y. (1978) Peroxisomal localization of serine:pyruvate aminotransferase in human liver. J. Biol. Chem. 253: 7598-7600

Noguchi, T. (1987) Amino acid metabolism in animal peroxisomes. In: Fahimi, H.D. and Sies, H. (eds.): Peroxysomes in Biology and Medicine, Springer-Verlag, Berlin, Heidelberg, pp. 234-243

Oda, T., Yanagisawa, M., and Ichiyama, A. (1982) Induction of serine:pyruvate aminotransferase in rat liver organelles by glucagon and a high-protein diet. J. Biochem. 91: 219-232

Oda, T., Miyajima ,H., Suzuki, Y., and Ichiyama, A. (1987) Nucleotide sequence of the cDNA encoding the precursor for mitochondrial serine:pyruvate aminotransferase of rat liver. Eur. J. Biochem. 168: 537-542

Oda, T., Miyajima, H., Suzuki, Y., Ito, T., Yokota, S., Hoshino, M., and Ichiyama, A. (1989) Purification and characterization of the active serine: pyruvate aminotranferase of rat liver mitochondria expressed in Escherichia coli. J. Biochem. 106: 460-467

Riggs, P. (1989) Expression and purification of maltose binding protein fusions. In: Ausubel, F. M., Brent, R., Kingston, R.E., Moor, D.D., Seidman, J.G., Smith, J.A., and Struhl, K. (eds.): Current Protocols in Molecular Biology, Vol. 2, Johon Wiley & Sons, New York, Chichester, Brisbane, Toronto, Singapore, 16. 6. 1-16. 6. 14

Rüegg, Th. and Rudinger, J. (1977) Reductive cleavage of cystine disulfides with tributylphosphine. Methods Enzymol. 47: 111-116

Simmaco, M., John, R.A., Barra, D., and Bossa, F. (1986) The primary structure of ornitine aminotransferase. Identification of active-site sequence and site of post-transrational proteolysis. FEBS Lett. 199: 39-42

Takada, Y. and Noguchi, T.(1982) Subcellular distribution, and physical and immunological properties of hepatic alanine:glyoxylate aminotransferase isoenzymes in different mammalian species. Comp. Biochem. Physiol. 72B, 597-604

Biochemistry of Vitamin B$_6$ and PQQ
G. Marino, G. Sannia and F. Bossa (eds.)
© 1994 Birkhäuser Verlag Basel/Switzerland

Pyridoxal Phosphate, GABA and Seizure Susceptibility

David L. Martin

Wadsworth Center for Laboratories and Research, New York State Department of Health, P.O. Box 509, Albany, NY 12201-0509 and Department of Environmental Health and Toxicology, State University of New York at Albany

Summary

Pyridoxal-P plays a major role in the short term regulation of γ-aminobutyric acid (GABA) synthesis in brain, as the GABA-synthesizing enzyme glutamate decarboxylase (GAD) is regulated in part by a tightly controlled cycle that interconverts the holo- and apoenzyme. This mechanism explains the sensitivity of brain GABA levels to vitamin B6 deficiency and very likely contributes to the enhanced seizure susceptibility that is a prominent symptom of vitamin B6 deficiency in animals and humans.

Introduction

Vitamin B6 deficiency produces pronounced neurological symptoms in both animals and humans. Prominent among these symptoms are overt seizures or enhanced seizure susceptibility (Coursin, 1969; Sharma et al., 1994). The importance of pyridoxal-P in the synthesis and degradation of GABA together with the great number of studies linking GABA-mediated synaptic transmission with seizures has led to the inference that a deficiency in GABAergic function is a major contributing factor to the seizures that accompany vitamin B6 deficiency. In this article, I will review the evidence that pyridoxal-P plays a central role in the regulation of GABA synthesis, and the evidence that GABAergic function is altered in vitamin B6 deficient animals.

γ-Aminobutyric acid (GABA) is the major inhibitory neurotransmitter in brain, and GABAergic neurons and nerve terminals are prominent features of virtually all brain regions. GABA has been studied extensively in connection with epilepsy and experimentally-induced seizures, and it has been clear for many years that manipulation of GABAergic function can induce seizures or markedly alter seizure susceptibility (Gale, 1985).

Pyridoxal-P plays a central role in the regulation of GABA metabolism

In brain the principal pathway for GABA synthesis is the conversion of glutamate to GABA by GAD, a pyridoxal-P-requiring enzyme. GABA is degraded to succinate in two enzymatic steps, the first of which is carried out by another pyridoxal-P requiring enzyme, GABA:2-oxoglutarate transaminase (GABA-T). From the point of view of understanding the regulation of GABA metabolism, most attention has been directed toward the control of GAD activity, because GAD determines the rate of GABA synthesis (Martin and Rimvall, 1993). GABA-T, which is a mitochondrial enzyme and is present in non-neuronal cells as well as in GABAergic neurons, is viewed as having a more passive role in GABA metabolism, so physiologic regulation of its activity has not received much attention. However, GABA-T has been a more promising target for pharmacologic intervention than GAD, because selective inhibitors of GABA-T can be used to manipulate brain GABA levels and seizure susceptibility (Gale, 1985).

GAD is present in brain in at least two forms termed GAD_{65} and GAD_{67} which are the products of two genes (Erlander et al., 1991). These two forms appear to differ somewhat in subcellular distribution as GAD_{65} appears to be more concentrated in synaptic terminals than GAD_{67}, whereas GAD_{67} appears more widely distributed within neurons including proximal dendrites (Kaufman et al., 1991; Esclapez et al., 1994). The expression of the two forms also is regulated by different mechanisms (Martin and Rimvall, 1993).

It has been known for many years that 50% or more of total GAD is present in brain as apoenzyme (apoGAD, enzyme without bound pyridoxal-P; Miller et al., 1977), and it is now thought that apoGAD serves as a reservoir of inactive enzyme that can be activated when additional GABA synthesis is required (Martin and Rimvall, 1993). For many years, pyridoxal-P was believed to be loosely bound to GAD, at least in contrast to GABA-T, but it is now clear that pyridoxal-P does not dissociate readily from GAD and that apoGAD is generated principally by an alternative transamination reaction carried out by GAD itself (Martin, 1987; Martin and Rimvall, 1993). Current knowledge of the mechanism of GAD is summarized in Figure 1. The principal reaction carried out by GAD is, of course, the decarboxylation of glutamate to produce GABA. However, the alternative transamination reaction occurs during a small fraction of

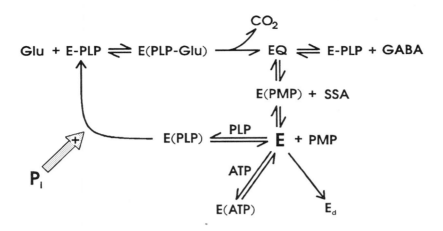

Figure 1. Cycle that converts holo- and apoGAD and its regulation by Pi and ATP. E, apoGAD; E-PLP, holoGAD; Ed, denatured GAD; PLP, pyridoxal-P; PMP, pyridoxamine-P; SSA, succinic semialdehyde.

turnovers, producing succinic semialdehyde (SSA) and pyridoxamine-P (PMP) thus yielding apoGAD. ApoGAD can be activated, of course, by pyridoxal-P thus regenerating holoGAD and completing a cycle of inactivation and reactivation. Each step of the cycle has been studied. As shown in Fig 1, GAD produces SSA and PMP in a 1:1 molar ratio when incubated with glutamate, and, as expected, GAD inactivates when it is incubated with glutamate or GABA in the absence of pyridoxal-P (Porter et al., 1985; Spink et al., 1985). Furthermore, the rate of inactivation is reduced when SSA is present, and apoGAD is activated when it is incubated with SSA and PMP (Porter et al., 1985).

The cyclic interconversion of apo- and holoGAD is strongly regulated by inorganic phosphate (Pi) and polyanions such as ATP. ATP is a potent competitive inhibitor of the activation of apoGAD by pyridoxal-P (Ki < 1 μM; Porter and Martin, 1988). Since the concentration of free ATP in the cytoplasm is at least 100-fold higher than the Ki, this inhibition appears to be physiologically important. In addition, ATP stabilizes apoGAD against thermal inactivation (Porter and Martin, 1988). This effect also appears to be physiologically important as apoGAD rapidly denatures at physiological temperatures. The inhibition of activation is not specific for ATP, as a variety of other polyanions including other nucleotides affect GAD similarly (Martin and Martin, 1982). Pi opposes the action of ATP at physiologic concentrations and strongly stimulates the activation of apoGAD by pyridoxal-P (Martin and Martin, 1979; Porter and Martin,

1988). The cycle of inactivation and reactivation together with the effects of ATP and Pi appear to account for the high levels of apoGAD in brain.

The preceding studies were carried out with purified brain GAD which was comprised principally of GAD_{65}. Although no detailed mechanistic comparison of GAD_{65} and GAD_{67} have appeared, the two forms do appear to differ in their interactions with the cofactor (Kaufman et al., 1991). To investigate which form of GAD accounts for the high level of apoGAD in brain, we developed a technique to specifically label the active site with [^{32}P]pyridoxal-P (Martin et al., 1990, 1991a,b). These experiments demonstrated that the great majority of apoGAD in brain is $apoGAD_{65}$. Furthermore, GAD was the major specifically-labeled protein in nerve endings and every brain region examined. Thus, GAD appears to be unusual if not unique among pyridoxal-P-dependent enzymes in being present in large amounts as apoenzyme in brain.

GABAergic function is altered in vitamin B6 deficiency

It has been clear for many years that brain GABA levels are reduced in vitamin B6 deficient animals (Tews, 1969) , and this fundamental finding has been replicated a number of times (e.g. Bayoumi et al., 1972; Sharma et al., 1994). The fact that GABA levels decrease rather than increase in deficient animals suggests that GABA synthesis is more sensitive to B6 deficiency than is GABA degradation. In keeping with this idea, the level of saturation of GAD by pyridoxal-P is substantially reduced in deficient animals while GABA-T is less affected (Bayoumi et al., 1972; Bayoumi and Smith, 1973; Martin and Martin, 1979). The effect on GAD is widespread in brain, as it occurs in several regions. While the reduced saturation of GAD should reduce the basal rate of GABA synthesis, the lower availability of pyridoxal-P should also reduce the cells' ability to increase the rate of GABA synthesis when neuronal activity increases. This inability to increase GABA synthesis in response to demand could lead to insufficient inhibitory function when deficient animals are challenged and thus help to explain the greater seizure susceptibility of vitamin B6 deficient animals whose behavior is otherwise stable.

While alterations in GABAergic function very likely contribute in a major way to the seizures observed in vitamin B6 deficiency, it would be simplistic to attribute these seizures solely to changes in the GABA system, as pyridoxal-P is involved in the metabolism of several transmitters. For example, brain glutamate levels are increased substantially in vitamin B6 deficient animals (Sharma et al., 1994). Since glutamate is a major excitatory transmitter in brain, this finding suggests that enhanced excitatory transmission may also contribute to the increased seizure susceptibility. Similarly, serotonin appears to be involved in some types of seizures (e.g. see Sharma et al., 1994).

Acknowledgement

This work was supported by grant MH-35664 from the USPHS/DHHS.

References

Bayoumi R.A., Kirwan J.R., and Smith W.R.D. (1972) Some effects of dietary vitamin B6 deficiency and 4-deoxypyridoxine on γ-aminobutyric acid metabolism in rat brain. *J. Neurochem.* 19: 569-576.

Bayoumi R.A. and Smith W.R.D. (1973) Regional distribution of glutamic acid decarboxylase in the developing brain of the pyridoxine deficient rat. *J. Neurochem.* 21: 603-613.

Coursin D.B. (1969) Vitamin B6 and Brain Function in Animals and Man. *Ann. N. Y. Acad. Sci.* 166: 7-15.

Erlander M.G., Tillakaratne N.J.K., Feldblum S., Patel N., and Tobin A.J. (1991) Two genes encode distinct glutamate decarboxylases. *Neuron* 7: 91-100.

Esclapez M., Tillakaratne N.J.K., Kaufman D.L., Tobin A.J., and Houser C.R. (1994) Comparative localization of two forms of glutamic acid decarboxylase and their mRNAs in rat brain supports the concept of functional differences between the forms. *J. Neurosci.* 14: 1834-1855.

Gale K. (1985) Mechanisms of seizure control mediated by γ-aminobutyric acid: Role of the substantia nigra. *Fed. Proc.* 44: 2414-2424.

Kaufman D.L., Houser C.R., and Tobin A.J. (1991) Two forms of the gamma-aminobutyric acid synthetic enzyme glutamate decarboxylase have distinct intraneuronal distributions and cofactor interactions. *J. Neurochem.* 56: 720-723.

Martin D.L. (1987) Regulatory properties of brain glutamate decarboxylase. *Cell. Mol. Neurobiol.* 7: 237-253.

Martin D.L., Wu S.J., and Martin S.B. (1990) Glutamate-dependent active-site labeling of brain glutamate decarboxylase. *J. Neurochem.* 55: 524-532.

Martin D.L., Martin S.B., Wu S.J., and Espina N. (1991a) Regulatory properties of brain glutamate decarboxylase (GAD): The apoenzyme of GAD is present principally as the smaller of two molecular forms of GAD in brain. *J. Neurosci.* 11: 2725-2731.

Martin D.L., Martin S.B., Wu S.J., and Espina N. (1991b) Cofactor interactions and the regulation of glutamate decarboxylase activity. *Neurochem. Res.* 16: 243-249.

Martin D.L. and Martin S.B. (1982) Effect of nucleotides and other inhibitors on the inactivation of glutamate decarboxylase. *J. Neurochem.* 39: 1001-1008.

Martin D.L. and Rimvall K. (1993) Regulation of γ-aminobutyric acid synthesis in the brain. *J. Neurochem.* 60: 395-407.

Martin S.B. and Martin D.L. (1979) Stimulation by phosphate of the activation of glutamate apodecarboxylase by pyridoxyl-5'-phosphate and its implications for the control of GABA synthesis. *J. Neurochem.* 33: 1275-1283.

Miller L.P., Walters J.R., and Martin D.L. (1977) Post-mortem changes implicate adenine nucleotides and pyridoxal-5'-phosphate in regulation of brain glutamate decarboxylase. *Nature* 266: 847-848.

Porter T.G., Spink D.C., Martin S.B., and Martin D.L. (1985) Transaminations catalysed by brain glutamate decarboxylase. *Biochem. J.* 231: 705-712.

Porter T.G. and Martin D.L. (1988) Stability and activation of glutamate apodecarboxylase from pig brain. *J. Neurochem.* 51: 1886-1891.

Sharma S.K., Bolster B., and Dakshinamurti K. (1994) Picrotoxin and pentylene tetrazole induced seizure activity in pyridoxine-deficient rats. *J. Neurol. Sci.* 121: 1-9.

Spink D.C., Porter T.G., Wu S.J., and Martin D.L. (1985) Characterization of three kinetically distinct forms of glutamate decarboxylase from pig brain. *Biochem. J.* 231: 695-703.

Tews J.K. (1969) Pyridoxine deficiency and brain amino acids. *Ann. N. Y. Acad. Sci.* 166: 74-82.

Biochemistry of Vitamin B_6 and PQQ
G. Marino, G. Sannia and F. Bossa (eds.)
© 1994 Birkhäuser Verlag Basel/Switzerland

Monoclonal antibodies to bovine brain GABA transaminase

Soo Young Choi[1], Sang Ho Jang[1], Byung Ryong Lee[1], Yong Kyu Kim[1], Sung-Woo Cho[2] and Eui Yul Choi[1]

[1]Department of Genetic Engineering, College of Natural Sciences, Hallym University, Chunchon, Korea 200-702
[2]Department of Biochemistry, College of Medicine, University of Ulsan, Seoul, Korea 138-040

Summary

Monoclonal antibodies(mAbs) have been produced to bovine brain GABA transaminase(GABA-T). The antibodies recognized a single band of molecular weight of 50kDa on an immunoblot with purified GABA-T and whole homogenates proteins of bovine brain. Cross-reactivities among mammalian including human and avian brain GABA-T with the antibodies were tested by Western-blot. The immunoreactive bands on Western blots appeared as a single protein band of Mr 50 kDa and were the same in all animal tested except in chicken. This result suggests that the brain GABA-T among the mammalians share a common epitope and they seemed to be similar in protein structure, while avian brain GABA-T is immunologically distinct from those of the mammalian brain. Only two mAbs of five clones have shown the cross-reactivities with human brain homogenate suggesting that human brain GABA-T is immunologically distinct from those of other mammalian brain at least on one epitope.

Introduction

4-Aminobutyric acid(GABA) is present in many tissues of mammalians and is believed to be a major imhibitory chemical neurotransmitter in the central nervous system. The metabolic degradation of GABA is brought about by the action of GABA-T which catalyzes the reversible transamination of the neurotransmitter GABA in mammalian brain to yield succinic semialdehyde and glutamic acid. We report here the monoclonal antibodies(mAbs) to bovine brain GABA-T have been produced, which specifically react with the purified enzyme on Western blot. Using the mAbs as specific probes, we compared the cross-reactivities among GABA-T enzymes from mammalian including human and avian brains.

Results and Discussion

Purification of GABA transaminase from bovine brain

GABA transaminase from bovine brain was purified for the first time to homogeneity by heat treatment, ammonium sulfate fractionation, CM-Sephadex, DEAE-Sephadex and hydroxyapatite chromatographic methods. The bovine brain GABA-T had different electrophoretic mobility when compared with that of pig brain enzyme by native PAGE. The result from the HPLC Superose-6 gel filtration gave an estimated molecular mass for the native enzyme of 100,000, which dessociates into subunits of 50,000 under reducing condition on SDS-PAGE (Fig.1). These results indicate that the enzyme is a dimer with identical subunits.

350

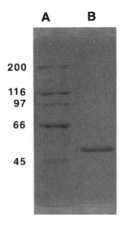

A B

200

116
97

66

45

Fig.1 SDS-PAGE of GABA transaminase
isolated from bovine brain.

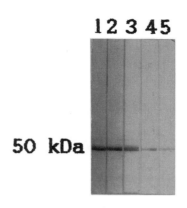

1 2 3 4 5

50 kDa

Fig.2 Immunoblots probed with five
representative mAbs to bovine brain
GABA-T enzyme was separated in on
SDS gel immunoblots.
1; mAbs GT8, 2; mAb GT17,
3; mAb GT146, 4; mAb GT187
5; mAbs GT347.

Production and partial characterization of mAbs to GABA-T

From two batches of fused cells, we initially obtained a total of 16 mAbs recognizing bovine brain GABA-T on immunodot blot. The hybridoma cells from positive wells were transfered on to 6-well plate and expanded, and the supernatant from the wells was further tested for immunoreactivity by the Western blot. Since some of the hybridoma clones either lost the ability to produce mAbs reacting with the antigen weakly on the immunoblot after cloning by limiting dilution, we finally selected 5 mAbs showing strong reactivity for further study. The immunoreactivities of 5 mAbs with purified GABA-T are shown in Fig.2.

Cross-reactivities among mammalian including human and avian GABA-T enzymes

In order to know the cross-reactivity of the mAbs with other mammalian and avian GABA-T enzymes, several animal brains from dog, cat, bovine, pig, rat, and chicken were removed and total proteins of brain homogenate were separated, transferred, and probed with the mAbs (Fig.3). The immunoreactive bands on Western blot appeared as a single protein band of 50 kDa and were the same in all animals tested except in chicken. The mAbs did not reacted with any protein band in chicken. This result suggests that the brain GABA-T proteins among the mammalians share a common epitope and they seemed to be simmilar in protein structure, while avian brain GABA-T is immunologically distinct from those of the mammalian brain.
The two mAbs(GT17, GT347) have shown the cross-reactivities with human brain homogenate, while GT8, GT146 didn't react with them suggesting that human brain

GABA-T is immnologically distinct from those of other mammalian brain at least on one epitope(Fig.4). Previous studies revealed that the molecular weight of GABA-T were different, depending on animal species, in the range of 50-52 kDa. The immunoblot result in this study confirms that all mammalian brain including human GABA-T enzymes are the same and the subunit molecular weight may be 50 kDa.

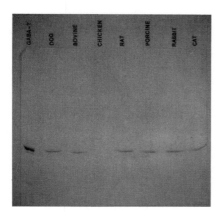

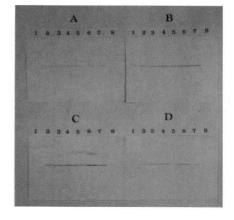

Fig.3 Cross-reactivities of GABA-T enzymes from mammalian and avian brain sorces with mAb GT17. Animal brains were removed and the total proteins of brain homogenates were immunoblotted with mAb GT17. The mAb recognized all GABA-T enzymes in animals tested except in chicken.

Fig.4 Cross-reactivities of GABA-T from various mammalian whole brain tissue with mAbs to bovine brain tissues with mAbs to bovine brain GABA-T. A:mAb GT8, B:mAb GT17 C:mAb GT146, D:mAb GT347 1:human 2:bovine 3:porcine 4.cat 5:rat 6:rabbit 7:dog 8:chicken brain

References

1.Choi,E.Y., and Jeon,K.W.(1989).*Exp.Cell.Res.*185,154-165
2. Choi,S.Y.,Kim,I.,Jang,S.H.,Lee,S.J.,Song,M.S.,Lee,Y.S. and Cho,S.W. (1993).*Mol.Cell.*3,397-401
3. Towbin,H.,Staehelin,T., and Gordon,J.(1979).*Proc.Natl.Acad.Sci.*76,4350-4354

Acknowledgement

This work was supported by a grant of Genetic Engineering Program from the Korean Ministry of Education, 1994 and partial grant of New Drug Development Program of the Korean Ministry of Health and Social Affairs, 1994.

Biochemistry of Vitamin B$_6$ and PQQ
G. Marino, G. Sannia and F. Bossa (eds.)
© 1994 Birkhäuser Verlag Basel/Switzerland

Effect of pyrroloquinoline quinone (PQQ) on the SLE-like (Systemic Lupus Erythematosus) disease in MRL-lpr/lpr mice

B. J. Weimann

F. Hoffmann - La Roche Ltd, Vitamins and Fine Chemicals Division, CH-4002 Basel, Switzerland

Summary

In MRL-lpr/lpr (MRL/1) mice developing the SLE-like autoimmune disorder, PQQ can modulate many features of the pathological process including immune functions. The mean survival time was extended; enlargements of lymphoid organs and also of the liver were reduced; titres of anti-double stranded (ds) DNA antibodies and concentrations of serum amyloid P component (SAP) were reduced; serum IgG levels were not changed; T cell mitogenic responses to concanavalin A (con A) were enhanced, whereas B cells stimulated with lipopolysaccharide (LPS) were not. The results suggest that PQQ partly inhibits the development of the SLE-like disease in MRL/1 mice, probably by reducing inflammation and influencing T cell differentiation.

Introduction

In humans SLE is an autoimmune disease of unknown aetiology. The cause depends on genetic and environmentally acquired factors, and preferentially occurs in females. MRL/1 mice develop a spontaneous SLE-like disease associated with pathologic expressions similar to the human disease (e. g. skin lesions, lymphadenopathy, multiple autoantibodies, inflammatory manifestations including glomerulonephritis, arthritis, vasculitis, etc.). A central question in autoimmune diseases is the origin of antibodies binding to a variety of self antigens. One factor in the progress of autoimmune diseases is related to the oxidative modification of cell structures by reactive oxygen intermediates (ROI), being continuously produced in the course of the normal aerobic metabolism. Due to genetic predisposition in affected individuals, ROI might not be as effectively inactivated as in normal individuals. Accordingly, the progress of autoimmune diseases would partly depend on ROI and conversely on the amounts of antioxidants at critical sites, such as mitochondria, nuclear and plasma membranes.

PQQ (4,5-dihydro-4,5-dioxo-1H-pyrrolo-[2,3-f]-quinoline-2,7,9-tricarboxylic acid) is synthesised in a variety of bacteria and functions as a cofactor in several oxidoreductases. Free PQQ was found in mammalian fluids and tissues (Flückiger et al., 1992). In mice it is an essential nutrient with an estimated daily need of about 1 µg (Killgore et al., 1989). In rats inflammatory reactions can be inhibited by PQQ (Hamagishi et al., 1990). Furthermore, PQQ serves as high affinity substrate for erythrocyte-NADPH-dependent methaemoglobin reductase and probably also for a similar enzyme isolated from liver. In addition, it protects heart tissue from reoxygenation damage after hypoxia (Xu et al., 1993). The present paper suggests that PQQ may inhibit the autoimmune pathology characteristic for MRL/1 mice.

Materials and Methods

MRL/1 mice had free access to a commercial diet and water without (control) or with 0.4 µg/ml PQQ from weeks 6 onwards. Assuming a daily water need of about 10 ml, mice would ingest roughly 4 µg PQQ. IgG, anti-dsDNA antibody titres and SAP were measured using corresponding ELISAs. Values are given as means ± SD and were analysed for statistically significant differences using analysis of variance.

Results and Discussion

In MRL/1 mice visible symptoms are necrotising lesions on the back and the ears probably reflecting cryoglobulin deposition in small and medium-sized arteries. Treatment with PQQ reduced the massive skin lesions. The fur coat was smoother than that of unsupplemented mice. The mean survival time was increased from 148 days in the control (n = 20) to 185 days in the PQQ-supplemented group (n = 17) corresponding to 25% of life extension. MRL/1 mice develop enlargements of lymphoid organs at 6 - 8 weeks of age, which progress rapidly thereafter. PQQ prevented the massive lymphoproliferation. The following organ weights were determined at week 16 (control vs PQQ supplement): spleens 505 ± 332 mg vs. 237 ± 66 mg (p = 0.04); axillary lymph nodes 448 ± 202 mg vs. 195 ± 83 mg (p = 0.006); thymus 268 ± 89 mg vs. 203 ± 65 mg (p = 0.12). A significant reduction of the liver weight was also found, 2,343 ± 417 mg vs. 1,716 ± 212 mg (p = 0.002, n = 8).

The capacity of MRL/1 mice to respond to exogenous stimulation is impaired. Responses to T cell mitogenic or antigenic stimuli and antibody response to foreign antigens and polyclonal activators seem to be defective (Cohen and Eisenberg, 1991). Proliferation of cultured splenocytes stimulated with LPS (B cell mitogen) was not affected by PQQ (253,909 ± 21,736 cpm vs. 256,604 ± 47,677 cpm, n = 8). Similarly, no effect was found when PQQ between 10^{-5} and 10^{-10} M was added to spleen cell cultures of unsupplemented mice. Proliferation increased, however, when cultures from PQQ-treated mice were stimulated with con-A (T cell mitogen, 186,587 ± 98,036 vs. 13,672 ± 7,460; p = 0.01). *In vitro* addition of PQQ to con A-stimulated cultures of splenocytes from unsupplemented mice resulted in a small, but statistically insignificant increase.

Amongst other abnormalities, MRL/1 mice develop elevated IgG concentrations in the serum. PQQ supplementation did not influence serum IgG levels. At week 16, they were 14.35

± 4.17 mg (n = 14) in the control, and 13.24 ± 3.07 mg (n = 6) in the PQQ-treated group. Among the autoantibodies against nuclear components, antibodies against dsDNA are specific for SLE in humans and mice as well. They occur relatively late, but then increase rapidly and correlate with the development of the disease and the death rate. Together with the antigen dsDNA they form soluble immune complexes, which adhere to the vasculature causing vasculitis and glomerulonephritis. At week 8, titres of anti-dsDNA antibodies were 178 ± 17 which increased to 1219 ±1592 (n = 14) at week 16. After PQQ supplementation a reduction of the titres to 347 ± 189 (p = 0.02, n = 19) was observed. It may be possible that PQQ partly corrects the aberrant T cell differentiation in the thymus as shown for vitamin E (Weimann, B. J., in press).

Acute phase proteins are rapidly synthesised in response to tissue injury, inflammation or infection, leading to increased amounts of proteins in the circulation. In MRL/1 mice a continuous increase of SAP levels was observed with increasing age. At week 16, concentrations of 345 µg/ml were found which were lower in PQQ-supplemented mice (246 µg/ml). Although the biological properties remain largely unknown, it seems that acute phase proteins limit the extent of inflammation and protect, e. g. against lethal effects of LPS, TNF or IL-1 (Tilg et al., 1993). C-reactive protein binds to chromatin and activates complement, resulting in solubilization and removal of chromatin by complement-mediated phagocytosis (Robey et al., 1984). ROI are activators of transcription (Meyer et al., 1993) and may also be mediators of apoptosis (Buttke and Sandstrom, 1994). Assuming PQQ protects cells from destruction due to its antioxidant properties, the amount of chromatin fragments and most likely of oxidatively modified DNA which may be present at sites of tissue damage would be decreased, resulting in diminished presentation of self-antigens to the immune system. This, in turn, would limit antibody production, immune complex formation and tissue deposition. The reduction of high SAP levels suggests that PQQ may down-regulate inflammatory processes by limiting oxidative processes and hence tissue destruction.

PQQ caused a definite amelioration of the disease (reduction of lymphoadenopathy and auto-antibody titres), but not an absolute cure of the chronic SLE-like disease in MRL/1 mice. The genetic pressure of the lpr mutation is most likely so strong that PQQ can retard, but not eliminate the disease completely. An improvement of all aspects of the lupus-like disease was also reported in mice infected with a recombinant vaccinia virus expressing interleukin-2 (Gutierrez-Ramos et al., 1990) or with a novel immunomodulator (Spetz-Hagberg et al., 1990). Reduction lymphadenopathy without suppressing levels of autoantibodies or circulating immune complexes (separation of autoimmune phenomena from lymphadenopathy) could be

356

shown in mice either expressing the transgenic αβ T cell receptor for the male antigen HY (Mountz et al., 1990) or after treatment with cyclosporin A (Mountz et al., 1987). The central process of clonal deletion of autoreactive T cells in the thymus probably functions only for potent or easily accessible self-antigens. It is also possible that this elimination is not effective for antigens being only present in minute amounts or not at all during embryonal development or in young growing animals because they are generated later in life because of continuous oxidative modifications. Due to the deterioration of the thymus with increasing age, the efficiency of the thymus to eliminate autoreactive T cells is reduced. Since humoral and cell-mediated immune responses decline with age and the incidence of autoantibodies increases both in humans and mice, autoimmunity seems to be strongly related to the ageing processes. The modulation of progressive autoimmune diseases and also of the ageing immune system by dietary manipulations (e. g. antioxidants such as PQQ) should lead to improved immune functions and extended life expectancy.

References

Buttke, T. M., and Sandstrom, P. A. (1994) Oxidative stress as a mediator of apoptosis. Immunol Today 15: 7 - 10.

Cohen, P. L., and Eisenberg, R. A. (1991) Lpr and gld: Single gene models of systemic autoimmunity and lymphoproliferative disease. Ann. Rev. Immunol. 9: 243 - 269.

Flückiger, R., Paz, M. A., Henson, E., Gallop, P. M., and Bergethon, P. R. (1992) Glycine-dependent redox cycling and other methods for PQQ and quinoprotein detection. In: V. L. Davidson (ed.): Principles and application of quinoproteins, Marcel Dekker Inc, New York, pp 331 -341.

Gutierrez-Ramos, J. C., Andreu, J. L., Revilla, Y., Vinuela, E., and Martinez, C. (1990) Revovery from autoimmuninity of MLR/lpr mice after infection with an interleukin-2/vaccinia recombinant virus. Nature 346: 271 - 274.

Hamagishi, Y., Murata, S., Kamei, H., Oki, T., Adachi, O., and Ameyama, M. (1990) New biological properties of pyrroloquinoline quinone and its related compounds: Inhibition of chemiluminescence, lipid peroxidation and rat paw edema. J. Pharmacol. Exp. Ther. 255: 980 - 985.

Killgore, J., Smidt, C., Duich, L., Romero-Chapman, N., Tinker, D., Reiser, K., Melko, M., Hyde, D., and Rucker, R. B. (1989) Nutritional importance of pyrroloquinoline quinone. Science 245: 850 - 852.

Meyer, M., Schreck, R. and Baeuerle, P. A. (1993) H_2O_2 and antioxidants have opposite effects on activation of NF-κB and AP-1 in intact cells: AP-1 as secondary antioxidant-responsive factor. EMBO J.: 2005 - 2015.

Mountz, J. D., Smith, H. R., Wilder, R. L., Reeves, J. P., and Steinberg, A. D. (1987) Cs-A therapy in MRL-lpr/lpr mice: amelioration of immunopathology despite autoantibody production. J. Immunol. 138: 157 - 163.

Mountz, J. D., Zhou, T., Eldridge, J., Berry, K., and Blüthmann, H. (1990) Transgenic rearranged T cell receptor gene inhibits lymphadenopathy and accumulation of CD4$^-$CD8$^-$B220$^+$ T cells in lpr/lpr mice. J. Exp. Med. 172:
1805 - 1817.

Robey, F. A., Jones, K. D., Tanaka, T., and Liu, T. Y. (1984) Binding of c-reactive protein to chromatin and nucleosome core particles A possible physiological role of C-reactive protein. J. Biol. Chem. 259: 7311 - 7316.

Spetz-Hagberg, A. L., Goldschmidt, T. J., Stalhandske, T., and Larsson-Sciard, E. L. (1990) Amelioration of intrathymic T cell development and peripheral T cell reactivities in autoimmune mice undergoing therapy with a novel immunomodulator. Int. Immunol. 2: 645 - 650.

Tilg, H., Vannier, E., Vachino, G., Dinarello, C. A., and Mier, J. W. (1993) Anti inflammatory properties of hepatic acute phase proteins: Preferential induction of interleukin 1 (IL-1) receptor antagonist over IL-1ß synthesis by human peripheral blood mononuclear cells. J. Exp. Med. 178: 1629 - 1636.

Xu, F., Mack, C. P., Quandt, K. S., Shlafer, M., Massey, V., and Hultquist, D. E. (1993) Pyrroloquinoline quinone acts with flavin reductase to reduce ferryl myoglobin in vitro and protects isolated heart from re-oxygenation injury. Biochem. Biophys. Res. Commun. 193: 434 - 439.

Conclusions

Francesco Bossa

Dipartimento di Scienze Biochimiche "A. Rossi Fanelli", Università di Roma "La Sapienza", Italy

Since I have the privilege of co-chairing the last session of the Symposium, I shall take the opportunity to say a few words about an important observation which was communicated to me yesterday evening by Rob John and which seems particularly appropriate after hearing the lecture by Philipp Christen on the molecular evolution of PLP dependent-enzymes. There was already an obscure report in the specialized literature on the occurrence of the following specific PLP-binding motif:

MXRIN

You can observe this consensus sequence in some *bona fide* PLP-dependent types, such as

YOSHIMASA<u>MO</u>RINO
MA<u>RIN</u>OMARTINEZCARRION
GENNARO<u>MA</u><u>RIN</u>O

Exon shuffling is clearly responsible for positioning specific domains either on the C- or N-terminal side of the common PLP-binding motif.

Having made this seminal observation, we asked ourselves a question concerning the compartments where these and other PLP dependent types meet periodically to perform a concerted action. Is there in these compartments some receptor whose structure is somehow related to the PLP-dependent motifs? The results of a preliminary survey of the present and future receptors are encouraging:

MA<u>RIN</u>AGRANDEDICAPRI
UNITEDSTATESOFA<u>MERI</u>CA

In order to establish whether the relationships between the structure of the PLP-dependent types and that of the receptors was of real significance and not just coincidental, we tried to reconstitute a functional system *in vivo* by mixing

GENNARO<u>MA</u><u>RIN</u>O with **MA<u>RIN</u>AGRANDEDICAPRI**

Nothing, or very little, happened. Obviously, to obtain a functional system, one or more additional factors are needed. The most important of these factors has been identified, isolated and analysed. The sequence is distinctively rich in asparagines and apparently unrelated to the previous ones.

GIOVANNISANNIA

The next experiment will be the cloning and amplification of this important molecule.

Many other active factors were obviously involved in bringing about this most recent and highly profitable interaction between PLP dependent types and the CAPRI receptor. Without knowing their precise sequences we have nevertheless appreciated their great functional efficiency as well as the immediate and obvious appeal of their three-dimensional structures.

Finally, we have some recommendations for those of you who wish to make further progress along this line of research: sophisticated algorithms and powerful computers are not needed, but it is important to reproduce exactly the experimental conditions. For example, aqueous buffers are not good. The addition of some ethanol is critical: not too little, not too much. You should also add to the mixture a special reagent, of which unfortunately I cannot give you the chemical formula since there is a patent pending:

TARALLO™

Subject index

(The page numbers refer to the initial page of the article in which the keyword occur)

Retinoids:
From Basic Science to Clinical Applications

Edited by
M.A. Livrea
University of Palermo, Institute of Biological Chemistry, Policlinico, Palermo, Italy
G. Vidali
National Cancer Institute, Laboratory of Molecular Biology,Genova, Italy

1994. 396 pages. Hardcover • ISBN 3-7643-2812-6
(MCBU)

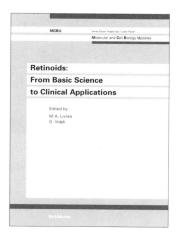

This book examines subjects from a variety of disciplines to report on the most recent experimental observations in basic as well as in applied research of natural and synthetic retinoids.

Written by leading scientists in this field, the chapters offer an extensive overview covering such areas as metabolism, nutrition, molecular and cell biology, and developmental biology, pharmacology and therapeutic use of vitamin A and its derivatives.

Basic investigators as well as clinicians will find this volume valuable both as a summary of recent research and as a stimulus for future experimental work in this continuously expanding field.

Birkhäuser Verlag • Basel • Boston • Berlin

BIRKHÄUSER

Carotenoids

Edited by
G. Britton, *University of Liverpool, UK*
S. Liaaen-Jensen, *University of Trondheim, Norway*
Pfander, H., *University of Berne, Switzerland*

The first volume of a new series, *Carotenoids*, provides an introduction to the fundamental chemistry of these compounds and detailed accounts of the basic methods used in carotenoid work. It is published in two parts, part A covering the general methods of isolation and analysis, and part B the application of spectroscopic techniques to identification and structure elucidation.

The books are designed primarily to pass on a wealth of practical experience of carotenoid work. A novel feature is the inclusion of a collection of Worked Examples of the isolation and analysis of carotenoids from the most important natural sources as established procedures that newcomers to carotenoids can easily follow.

All chapters are written by leading experts in the field and provide not only up-to-date information on specialized topics for experienced carotenoid researchers but, especially, practical guidance to workers in plant physiology, photosynthesis, taxonomy, biotechnology, food science, nutrition and medicine who wish to venture into the carotenoid field.

Volume 1A:
Isolation and Analysis

1994. Approx 400 pages. Hardcover
ISBN 3-7643-2908-4

Contents: Scope of the series • History of carotenoid research • Carotenoids today and challenges for the future • Structures and nomenclature • Isolation and analysis • Chemical derivatization • Chromatography • General Aspects, LCC, TLC, HPLC, SFC
Worked examples, describing the isolation and analysis of carotenoids from various sources (higher plants, algae, bacteria, invertebrates, fish, egg yolk, human plasma, feed) as well as the analysis of special groups of carotenoids (geometrical isomers, glycosides and glycosyl esters, carotenoid sulphates and carotenoid proteins).
Appendix to the handbook Key to Carotenoids

Volume 1B:
Spectroscopy

1994. Approx. 450 pages. Hardcover
ISBN 3-7643-2909-2

Contents: Electronic spectra: UV/visible spectroscopy • IR spectroscopy • Raman spectroscopy • NMR spectroscopy • Circular dichroism • Mass spectrometry • X-Ray • Integrated approach to structure elucidation

Set Volumes 1A and 1B
ISBN 3-7643-2910-6
Set Volumes 1A and 1B and Key to Carotenoids
ISBN 3-7643-2936-X

Birkhäuser Verlag • Basel • Boston • Berlin

ADVANCES IN LIFE SCIENCES

This topical volume comprises review articles written by leading experts on recent advances in metallothionein research. Attention is focused on the biological roles and medical implications of metallothionein in addition to chemical and biochemical developments.

Metallothionein III
Biological Roles and Medical Implications

Edited by
K.T. Suzuki, *Chiba University, Inage, Japan*
N. Imura, *Kitasato University, Tokyo, Japan*
M. Kimura, *Keio University, Tokyo, Japan*

1993. 496 pages. Hardcover • ISBN 3-7643-2769-3 (ALS)

Metallothioneins play a pivotal role in regulating the flow of the essential trace elements zinc and copper through the cell, and in modulating the harmful environmental influences of toxic metals and of various stress conditions.

This topical volume focusses on the biological roles and medical implications of metallo-thioneins, and related chemical and biochemical developments. Leading experts present and discuss new findings on the roles of metallothioneins in various kinds of stress conditions including exposure to heavy metals, organic and inorganic chemicals and the physical environment as well as in homeostatic regulation of essential heavy metals, copper and zinc.

Of special interest is the ability of metallothioneins to scavenge for free radicals and active oxygen species in the context of resistance mechanisms in anti-cancer reagents such as adriamycine, and reduction of site-specific side- effects by anti-cancer reactions such as cisplatin.

In addition, this volume deals with the possible role of metallothioneins in cell differentiation and proliferation, the induction mechanisms by cytokines and hormones, a possible new class of metallothionein found as growth inhibitory factor (GIF) in neuronal cells, a marker protein to monitor the environmental contamination by heavy metals, phytochelatin (g-EC peptide, cadystine) and the coordination chemistry for metal-thiolate cluster.

Topics include:
A possible new class of metallothionein found as growth inhibitory factor (GIF) in neuronal cells • Sequestration of free radicals and active oxygen species • Reduction of site-specific side effects by anti-cancer reagents such as cisplatin • Resistance mechanisms for anti-cancer reagents such as adriamycin • Possible roles in cell differentiation and proliferation • Coordination chemistry for metalthiolate cluster • Detoxification of heavy metals • Homeostatic regulation of essential heavy metals, copper and zinc • A marker protein to monitor the environmental contamination by heavy metals • Phytochelatin (g-EC peptide, cadystine)

Birkhäuser Verlag • Basel • Boston • Berlin

DATE DUE

DEC 0 8 1995	